The Roy Adaptation Model

The Definitive Statement

The Roy Adaptation Model

The Definitive Statement

Heather A. Andrews
R.N., Ph.D.
Vice President—Nursing
University of Alberta Hospitals
Edmonton, Alberta, Canada

Sister Callista Roy
R.N., Ph.D., FAAN`
Professor and Nurse Theorist
School of Nursing
Boston College
Chestnut Hill, Massachusetts

APPLETON & LANGE
Norwalk, Connecticut/San Mateo, California

Notice: Our knowledge in clinical sciences is constantly changing. As new information becomes available, changes in treatment and in the use of drugs become necessary. The authors and the publisher of this volume have taken care to make certain that the doses of drugs and schedules of treatment are correct and compatible with the standards generally accepted at the time of publication. The reader is advised to consult carefully the instruction and information material included in the package insert of each drug or therapeutic agent before administration. This advice is especially important when using new or infrequently used drugs.

Copyright © 1991 by Appleton & Lange
A Publishing Division of Prentice Hall
© 1986 by Appleton-Century-Crofts

91 92 93 94 95 / 10 9 8 7 6 5 4 3 2 1

Prentice Hall International (UK) Limited, *London*
Prentice Hall of Australia Pty. Limited, *Sydney*
Prentice Hall Canada, Inc., *Toronto*
Prentice Hall Hispanoamericana, S.A., *Mexico*
Prentice Hall of India Private Limited, *New Delhi*
Prentice Hall of Japan, Inc., *Tokyo*
Simon & Schuster Asia Pte. Ltd., *Singapore*
Editora Prentice Hall do Brasil Ltda., *Rio de Janeiro*
Prentice Hall, *Englewood Cliffs, New Jersey*

Library of Congress Cataloging-in-Publication Data
Roy, Callista.
    The Roy adaptation model : the definitive statement / Callista Roy,
Heather A. Andrews,
        p.   cm.
    Rev. ed. of: Essentials of the Roy adaptation model / Heather A.
Andrews, Callista Roy.
    Includes bibliographical references.
    Includes index.
    ISBN 0-8385-2272-6
    1. Roy adaptation model.   2. Nursing—Psychological aspects.
3. Nurse and patient.   I. Andrews, Heather A.   II. Andrews, Heather
A. Essentials of the Roy adaptation model.   III. Title.
    [DNLM: 1. Adaptation, Psychological.   2. Models, Theoretical.
3. Nursing.   WY   100 R888r]
RT84.5.R66   1991
610.73'019—dc20
DNLM/DLC
for Library of Congress   90-1271
                                                                      CIP

Production Assistance: Tage Publishing Service
Acquisitions Editor: Marion K. Welch

PRINTED IN THE UNITED STATES OF AMERICA

Contributing Authors

Heather A. Andrews, R.N., Ph.D.   (Chapters 1, 2, 3, 13, 16)
Vice President—Nursing
University of Alberta Hospitals
Former Assistant Director
Royal Alexandra Hospitals School of Nursing
Edmonton, Alberta, Canada

Marjorie Buck, R.N., M.N.   (Chapters 14 and 15)
Nurse Clinician
A Child's Garden School
Albuquerque, New Mexico
Former Instructor, Department of Nursing
Mount St. Mary's College
Los Angeles, California

Zona Chalifoux, R.N., M.N.   (Chapter 12)
Doctoral Student
University of Virginia
Charlottesville, Virginia
Former Lecturer, Department of Nursing
Mount St. Mary's College
Los Angeles, California

Joan Seo Cho, R.N., M.N.   (Chapter 7)
Assistant Professor, Department of Nursing
Mount St. Mary's College
Los Angeles, California

Joanne Gray, R.N., M.S.N.   (Chapter 20)
Nursing Consultant
Anaheim, California

Karen Jensen, R.N., M.N.   (Chapter 10)
Assistant Professor
Department of Nursing
Mount St. Mary's College
Los Angeles, California

Kathleen Nuwayhid, R.N., M.N.   (Chapter 17)
Instructor
Department of Nursing
Vanier College, Vanier St. Laurent
Quebec, Canada
Former Instructor, Department of Nursing
Mount St. Mary's College
Los Angeles, California

Donna Romyn, R.N., B.Sc.N., M.N.   (Case Studies, Parts 2 and 3)
Assistant Director
Royal Alexandra Hospitals School of Nursing
Edmonton, Alberta, Canada

Sister Callista Roy, R.N., Ph.D., F.A.A.N.   (Chapters 1, 2, 3, 7, 9,
   11, 21)
Professor and Nurse Theorist
School of Nursing
Boston College, Chestnut Hill, Massachusetts
Neuroscience Nursing Staff Privileges
Beth Israel Hospital Nursing Service
and
Center for the Advancement of Nursing Practice
Boston, Massachusetts
Research Professor in Nursing
Mount St. Mary's College
Los Angeles, California

Marsha Keiko Sato, R.N., M.N.   (Chapter 8)
Assistant Professor
Department of Nursing
Mount St. Mary's College
Los Angeles, California

Jane Servonsky, R.N., M.S.N. (Chapters 5, 6, 19)
Associate Professor
Department of Nursing
Norfolk State University
Norfolk, Virginia
Former Associate Professor, Department of Nursing
Mount St. Mary's College
Los Angeles, California

Mary Poush Tedrow, R.N., Ed.D (Chapters 18, 19)
Associate Professor
California State University
Dominges Hills, California
Former Assistant Professor, Department of Nursing
Mount St. Mary's College
Los Angeles, California

Catherine Rivera Thompson, R.N., M.N. (Chapter 4)
Coordinator Sophomore Year
Department of Nursing
Mount St. Mary's College
Los Angeles, California

Contents

Preface

The Roy Adaptation Model: The Definitive Statement is an introduction
to the Adaptation Model for nursing and clinical nursing practice based
on the model developed by Sister Callista Roy. The purpose of this new
book is to assume the role of the definitive text on the model. The authors
have designed a compact, consistent, updated, and easy-to-use text that
describes the key concepts of the model. Each element of the model is
addressed in a way that identifies and analyzes substantive nursing
knowledge for clinical practice.

Textbooks that use nursing models have proliferated in the past decade. Many nurse theorists have provided texts that explain the philosophical, theoretical, and conceptual bases for their given view of the
phenomenon of nursing and its use in education, practice, and research.
Clinical specialty textbooks have been influenced by these theoretical
developments. Some use a nursing process approach, emphasizing the
basis for clinical judgments. Others present one or several nursing models
and examples of their application. Still, no other text on a nursing model
has had the advantage of unifying and presenting model-based knowledge by authors who have taught and practiced for 20 years with that
model. The contributing authors in this text have been associated with
the Roy model over these years since its introduction by the theorist at
Mount St. Mary's College in Los Angeles.

This book builds on the four previous books on the Roy Adaptation
Model authored by Roy. It updates the essential components presented
earlier (Andrews and Roy, 1986) for use in the 1990s. For example, there
is a consistent link from the introduction of the philosophical assumptions to the understanding of persons within the environment. Contextual stimuli reflect today's social setting, and a perspective is maintained
on issues relative to the freedom of the individual with awareness of
common social concerns. This text emphasizes a basic premise of the

model that all nursing care planning takes place within the nurse–patient relationship. Of particular note is that the model's view of the person and of health leads to the conclusion that a typology of positive life processes is key to nursing judgment and diagnosis. While others debate a typology of diagnoses for health, this text offers the model's first typology of indicators of positive adaptation.

The organization of knowledge of processes leading to the indicators of positive adaptation, begun in the two introductory texts (Roy, 1976 and Roy, 1984), is continued with some new foci in both content and format. The content of this book focuses on the theoretical background for each of the components of the adaptive modes. This is particularly strengthened in the section in which the physiological mode is introduced. Benefiting from Roy's postdoctoral studies as a Robert Wood Johnson Clinical Nurse Scholar in the neurosciences (with Dr. Connie Robinson at the University of California at San Francisco), ongoing work on integrated cognator and regulator processes is explained.

For each of the other adaptive modes—self concept, role function, and interdependence—focus is on basic understanding of the mode, its use in nursing practice, and on interrelations between and among the four adaptive modes. This expanded text benefits from the substantial knowledge development work done by key authors working with the model. The essence of two decades of their work is presented, making it possible for this text to be used alone.

In format, this expanded text maintains the diagrammatic conceptualizations of the model that were developed at the Royal Alexandra Hospitals School of Nursing, Edmonton, Alberta, Canada, while Andrews worked with faculty on curriculum revision. These have been useful to many readers in illustration of the essentials of the model and their interrelationships. Other key figures and tables have been added to further highlight essential content. In moving from the 1976 and 1984 introductory text to *The Roy Adaptation Model,* the aim is to have a unified and compact format, as well as consistent, substantive, and updated content.

Each chapter of Parts I through V follows a similar topical outline. Ample use of illustrations and clinical examples of the basic concepts of the model continue the focus on the essentials, but with greater depth. The use of objectives and definitions of key concepts helps to focus the reader, while exercises for application, assessment of understanding, and feedback provide for further understanding and for achievement of the identified objectives. Both an introduction and summary are provided for each chapter to give an overview and a review of the content. References used in the chapter are followed by additional references for readers wanting supplementary material.

Chapter 20 of Part VI adds significantly to other publications on applications of models by describing and comparing five implementation projects conducted by one author who has used Roy and other faculty from Mount St. Mary's College as consultants since the 1970s. The final chapter, Chapter 21, focuses on research. The in-depth theoretical work done on the Roy Adaptation Model (Roy and Roberts, 1981) is followed here by a new vision of the structure of knowledge based on the model. The decade between these works has seen great growth in the literature on the epistemology of nursing. One can now see connections between where the 1981 text left off with a middle-range systems theory approach and the current emphasis on processes and patterns, interrelatedness and integration, and stability and change. Chapter 21 includes the updated structure for a basic nursing science and the clinical nursing science as well as illustrations of specific research projects based on the model within both branches of nursing knowledge.

This text is intended primarily for use in agencies and educational institutions that are using the Roy Adaptation Model as a basis for nursing practice and education. It can provide the essential content needed for diploma, associate degree, and baccalaureate degree students. Masters level students will find the clarity of presentation an efficient method to become acquainted with the essentials as a basis for more in-depth analysis and application of concepts. Doctoral students can increasingly find in the essentials of the model the basis for asking significant research questions and for adding to basic and clinical knowledge development. Similarly new applications of the model for communities, for families, and for nursing service organizations can be derived from the essentials described here and referred to in the references. This text is also a useful orientation tool for nursing service personnel and faculty.

As the health care profession gropes with problems without answers and issues without responsibilities, nurses continue to articulate to the public, to other disciplines, and among themselves, the essence of nursing's position. Clear, nonpolemic presentations of nursing's unique perspective, its role, and implications of what that role means are needed. This text makes every effort to contribute to this important but difficult task faced by all members of the discipline.

The authors are indebted to those who have encouraged and assisted with the development of this text. First, we appreciate deeply those who have contributed to and offered stimulation to the development of the model through the years, especially at both of our home institutions. The nurses in practice, graduate students, and audiences, from near and far, who comment and raise questions have continued to play an important role in shaping this scholarly work within practice parameters. Sister Callista Roy offers special mention to her clinical mentors in neuroscience at University Hospitals and San Francisco General Hospital. We acknowledge, too, the courage of our editor, Marion Kalstein-Welch, who listened, then supported the idea that we could take two good books, one introductory and one on essentials, and make them into one better book.

We hope, then, to add to the collection at a later time a text on clinical nursing that could satisfy new needs for looking at more complex adaptation situations and advanced practice. Finally, each of us has a long list of family, friends, and colleagues who have left their mark on us and on this work and we are grateful to all.

Sister Callista Roy
Heather A. Andrews

Part I

Introduction to the Roy Adaptation Model

The Roy Adaptation Model is currently one of the most highly developed and widely used conceptual descriptions of nursing. Formal development of the model began in the late 1960s and, since that time, nurses in the United States and around the world have helped Roy in clarifying, refining, and extending the basic concepts to the stage of development presented in this text. The major concepts associated with nursing models— the person, the environment, health, and nursing—are introduced in this section and discussed in further detail throughout the text.

Chapter One ────────────

Essentials of the Roy Adaptation Model

Heather A. Andrews and
Sister Callista Roy

The first formal descriptions of the Roy Adaptation Model were made by Sister Callista Roy while she was a graduate student in the School of Nursing at the University of California at Los Angeles. The roots of the model lie in Roy's own personal and professional background. Roy is committed to philosophic assumptions characterized by the general principles of humanism and veritivity (a term coined by Roy). The assumptions associated with systems theory and adaptation-level theory form the scientific basis for the model.

Under the mentorship of Dorothy E. Johnson, Roy became convinced of the importance of defining nursing. She was influenced also by studies in the social sciences, and clinical practice in pediatric nursing provided experience with the resiliency of the human body and spirit. Roy began to seek ways to express her beliefs about nursing and to explore these further in her studies. The first publication on the Roy Adaptation Model appeared in 1970. (See Roy 1970.) By that time, Roy was on the faculty of the baccalaureate nursing program of a small liberal arts college. There she had the opportunity to lead the implementation of this model of nursing as the basis of the nursing curriculum. During the next decade, more than 1500 faculty and students at Mount St. Mary's College helped to clarify, refine, and extend the basic concepts of the Roy Adaptation Model for nursing.

This chapter provides an overview of the major concepts of the model and the associated philosophic and scientific assumptions.

OBJECTIVES

After studying this chapter, the reader will be able to do the following:

1. Describe the scientific and philosophic assumptions underlying the Roy Adaptation Model.
2. Identify the key terms in Roy's description of the person.
3. State the difference between adaptive and ineffective responses.
4. Differentiate the three classes of stimuli.
5. Define adaptation level.
6. Identify specific behaviors as indicative of cognator or regulator activity.
7. Define health in terms of the Roy Adaptation Model.
8. Describe the goal of nursing in terms of the Roy Adaptation Model.

KEY CONCEPTS DEFINED

- *Adaptation level:* a changing point that represents the person's ability to respond positively in a situation.
- *Adaptive responses:* responses that promote integrity in terms of the goals of the human system.
- *Behavior:* internal or external actions and reactions under specified circumstances.
- *Cognator subsystem:* a major coping process involving four cognitive-emotive channels: perceptual/information processing, learning, judgment, and emotion.
- *Contextual stimulus:* all other stimuli present in the situation that contribute to the effect of the focal stimulus.
- *Coping mechanisms:* innate or acquired ways of responding to the changing environment.
- *Focal stimulus:* the internal or external stimulus most immediately confronting the person.
- *Goal of nursing:* the promotion of adaptation in each of the four modes, thereby contributing to the person's health, quality of life, and dying with dignity.
- *Health:* a state and a process of being and becoming an integrated and whole person.
- *Humanism:* the broad movement in philosophy and psychology that recognizes the person and subjective dimensions of the human experience as central to knowing and valuing (Roy 1988).
- *Ineffective responses:* responses that do not contribute to integrity in terms of the goals of the human system.
- *Person:* as an adaptive system, the individual is described as a whole comprised of parts that function as a unity for some purpose.
- *Regulator subsystem:* a major coping process involving the neural, chemical, and endocrine systems.
- *Residual stimulus:* an environmental factor within or without the person whose effects in the current situation are unclear.

- *Stimulus:* that which provokes a response.
- *Veritivity:* a principle of human nature that affirms a common purposefulness of human existence (Roy, 1988).

OVERVIEW OF THE ROY ADAPTATION MODEL

Nursing models, as conceptual descriptions of nursing, are based on both scientific and philosophic assumptions. Knowledge development for any field reflects and moves forward the philosophic and scientific thinking of the day. So, too, nurse theorists identify the beliefs, values, and knowledge on which they base their work. For the Roy Adaptation Model, the scientific assumptions reflect the von Bertalanffy (1968) general systems theory and Helson's (1964) adaptation-level theory; the philosophic assumptions on which the model is based are associated with humanism and veritivity. The manner in which the major concepts of the model have been developed evidences the pervasive influence of each of these perspectives.

Within the context of these four major scientific and philosophic perspectives, specific assumptions underlying the Roy Adaptation Model can be identified. These are illustrated in Table 1–1. The contribution of systems theory to the scientific foundation of the Roy Model is evident in the description of the person as an adaptive system. Roy views the individual as functioning with interdependent parts acting in unity for some purpose. Control mechanisms are central to the functioning of the human system. The systems theory concepts of inputs (stimuli) and outputs (behavior) also contribute to important concepts in the model.

Adaptation-level theory (Helson 1964) forms the basis for the under-

TABLE 1–1. ASSUMPTIONS UNDERLYING THE ROY ADAPTATION MODEL

SCIENTIFIC	
Systems Theory	**Adaptation-Level Theory**
Holism	Behavior as adaptive
Interdependence	Adaptation as a function of stimuli and adaptation level
Control processes	
Information feedback	Individual, dynamic adaptation levels
Complexity of living systems	Positive and active processes of responding

PHILOSOPHIC	
Humanism	**Veritivity**
Creativity	Purposefulness of human existence
Purposefulness	Unity of purpose
Holism	Activity, creativity
Interpersonal process	Value and meaning of life

standing that the individual as a system has the capacity to adapt to and create changes in the environment. The ability to respond positively to these changes is a function of the person's *adaptation level*—a changing point influenced by the demands of the situation and the person's internal resources, including capabilities, hopes, dreams, aspirations, motivations, and all that makes the person constantly move toward mastery (Roy 1990).

Roy (1988) has identified eight specific assumptions associated with the two philosophic principles of humanism and veritivity. *Humanism,* defined by Roy (1988) as the broad movement in philosophy and psychology that recognizes the person and subjective dimensions of the human experience as central to knowing and valuing, serves as the basis for the following four specific assumptions. In humanism, it is believed that the individual (a) shares in creative power, (b) behaves purposefully, not in a sequence of cause and effect, (c) possesses intrinsic holism, and (d) strives to maintain integrity and to realize the need for relationships.

Veritivity, a term coined by Roy (1988), pertains to the principle of human nature that affirms a common purposefulness of human existence. In veritivity, it is believed that the individual in society is viewed in the context of the (a) purposefulness of human existence, (b) unity of purpose of humankind, (c) activity and creativity for the common good, and (d) value and meaning of life. Further articulation of the philosophical assumptions underlying the Roy Model can be found in Roy (1988).

These assumptions have constituted the basis for and are evident in the specific description of the following major concepts of the Roy Adaptation Model—the person, the environment, health, and nursing.

THE ADAPTIVE SYSTEM AS THE FOCUS OF NURSING

Typically, nurses are viewed as caring for individuals. The recipient of nursing care may be an individual, a family or group, a community, or society as a whole. Since the basis for any family, group, community, or society is the individual, the discussion in this text will focus on the person and the concepts involved in relating on a one-to-one basis in a nursing capacity. It should be noted, however, that in more advanced levels of nursing practice, the principles inherent in this view of the person can be applied to families, groups, communities, and society as a whole. (See Roy 1983, 1984a, and Roy and Anway 1989.)

The Person as an Adaptive System

Roy describes the recipient of nursing care in terms of a holistic adaptive system (Roy 1984b). The term *holistic* stems from the humanistic philosophic assumptions underlying the model and pertains to the idea that the human system functions as a whole and is more than the mere sum of

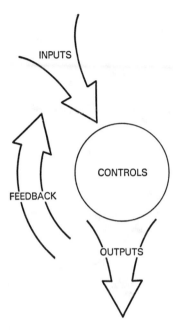

Figure 1–1. Diagrammatic representation of a simple system

its parts. The term *adaptive* is an integral concept in the scientific assumptions underlying the model and means that the human system has the capacity to adjust effectively to changes in the environment and, in turn, affects the environment.

In order to understand persons as adaptive systems, it is important to grasp the meaning of the term *system*. Broadly defined, a *system* is a set of parts connected to function as a whole for some purpose, and it does so by virtue of the interdependence of its parts. In addition to having wholeness and related parts, systems also have *inputs, outputs,* and *control* and *feedback* processes. This is illustrated in Fig. 1–1.

Roy has applied this general systems theory in her description of the person. As illustrated in Fig. 1–2, inputs for the person have been termed stimuli and may come externally from the environment (external stimuli) and internally from the self (internal stimuli). Certain stimuli pool to make up a specific input, the person's adaptation level. The person's response (output) is thus a function of the input stimuli and the person's individual adaptation level. This level is significant as the person processes environmental changes. Roy has termed the major mechanisms for coping the regulator and the cognator mechanisms. The person's behavior results from cognator and regulator processing.

The individual's behavior as the output of the human system takes the form of adaptive responses and ineffective responses. These responses act as feedback or further input to the system, allowing the person to decide whether to increase or decrease efforts to cope with the

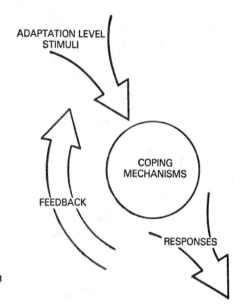

Figure 1–2. The person as a system

stimuli. As will be evident as the view of the person according to the Roy Adaptation Model is explored further, all of the various aspects of the person are interrelated and anything happening to one aspect will have an effect on the others.

It has been noted that the person as an adaptive system is affected by the world around and within. In the broadest sense, this world is called the environment. According to the Roy Adaptation Model for Nursing, the environment is more specifically known as stimuli: focal, contextual, and residual. It is the pooling of these stimuli that make up the adaptation level, or the ability of the person to cope with the changing environment. Based on the environment and the current adaptation level, the person makes a response. Responses can be adaptive or ineffective.

The nurse soon learns that the person never acts in isolation, but is influenced by the environment and in turn affects the environment. Understanding this ongoing interaction and its effect on adaptation is important to nursing practice according to the Roy Adaptation Model for Nursing.

Stimuli. The Roy Adaptation Model for Nursing describes three classes of stimuli that form the person's environment (Roy 1984b). The naming of these stimuli and their original descriptions are based on the work of a physiological psychologist, Harry Helson (1964). The use of these categories by thousands of nurses has clarified their meaning within the nursing framework.

The *focal stimulus* is the internal or external stimulus most immediately confronting the person; the object or event that attracts one's attention. For example, a person may turn around quickly when a loud noise comes from behind or be annoyed by an internal buzzing sound. The person focuses on the stimulus and spends energy dealing with it. In this example of internal or external noise, the person tries to find its source to decide how to handle it.

With the environment constantly changing, many stimuli never become focal; that is, they never immediately confront the person. We generally do not pay attention to the weather unless it is particularly pleasant or unpleasant or is changing. Similarly, positive or negative changes in the environment can become focal, or confront the person, and require a response.

As the nurse using the Roy Adaptation Model views the patient, she will note the many stimuli that may be focal. For the surgical patient, pain may be a focal stimulus, the one on which the patient focuses attention and energy. For the pediatric patient, being away from home may be the focal change. When the nurse is working in the home with the elderly patient who is recovering from a stroke, she may find that the person focuses mainly on the fear of another stroke.

Contextual stimuli are all other stimuli present in the situation that contribute to the effect of the focal stimulus. That is, contextual stimuli are all the environmental factors that present to the person from within or without but which are not the center of the person's attention and/or energy. These factors will influence how the person can deal with the focal stimulus. In our common experience with the weather, it is not the temperature alone that makes us react to the heat or cold. When high humidity is added to high temperatures, the heat is less tolerable, and when a wind chill is added to cold temperatures, one is more affected by the cold. While more attention is devoted to the focal stimulus, the contextual stimuli are those that also can be identified as affecting the situation.

Just as a patient may have many environmental changes that can be focal, so each of those situations can have many contextual stimuli. The person in pain may be more distressed by pain when the cause of it is unknown. Similarly, pain may be better tolerated when the person knows what is expected and that it is temporary. A little girl may handle being away from home more easily when she can have her own toys with her and expects her parents to return. The man who fears another stroke may find that this fear is intensified by memories of his own stroke and of the death of a brother from a stroke. In these examples, it can be seen that the contextual stimuli are also within or outside the person and that they can be positive or negative factors.

Residual stimuli are environmental factors within or without the person whose effects in the current situation are unclear. The person may not be aware of the influence of these factors, or it may not be clear to the observer that they are having an effect. For example, a person who is frightened in a storm may have forgotten being lost once in a storm as a child. A friend who observes that the person is very frightened may have a hunch that there has been a bad experience in the past. However, in describing what is causing the fright, the observer can only consider this as a possibility since the person has never mentioned such an experience.

In looking at what is affecting the person in a given nursing situation, it is useful for the nurse to consider *possible* influencing stimuli and, in this way, can further describe the situation. For example, a nurse may observe the child's reaction to being away from home and consider that this might be the child's first separation from his or her parents. The nurse frequently uses the category of residual stimuli to place general knowledge about what influences the type of behavior observed. Then the nurse gets to know the individual well enough to decide whether that stimulus is focal, contextual, or perhaps not applicable to the patient. By using the category of residual stimuli, one has a place to include even uncertain influencing stimuli and the nurse's intuitive impressions.

The nurse recognizes that focal, contextual, and residual stimuli change rapidly. The environment is changing constantly and the significance of any one stimulus is changing. What is focal at one time soon becomes contextual and what is contextual may slip far enough into the background to become residual, that is, just a possible influence. For example, a person watching a national weather report may be vaguely aware of the weather patterns in another part of the country. However, if that person will be travelling to that area soon, attention is focused on what is being said. Throughout this text, there are examples of the three types of stimuli and their importance in providing nursing care according to the Roy Adaptation Model.

Adaptation Level. The focal, contextual, and residual stimuli pool to make up the person's adaptation level. *Adaptation level* is the name given to the changing point that represents the person's ability to respond positively in a situation. Helson (1964) first used this term in a technical sense related to how the person's ability to deal with a situation comes from two aspects—the demands of the situation, and the person's current internal conditions. An example from Helson's work pertains to a person lifting a series of varying lead weights. The person's response to each weight is influenced by the actual weight of the object, the heaviness of the previous weight, and other factors in the situation—physical fitness relative to weight lifting, for example. Thus, ability to respond positively depends on all three types of stimuli and their current effect on the person. The focal stimulus is judged to have the greatest effect, but there may be many relevant contextual stimuli and any number of residual stimuli that can be considered.

As the concept has been further developed in nursing, the notion of adaptation level conveys that the person is not passive in relation to the environment. The person and environment are in constant interaction with each other. If a person's ability to deal with a new experience is limited, one may actively seek to learn about this experience. For example, in setting up a new household, the young adult may choose to take a short course on finances. In this way, persons can change their own adaptation level. Similarly, one can also change the external environment. For example, if a group of employees finds that a focal concern for them is the unrealistic demands of their employer, they may take positive action together to change the employer's expectations. In this way, the person is an active participant in the process of responding positively, or adapting to the environment. Individual opportunities for mastery and mutual enhancement of human beings and their environment have become social issues in the postindustrial era.

When thinking of adaptation level in clinical terms, one should bear in mind that nurses meet persons who have varying levels of ability to cope with changing circumstances. These varying levels are made up of the pooled effect of the major relevant influencing stimuli. That is, at any given time, the person will respond on the basis of the combined effect of the internal and external environment. As has been noted, the current internal state includes a person's past experiences, even those of which the person may not be aware. The nurse is impressed often by the extent to which persons can cope with potentially overwhelming situations. Many parents of a child with birth defects respond with love, concern, and appropriate planning. This response is related to the pooled effect of all that these persons bring to this demanding situation and to the new levels of mastery they attain.

Adaptation level, then, is a concept that can be described by identifying the relevant focal, contextual, and residual stimuli in a situation. Together, these stimuli determine a range of coping for the person. Many positive life experiences may give a person a broad range of abilities to deal with life's changes. A changing situation may limit that range. For example, a single parent may have worked very hard to maintain a family and home and her broad range of coping is an example to all her friends and colleagues. However, recognizing that she is the sole support and parent of that family, she may find it unusually difficult to handle an illness that requires even a short hospitalization.

The nurse is aware of both the strengths and limitations of the persons with whom she deals whether they are patients or co-workers. She also recognizes minor fluctuations in her own changing adaptation level in situations of fatigue and anxiety. Furthermore, she knows that at times the challenges of her work can tax her own resources. For example, in working with dying patients, she must call on all her resources and sometimes those outside herself to deal with the physical and emotional demands of the situation. The nurse does not avoid these experiences, but can see them as new opportunities for growth, further extension of her inner resources, and the broadening of her adaptation range.

Responses. As has just been described, stimuli and adaptation level serve as input to the person as an adaptive system. After processing this input through control mechanisms, the person makes a response. Those familiar with the American Nurses' Association (1980) definition of nursing are aware of the focus therein on human responses to actual or potential health problems. The Roy Adaptation Model suggests a particular way of viewing these responses. Within the model, responses are not limited to problems but rather the model accommodates all responses of the adaptive system. These responses are called behavior.

Behavior is defined in the broadest sense as internal or external actions and reactions under specified circumstances. A person who responds to a loud noise, by walking toward the noise is making an external response. At the same time, the person's increased heart rate is an internal response. Behaviors can be observed, measured, or subjectively reported. For example, one can see the person walk across the room, a monitor can measure heart rate, or the person may say that he or she feels frightened.

As the nurse views the person as an adaptive system, the output behavior shows how well the person is adapting to environmental change. This observation is key to nursing assessment and intervention. The nurse's assessment of behaviors is discussed in detail in Chapter 2.

An important concern is whether the behavior is adaptive or ineffective. In general, the judgment about the effectiveness of the behavior is made in collaboration with the person and is specific to that person and the condition and circumstances. However, the Roy Adaptation Model provides broad guidelines for nursing judgments about adaptive behaviors.

Adaptive responses are those that promote the integrity of the person in terms of the goals of adaptation: survival, growth, reproduction, and mastery. To drink water when one's body fluids are depleted is an adaptive response contributing directly to survival. Similarly, to seek out new educational experiences contributes to growth and mastery. The notion of reproduction includes the continuation of the human species by having children but it also involves the many ways that people procreate their own persons. For example, the Native American grandfather lives on in the life of his grandchild by instilling the values of the tribe in the child. One's personal contributions are propagated both through individuals and to the whole society. The cultural heritage left by poets and artists can be viewed as their own adaptive responses related to reproduction. Adaptive responses, then, promote the goals of adaptation and promote the integrity of the person. Furthermore, the person's adaptation has an effect on the broader society.

Ineffective responses, on the other hand, are those that neither promote integrity nor contribute to the goals of adaptation. That is, they may, in the immediate situation or if continued over a long time, threaten the person's suvival, growth, reproduction, or mastery. To refuse to eat for one day may not be a serious threat to survival, but to continue such a fast over many weeks may be a serious threat and is ineffective for survival.

In judging effectiveness, then, one looks at the effect of the behavior on the general goals of adaptation. At the same time, the person's individualized goals are a major consideration. For example, there has been much discussion of the right to die. In certain stages of illness, sheer survival may not be the person's highest goal. Rather, the person may choose to be free from medical intervention to enter the final developmental stage of life, that is, death. One author (Dobratz 1984) has described this developmental stage according to the Roy model as the person's life closure. Goals of reproduction, in the sense of legacy of self, and mastery are more prominent at this time. The total integrity of the person may be at its highest point as all of the experiences of life are brought together in this closure. Ineffective responses in this situation would be those that do not contribute to the person's own adaptive goals.

In addition to these broad guidelines for determining adaptive and ineffective responses, the nurse's understanding of the cognator and regulator mechanisms can offer further guidelines. In general, indications of adaptive difficulty can be observed in pronounced regulator activity and cognator ineffectiveness. For example, a person may have a rapid pulse and tense muscles, but may deny that anything is bothering him. The nurse recognizes that the body is automatically responding to some threat, but the person is not effectively using his cognitive and emotional processes to deal with the situation. The response that nothing is bothering him is ineffective in handling the threat. Chapter 2 includes further discussion of the nurse's assessment of adaptive and ineffective behavior and how the basic concepts of the Roy Adaptation Model are used in conjunction with established norms.

Responses, then, are the person's behavior as an adaptive system. They can be observed, intuitively perceived, measured, or subjectively reported. As the nurse helps the person promote adaptation, she assesses the person's current responses and their effectiveness.

Coping Mechanisms. In a simple system, the control process comes from an internal mechanism. Roy has conceptualized the complex controls within the person as the *coping mechanisms* and has broadly categorized these mechanisms as the regulator subsystem and the cognator subsystem.

Coping mechanisms are defined as innate or acquired ways of responding to the changing environment. *Innate* coping mechanisms are genetically determined or common to the species and are generally viewed as automatic processes; the person does not have to think about them. An example of innate coping mechanism is a person's ability to adapt visually to changing intensity of light. When a person enters a darkened room, the iris in the eye automatically dilates to permit the entrance of more light, thus enhancing visual acuity. This response is automatic, unconscious, and innate.

Acquired coping mechanisms are developed through processes such as learning. The experiences encountered throughout life contribute to customary responses to particular stimuli. A child, soon learns an appropriate response to a ringing telephone; the ringing (stimulus) activates acquired coping mechanisms that result in a series of actions to answer the phone (response). This response is deliberate, conscious, and acquired.

Roy further categorizes these innate and acquired coping mechanisms into two major subsystems, the regulator and the cognator subsystems. A basic type of adaptive process, termed by Roy the *regulator subsystem,* responds automatically through neural, chemical, and endocrine coping processes. Stimuli from the internal and external environment (through the senses) act as inputs to the nervous system and affect the fluid and electrolyte and endocrine systems. The information is channeled automatically in the appropriate manner and an automatic, unconscious response is produced. At the same time, inputs to the regulator subsystem have a role in the forming of perceptions.

A mother in labor provides an example of regulator subsystem activity. During the birth process internal stimuli, both chemical and neural, initiate endocrine and central nervous system activity to produce physiological responses of labor such as uterine contraction and opening of the cervix to permit birth of the baby. External stimuli, such as medications administered during labor (for example, a drug whose action is to intensify the uterine contractions), would also affect regulator subsystem activity and, subsequently, body response.

All aspects of the regulator subsystem are so interrelated that one cannot isolate any one system as being the only active system in a particular process. As in this example, both chemical and neural processes are involved. These complex interrelationships are further evidence of the holistic nature of the person.

The second major coping process is termed the *cognator subsystem.* This subsystem responds through four cognitive-emotive channels: perceptual/information processing, learning, judgment, and emotion. Perceptual/information processing includes the activities of selective attention, coding, and memory. This component of the cognator is discussed further in Chapter 11. Learning involves imitation, reinforcement, and insight whereas the judgment process encompasses such activities as problem solving and decision making. Through the person's emotions, defenses are used to seek relief from anxiety and to make affective appraisal and attachments.

An example that illustrates all four cognitive-emotive channels is that of a person driving a car. Learning (imitation, reinforcement, and insight) is involved in mastering the skills needed to operate the vehicle. When gearshifting is required, insight as to the position and function of the various gear ratios and correct positioning of the gearshift is essential. The *rules of the road* and their application are handled by perceptual/information processing and the judgment process is consistently active, although at some times it may be more effective than at others. Even the emotions are called into action, especially when another driver has suddenly cut into the line of traffic.

As with the regulator subsystem, internal and external stimuli including psychological, social, physical, and physiological factors act as inputs to the cognator subsystem. This information is processed through the four channels mentioned previously, and responses are produced.

Thinking again of our driver, the traffic light ahead has just turned yellow, and he is already 10 minutes late for an appointment (external and internal stimuli). Through the judgment process, the driver decides to go through the yellow light instead of stopping. His response would probably be to step a little harder on the accelerator.

The examples have been simplified for the purposes of illustration. Roy and Roberts (1981) have described possible ways to conceptualize the interrelationships of the regulator and cognator subsystems. The complex relationships within and between cognator and regulator further illustrate the holistic nature of the person as an adaptive system.

The Adaptive Modes

Although it has been possible to identify specific processes inherent in the regulator and cognator subsystems, it is not possible to observe directly the functioning of these systems. Only the responses that are produced can be observed.

The behaviors that result from the regulator and cognator mechanisms can be observed in four categories or adaptive modes, developed by Roy to serve as a framework for assessment (Roy 1988). These four modes have been termed the psychological, the self-concept, the role function, and the interdependence modes. It is through these four major categories that responses are carried out and adaptation level can be observed. These four adaptive modes are discussed in greater detail in later chapters, however, a definition of each is provided here.

Physiological Mode. The physiological mode as described in the Roy Adaptation Model is associated with the way the person responds as a physical being to stimuli from the environment. Behavior in this mode is the manifestation of the physiological activities of all the cells, tissues, organs, and systems comprising the human body. As with each of the adaptive modes, stimuli activate the coping mechanisms producing adaptive and ineffective behavior. In this case, the coping mechanisms are those associated with physiological functioning and the responses produced are physiological behaviors. It is the person's physiological behavior that indicates whether the coping mechanisms are able to adapt to the stimuli affecting them.

Five needs are identified in the physiological mode relative to the basic need of **physiological integrity:** oxygenation, nutrition, elimination, activity and rest, and protection. Also inherent in a discussion of physiological adaptation are complex processes involving senses, fluids and electrolytes, neurological function, and endocrine function. These can be viewed as mediating regulatory activity and encompassing many physiological functions of the person. These nine components are described within the model as a basis for nursing assessment of the physiological mode.

Self-Concept Mode. The self-concept mode is one of three psychosocial modes, and it focuses specifically on the psychological and spiritual aspects of the person. The basic need underlying the self-concept mode has been identified as **psychic integrity**—the need to know who one is so that one can be or exist with a sense unity. Psychic integrity is basic to health and adaptation problems in this area may interfere with the person's ability to heal or to do what is necessary to maintain other aspects of health. It is important for the nurse to have knowledge about the self-concept mode in order to be able to assess behaviors and stimuli influencing the person's self-concept.

Self-concept is defined as the composite of beliefs and feelings that a person holds about him or herself at a given time. Formed from internal perceptions and perceptions of others, self-concept directs one's behavior.

The self-concept mode is viewed in the Roy Adaptation Model as having two components: the **physical self** including body sensation and body image and the **personal self** comprised of self-consistency, self-ideal, and moral-ethical-spiritual self. Some examples of these components include the statement, "I look terrible!"—a behavioral statement related to body image. The statement, "I know I can win this game," illustrates self-ideal behavior.

Role Function Mode. The role function mode is one of two social modes and focuses on the roles the person occupies in society. A *role,* as the functioning unit of society, is defined as a set of expectations about how a person occupying one position behaves toward a person occupying another position. The basic need underlying the role function mode has been identified as **social integrity**—the need to know who one is in relation to others so that one can act.

A classification of roles as primary, secondary, and tertiary has been adapted for use in the Roy Adaptation Model. Associated with each role are **instrumental behaviors** and **expressive behaviors,** assessment of which provides an indication of social adaptation relative to role function. Each type of behavior can be illustrated with the role of mother. Caring for the baby's physical needs involves instrumental behaviors; holding and cuddling the baby are expressive behaviors. The manner in which the person fulfills these role expectations is an indication of role functioning.

Interdependence Mode. The interdependence mode is the final adaptive mode Roy describes. It focuses on interactions related to the giving and receiving of love, respect, and value. The basic need of this mode is termed **affectional adequacy**—the feeling of security in nurturing relationships.

Two specific relationships are the focus of the interdependence mode: **significant others**, persons who are the most important to the individual, and **support systems**, that is, others contributing to the meeting of interdependence needs. In relation to these specific relationships, two major areas of interdependence behavior have been identified (Randell, Tedrow, and VanLandingham 1982): **receptive behavior** and **contributive behavior**, applying respectively to the receiving and giving of love, respect, and value in interdependent relationships. For example, a significant other for a child would be the mother. In this interdependent relationship, receptive behavior on the child's part would be allowing mother to comfort when hurt, and contributive behavior would be giving Mom a hug and a kiss on leaving for school. The assessment of receptive and contributive behaviors provides an indication of social adaptation relative to the interdependence mode.

Each person's behavior is viewed in relation to the four adaptive modes; they provide a particular form or manifestation of cognator and regulator activity within the adaptive process. Although these modes are frequently viewed separately for teaching and assessment purposes, it must be remembered that they are interrelated. In Fig. 1–3, the four modes are depicted as four overlapping circles, central to which is a circle representing the coping mechanisms. As an illustration of interrelationships, it can be noted that the physiological mode in the diagram is intersected by each of the other three modes. Behavior in the physiological mode may have an effect on or act as a stimulus for one or all of the other modes. In addition, a given stimulus may affect more than one mode or a

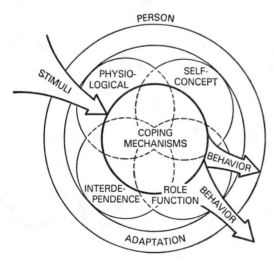

Figure 1–3. The person as an adaptive system

particular behavior may be indicative of adaptation in more than one mode. Such complex relationships among modes further demonstrate the holistic nature of the person. Roy has used the kaleidoscope as an image of the multifaceted interrelations.

ENVIRONMENT

Environment is the second major concept of a nursing model and it is understood as the world within and around the person. According to the Roy Adaptation Model, the changing environment stimulates the person to make adaptive responses. For human beings, life is never the same. It is constantly changing and presenting new challenges. The person has the ability to make new responses to these changing conditions. As the environment changes, the person has the continued opportunity to grow, to develop, and to enhance the meaning of life for everyone. One example of a positive response to changing circumstances is the patient who reorders life's priorities after suffering a near-fatal heart attack. Altering a style of living can provide a more satisfying life for the person and his family. For example, the person may make a decision to spend more of his time and energy with his wife and children and less at work.

In describing the environment, Roy has drawn upon the work of Helson (1964). This physiological psychologist describes *adaptation* as a function of the degree of change taking place and the person's adaptation level. The three types of stimuli described previously pool to make up the person's adaptation level. Those immediately confronting the person are termed **focal stimuli**. All other stimuli present that can be identified as influencing the current situation are called **contextual stimuli**. The **residual stimuli** are those that may influence the adaptation level, but whose effect has not been confirmed.

According to Roy, *environment* includes all conditions, circumstances, and influences that surround and affect the development and behavior of the person. These influencing factors are categorized as focal, contextual, and residual stimuli.

HEALTH

An understanding of the description of health as presented in the Roy Adaptation Model is contingent on an understanding of the concepts of the person and the environment as presented earlier in this chapter. The concept of health as articulated in the model is in the developing stages. It is recognized that, with further consideration of the model from the theoretical perspective and its increasing use in practice, the clarity with which this concept can be described will be enhanced.

A universally accepted definition of health is that provided by the Constitution of the United Nations World Health Organization: Health is "a state of complete physical, mental, and social well-being and not merely the absence of disease or infirmity" (United Nations 1968). This statement describes optimum health—a state of being. Health also has been described as a continuum ranging from peak wellness to extreme poor health and death. Traditionally, health concerns were considered to be primarily physical in nature but it is becoming increasingly common to see definitions of health that encompass the more holistic perception of the person as reflected in the definition presented by the World Health Organization.

A working document of the Government of Canada (Lalonde 1975) emphasized the intention to give to human biology, the environment, and lifestyle as much attention as has been given to the financing of the health care organization so that all four avenues to improve health are pursued. Newman (1979) has developed the notion of health as the synthesis of disease and nondisease. Her later work (Newman 1986) has focused on health as expanding consciousness.

In viewing health from the nursing perspective, it is necessary to articulate a definition in terms of the related concepts of the nursing model. Earlier in the chapter, it was noted that a person was described as an adaptive system constantly growing and developing within a changing environment. A person's health can be described as a reflection of this interaction or adaptation. In this earlier discussion, successful adaptation was viewed in terms of the goals of the human system—survival, growth, reproduction, and mastery. Adaptive responses were said to promote integrity or wholeness relative to these goals—integrity implying soundness, an unimpaired condition leading to wholeness. Health can be viewed in light of individual goals and the purposefulness of human existence. The fulfillment of one's purpose in life is reflected in becoming an integrated and whole person. Thus, in the Roy Adaptation Model, *health* is defined as a state and a process of being and becoming an integrated and whole person. Lack of integration represents lack of health (Roy 1984).

Consider the following two situations: In the first case, a 28-year-old woman, as a result of an accident, is quadriplegic. Although confined to a wheelchair and assisted by mechanical devices, she has developed a fruitful and meaningful life as a wife, author, and painter. Her perspective on life is an encouragement to all those with whom she comes in contact.

In the second case, a 20-year-old male college student is becoming increasingly dependent on drugs to see him through his academic year. Where initially he was using them during stressful periods of examination, now he is finding that he cannot function on a day-to-day basis without their assistance. His grades are falling and he is considering withdrawing from the program.

In considering health as a reflection of adaptation with a goal of becoming an integrated and whole person, it is the first situation that exemplifies health. The woman is demonstrating the integration indicative of successful adaptation while the young man is responding ineffectively to his changing environment. The need for intervention is apparent.

GOAL OF NURSING

Generally speaking, nursing's goal is to contribute to the overall goal of health care, that is, to promote the health of individuals and society. To be meaningful within the context of a nursing model, the goal of nursing must be described in terms of the related concepts of the model.

Nursing activities, as discussed in depth in the next chapter, involve the assessment of behavior and the stimuli that influence adaptation. Nursing judgments are based on this assessment and interventions are planned to manage these stimuli. Nursing acts to enhance the interaction of the person with the environment—to promote adaptation.

Consider the situation of a first-time mother hospitalized for the birth of her child. Following the birth, nursing care for the mother would be directed towards helping her adapt to her new role. In addition to physiological concerns such as nutrition, elimination, and healing, goals would relate to the mother's ability to care for the child, the support systems that she may have in place when help is required, and the integrity of her self-concept throughout the adjustment period. In this case, the goal of nursing care is to assist the new mother in all aspects of adaptation. The nurse will identify the mother's level of adaptation and coping abilities, identify difficulties, and intervene where necessary to promote the mother's adaptation. In this manner, the integrity of the newborn child is maintained, as well.

Thus, Roy defines the *goal of nursing* as the promotion of adaptation in each of the four modes, thereby contributing to the person's health, quality of life, and dying with dignity. It must be recognized that complete physical, mental, and social well-being, the common understanding of optimal health is not possible for every person. It is the nurse's role to promote adaptation in situations of health and illness; to enhance the interaction of the person with their environment, thereby promoting health.

SUMMARY

In summary, the Roy Adaptation Model defines the person as an adaptive system with cognator and regulator coping mechanisms acting to maintain adaptation with respect to the four adaptive modes. This concept of the person was depicted in Fig. 1–3. Stimuli from the internal and external environment activate the coping mechanisms, the regulator and cognator subsystems, which in turn produce behavioral responses relative to the physiological, self-concept, role function, and interdependence modes. These responses may be either adaptive and thus promoting the integrity or wholeness of the person (as depicted by the arrow remaining with the adaptation circle) or ineffective and not contributing to the goals of the person (arrows extending beyond the adaptation circle). Although, for descriptive purposes, it has been necessary to present each aspect of the person as a separate entity, the model is based on the belief that the person functions in a holistic manner with each aspect related to and affected by the others.

Health is a state and a process of being and becoming an integrated and whole person. It is a reflection of adaptation, that is, the interaction of the person and the environment. Nursing acts to promote this adaptation. The goal of nursing is stated as the promotion of adaptation in each of the four modes. In promoting adaptation, the nurse contributes to the person's health, quality of life, and dying with dignity.

The scientific and philosophic assumptions that form the basis for these ideas are systems theory, adaptation-level theory, humanism, and veritivity. As the major concepts of the model are explored in more depth, the influence of these foundational assumptions will become increasingly evident.

EXERCISES FOR APPLICATION

1. Imagine yourself in rush-hour traffic approaching an intersection at which the light for your direction of traffic has just turned to yellow. Suggest focal, contextual, and residual stimuli that might have an effect on your judgment as to what action to take.

2. From your personal experience in writing an important examination, suggest focal, contextual, and residual stimuli that serve (a) to broaden your adaptation level or range of coping abilities, and (b) to limit that range.

3. In considering your own behavioral responses during the last minute, suggest two responses that can be (a) observed, (b) measured, and (c) subjectively reported.

4. Suggest two behavioral responses that would be considered adaptive in promoting your mastery of the content presented in this chapter and two that would be considered ineffective. An example of an adaptive response would be "underlining important concepts"; an ineffective response would be "daydreaming."

5. Jot down phrases that are descriptive of your personal perception of health. Compare them to the definition of health identified in the Roy Adaptation Model.

ASSESSMENT OF UNDERSTANDING

Questions

1. Associate the specific assumptions in Column A with the appropriate major scientific and philosophic perspectives in Column B.

   Column A
   ___ a. The individual possesses intrinsic holism.
   ___ b. Control mechanisms are central to human functioning
   ___ c. The individual behaves purposefully
   ___ d. There is unity of purpose of humankind
   ___ e. Environmental changes can be focal, contextual, or residual

   Column B
   1. Systems theory
   2. Adaptation-level theory
   3. Humanism
   4. Veritivity

2. Fill in the missing words.
   In a human system, inputs have been termed _____ and _____. The controls or _____ _____ are central to function and their activity is manifest by _____ which act as feedback and further input to the system.

3. Label each of the following descriptions according to whether it indicates an adaptive (A) or ineffective (I) response.
   (a) _____ Disrupts integrity
   (b) _____ Does not contribute to survival, growth, reproduction, or mastery
   (c) _____ Promotes integrity
   (d) _____ Contributes to the goals of the human system

4. Situation: A four-year-old child is having a plaster cast changed. He has been wearing casts on his left ankle since he was six months old in order to correct a congenital problem. The second the plaster saw comes into view, he begins to scream, calling for his mother. On previous occasions, the staff doing the procedure have had to restrain him and proceed as quickly as possible with their task.
   Label the following stimuli as focal (F), contextual (C), or residual (R).
   (a) _____ past experience with cast removal
   (b) _____ the sight of the plaster saw
   (c) _____ previous cut due to saw blade

5. Which of the following statements apply to *adaptation level*?
   (a) It is a changing point.
   (b) It is a person's state of health.

(c) It is the person's ability to respond positively.

(d) It is the pooled effect of three types of stimuli.

6. Classify the underlined behaviors in the following situation as being indicative of regulator or cognator activity.

As a young woman was <u>driving calmly down the street</u>, smelling fresh spring air, a small child suddenly ran out in front of her car. She <u>slammed on the brakes</u> and <u>swerved to the left</u> to avoid hitting him. As the child ran off, oblivious to the near accident, she was left in silence with the fierce <u>pounding of her heart</u> in her chest and her <u>body shaking</u> with fright.

7. Insert the appropriate words in the following description of health according to the Roy Adaptation Model.

Health is a _____ and a _____ of being and becoming an _____ and _____ person.

8. Which of the following statements pertain to the goal of nursing as described in the Roy Adaptation Model?

Roy's goal of nursing is

(a) to achieve the health of individuals and society.

(b) to enhance the interaction of the person and the environment.

(c) to promote adaptation.

(d) to promote complete physical, mental, and social well-being for every person.

Feedback

1. (a) 1 and 3
   (b) 1
   (c) 3 and 4
   (d) 4
   (e) 2
2. Stimuli, adaptation level, coping mechanisms, responses or behaviors.
3. (a) I
   (b) I
   (c) A
   (d) A
4. (a) C
   (b) F
   (c) R
5. a, c, d
6. Behaviors indicative of regulator activity: pounding of her heart, body shaking. Behaviors of cognator activity: driving calmly down the street, slammed on the brakes, swerved to the left.
7. state, process, integrated, whole.
8. b, c

REFERENCES

American Nurses' Association. *Nursing: A Social Policy Statement.* Kansas City: American Nurses' Association, 1980.

Dobratz, M.C. Life closure, in *Introduction to Nursing: An Adaptation Model* (2nd ed.), Sr. C. Roy, pp. 497–518. Englewood Cliffs, N.J.: Prentice-Hall, 1984.

Helson, H. *Adaptation Level Theory.* New York: Harper & Row, 1964.

Lalonde, M. *A New Perspective on the Health of Canadians.* Ottawa: Information Canada, 1975.

Newman, M. *Theory Development in Nursing.* Philadelphia: F.A. Davis, 1979.

Newman, M. *Health as Expanding Consciousness.* St. Louis: The C.V. Mosby, 1986.

Randell, B., M. Tedrow, and J. VanLandingham. *Adaptation Nursing: The Roy Conceptual Model Made Practical.* St. Louis: The C.V. Mosby Company, 1982.

Roy, Sr. C. Adaptation: A conceptual framework for nursing, *Nursing Outlook* 18, no. 3 (March 1970): 43–45.

Roy, Sr. C. Roy Adaptation Model and application to the expectant family and the family in primary care, in *Family Health: A Theoretical Approach to Nursing Care,* eds. J. Clements and F. Roberts. pp. 255–278, 298–303, and 375–378. New York: John Wiley and Sons, 1983.

Roy, Sr. C. The Roy Adaptation Model in nursing: applications in community health nursing, in *Proceedings of the Eighth Annual Community Nursing Conference,* ed. M.K. Asay and C.C. Assler. University of North Carolina, Chapel Hill, North Carolina, May 22, 1984a.

Roy, Sr. C. The Roy Adaptation Model in nursing, in *Introduction to Nursing: An Adaptation Model* (2nd ed.), Sr. C. Roy, pp. 27–41. Englewood Cliffs, N.J.: Prentice-Hall, 1984b.

Roy, Sr. C. An explication of the philosophical assumptions of the Roy Adaptation Model, *Nursing Science Quarterly* 1(1) 1988: 26–34.

Roy, Sr. C. Theorist's response to "Strengthening the Roy Adaptation Model Through Conceptual Clarification," *Nursing Science Quarterly,* 3, no. 2 (1990): 64–66.

Roy, Sr. C., and J. Anway. Roy's Adaptation Model: Theories and propositions for administration, in *Dimensions and Issues of Nursing Administration,* B. Henry, C. Arndt, M. DiVincenti, and G. Marriner-Tomey. St. Louis: The C.V. Mosby, 1989.

United Nations. *Everyman's United Nations* (8th ed.), p. 509. New York: U.N. Office of Public Information (U.N. Publication E.67.I.2), March 1968.

von Bertalanffly, L. *General Systems Theory.* New York: Braziller, 1968.

Additional References

Buck, M.H. Self-concept: Theory and development, in *Introduction to Nursing: An Adaptation Model* (2nd ed.), Sr. C. Roy, pp. 255–283. Englewood Cliffs, N.J.: Prentice-Hall, 1984.

Fitzpatrick, J.J., and A.L. Whall. *Conceptual Models of Nursing: Analysis and Application.* Bowie, Md.: Brody Co., 1983.

Nuwayhid, K.A. Role function: Theory and development, in *Introduction to Nursing: An Adaptation Model* (2nd ed.), Sr. C. Roy, pp. 284–305. Englewood Cliffs, N.J.: Prentice-Hall, 1984.

Roy, Sr. C. Adaptation: A conceptual framework for nursing, *Nursing Outlook,* 18, (1970): 43–45.

Roy, Sr. C. The Roy Adaptation Model for nursing, in *Introduction to Nursing: An Adaptation Model* (2nd ed.), Sr. C. Roy, pp. 27–41, Englewood Cliffs, N.J.: Prentice-Hall, 1984.

Roy, Sr. C. An explication of the philosophical assumptions of the Roy Adaptation Model, in *Nursing Science Quarterly,* 1, no. 1 (1988): 26–34.

Roy, Sr. C., and S. Roberts. *Theory Construction in Nursing: An Adaptation Model.* Englewood Cliffs, N.J.: Prentice-Hall, 1981.

Tedrow, M.P. "Interdependence: Theory and Development," in *Introduction to Nursing: An Adaptation Model* (2nd ed.), Sr. C. Roy, pp. 306–322. Englewood Cliffs, N.J.: Prentice-Hall, 1984.

Chapter Two

The Nursing Process According to the Roy Adaptation Model

Heather A. Andrews and
Sister Callista Roy

Nursing is a scientific discipline that is practice oriented. The specific activities that distinguish nursing from other disciplines are collectively termed *the nursing process*. This nursing process is a problem-solving approach for gathering data, identifying person's needs, selecting and implementing approaches for nursing care, and evaluating outcomes of care being given.

The recipient of nursing care is the person—singly or in groups. Each person copes differently with changes in health status and it is the nurse's responsibility to help persons adapt to these changes. She must be able to identify the person's level of adaptation and coping abilities, to identify difficulties, and to intervene to promote adaptation.

The nursing process as described by Roy relates directly to the view of the person as an adaptive system. Six steps have been identified in the nursing process according to the Roy Adaptation Model.

1. Assessment of behavior
2. Assessment of stimuli
3. Nursing diagnosis
4. Goal setting
5. Intervention
6. Evaluation

This chapter will explore each of these steps and relate it to Roy's view of the person.

It is important to recognize that, although the steps of the nursing process have been separated and specified for ease of discussion, the process is ongoing and simultaneous. For example, the nurse would be assessing the person's behaviors in one respect while she is implementing an intervention in another. This is similar to the conceptualization of the person: Although it was necessary to present each aspect as a separate entity, one must bear in mind the belief that the person functions in a holistic manner with each aspect related to and affected by the others.

Collaboration with the person in each step of the nursing process is important. Individuals must be involved in observation of and decisions relative to their state of adaptation. They provide valuable insight that may assist the nurse in attempts to promote adaptation. The form the individual participation takes will vary. For example, how the person can communicate differs with age and level of consciousness.

OBJECTIVES

After studying this chapter, the reader will be able to do the following:

1. Given a situation, identify behaviors demonstrated.
2. Apply criteria to evaluate specified behaviors as adaptive or ineffective.
3. In a given situation, identify stimuli influencing designated behaviors.
4. Classify designated stimuli as being focal, contextual, or residual.
5. In a given situation, make a nursing diagnosis using each of the three methods.
6. Derive complete goal statements when provided with assessment data and nursing diagnoses.
7. In a given situation, identify actions that could serve to alter appropriately a specific stimulus.
8. Given goal statements, describe the evidence that would indicate that nursing interventions had been effective.

KEY CONCEPTS DEFINED

- *Adaptation problems:* broad areas of concern related to adaptation and describing difficulties related to the indicators of positive adaptation.
- *Behavior:* actions or reactions under specified circumstances.
- *Contextual stimuli:* all internal or external stimuli evident in the situation other than the focal stimulus.
- *Evaluation:* judging the effectiveness of the nursing intervention in relation to the person's behavior.
- *Focal stimulus:* the internal or external stimulus most immediately confronting the person.
- *Goal setting:* the establishment of clear statements of the behavioral outcomes of nursing care for the person.
- *Norms:* generally accepted guidelines, expectations used to guide judgment about the effectiveness of behavior.

- *Nursing diagnosis:* a judgment process resulting in a statement conveying the person's adaptation status.
- *Nursing process:* a problem-solving approach for gathering data, identifying the person's needs, selecting and implementing approaches for nursing care, and evaluating the outcomes of care being given.
- *Residual stimuli:* those stimuli having an undetermined effect on the person's behavior.

ASSESSMENT OF BEHAVIOR

The first step of the nursing process as described by the Roy Adaptation Model is the assessment of behavior. The goal of nursing activities is to promote adaptation. The one indicator of how a person is managing to cope with or adapt to changes in health status is behavior. Thus the first step in the nursing process involves gathering data about the person's behavior and the current state of adaptation. In Fig. 2–1 each step of the nursing process as it relates to Roy's description of the person is illustrated.

The Roy Adaptation Model views the person as a holistic, adaptive system. Input, in the form of stimuli from the internal and external environment, activates regulator and cognator coping mechanisms that act to maintain adaptation with respect to the four adaptive modes. The result is behavioral responses. These responses may be either adaptive or ineffective. The former promotes integrity of the person in terms of the goals of the human system, and the latter disrupts or does not contribute to this integrity.

The person's responses are the focus of the first step of the nursing process—assessment of behavior. Behavior has been defined as actions or reactions under specified circumstances. It may be observable or nonobservable. In an anxious situation, the phenomenon of "butterflies in the stomach" may occur. This is a nonobservable behavior. It must be reported or otherwise demonstrated by the person. On the other hand, observable behavior can be discerned by another. A scream by a frightened person would be an observable behavior.

Under normal circumstances, most people cope effectively with the changes that occur in their internal and external environments. However, there may be times—during an illness, for example—when there is stress placed on a person's coping abilities. The stimuli or changes being faced may be outside the person's zone of adaptation. It is often at these times that the nurse encounters the person.

In a nursing situation, the primary concern is a certain type of behavior, a behavior that requires further adaptive response as a result of environmental changes straining the person's coping mechanisms. Important aspects of nursing are knowing how to (1) assess these behav-

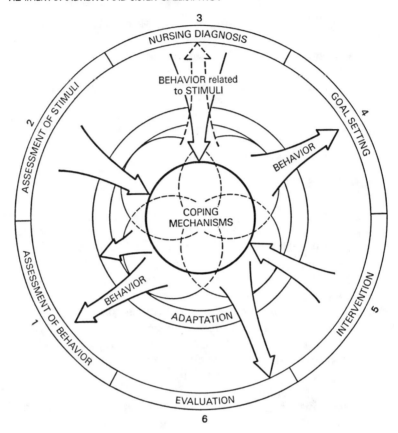

Figure 2—1. The nursing process as it relates to Roy's description of the person

iors, (2) compare them to specific criteria to evaluate their contribution to the maintenance of integrity, and (3) identify the strengths and strains of the coping process.

Gathering Behavioral Data

In assessing behavior, the nurse systematically looks at responses in each adaptive mode. As mentioned previously, the four adaptive modes (physiological, self-concept, role function, and interdependence) are a classification of ways of coping that manifest regulator and cognator activity. It is in relation to these four major categories that responses are carried out and that observable and nonobservable behaviors occur.

As described, all behavior is not directly obvious to another person. Nonobservable behavior must either be reported by the person or demonstrated in some other manner. Observable behaviors typically can be seen, heard, and/or measured. Thus, in assessing behavior in each adaptive mode, the nurse uses skills of observation, measurement, and interviewing to obtain behavioral data. The scope of this text permits only a brief look at each of these methods of behavioral assessment. Proficiency in their use is achieved through knowledge and practice of the principles involved.

The nurse, when applying observational skills, uses her senses to obtain data about the person's behavior. She may see cyanotic skin color, feel a weakened pulse, smell body odor, or hear unusual chest sounds. She may even "sense" a patient's discomfort even as the person denies this. The nurse's description of these observations would constitute behavioral data.

Behavioral responses can be measured and the measurements compared to preestablished criteria. The nurse may take a blood pressure reading, test a urine specimen, or have a person read an eye chart. The measured value becomes the behavioral data.

The nurse uses interviewing skills to listen to and purposefully question in order to obtain behavioral data. For example, a person's expression of pain should signal the nurse to ask questions regarding the nature of the pain. The person's verbal response becomes the behavioral data that the nurse identifies and records.

Effective communication between the nurse and the person for whom she is caring is important in each aspect of assessment of behavior and throughout the nursing process. Without effective communication and caring (Watson 1985, Benner and Wrubel 1989), the effectiveness of all nursing actions is questionable.

The process of data collection relative to behavior is a systematic process. In later chapters, specific behavioral data to be gathered relative to each of the adaptive modes are identified. On initial assessment, these specific data are gathered by means of skillful observation and sensitivity, accurate measurement, and purposeful interview within the nurse/ patient relationship. An initial nursing judgment is made as to whether the behavior is adaptive or ineffective. Criteria have been established to assist in this decision.

Tentative Judgment of Behavior

As presented in Chapter 1, adaptive responses are those that promote the integrity or wholeness of the person in terms of the goals of the human system (survival, growth, reproduction, and mastery). Ineffective responses are those that do not contribute to these goals and thereby disrupt integrity.

A person's individualized adaptive goals are a major consideration. Chapter 1 provided an example of the person in the final developmental stage—death. At this point, survival may not be the person's highest goal.

Although the parameters for the designation of adaptive responses are wide, in some areas normal values are available to guide judgment about the effectiveness of behavior. For example, based on data from large numbers of people, charts are available suggesting average weights and heights for specific age groups, and we know normal ranges for values of pulse, blood pressure, and temperature. In other areas, expectations or generally accepted guidelines are evident. When behavior does not align with these generally accepted norms, guidelines, or expectations, there is reason to suggest it may be ineffective. For example, there are some general expectations as to how a new mother behaves toward her baby. These are based on common cultural norms and nursing research.

In situations where *norms* are not available, Roy has hypothesized general indications of adaptation difficulty: pronounced regulator activity with cognator ineffectiveness. Some signs of pronounced regulator activity are

1. increase in heart rate or blood pressure,
2. tension,
3. excitement,
4. loss of appetite,
5. increase in serum cortisol.

Signs of cognator ineffectiveness include

1. faulty perception/information processing,
2. ineffective learning,
3. poor judgment,
4. inappropriate affect.

Such behaviors require energy that could be used more effectively to respond to other stimuli. Furthermore, they limit the full potential of the person and can affect integrity.

In making the initial judgment as to whether behavior is adaptive or ineffective, it is important that the nurse continually involve the person for whom she is caring. The person's perception of the effectiveness of the behavior is an integral consideration. For example, a nurse may observe that her patient slept soundly for eight hours during the night and determine that this behavior was adaptive in meeting the patient's need for rest. However, when she asks, "Do you feel well rested?" she learns that the patient was actually lying quietly awake and, in fact, had slept only two hours and is feeling very tired as a result. By validating her observation with the person, the nurse changes her judgment of behavior from *adaptive* to *ineffective*.

By initially evaluating behaviors as adaptive or ineffective the nurse has a basis on which to set priorities of concern. The primary concern would be the behaviors that are disrupting the person's integrity and not promoting the adaptation. However, the importance of identifying, maintaining, and enhancing adaptive behaviors is acknowledged, as well.

In this manner, the nurse obtains an indication of whether the person is coping effectively with changes in the internal and external environment and is able to set priorities with respect to the next level of the nursing process—assessment of stimuli.

ASSESSMENT OF STIMULI

As discussed in the previous chapter, it is change in the internal and external stimuli that places stress on the person's coping abilities. The individual's behavior manifests whether or not he or she is coping effectively with these changes. Whereas the first level of assessment in the nursing process involves the assessment of this behavior and a tentative judgment as to whether it is adaptive or ineffective; the second step of the nursing process involves the identification of internal and external stimuli that are influencing the behaviors.

The skills used in assessing stimuli are the same as those used in assessing behaviors, namely, astute and sensitive observation, measurement, and interview. Behavior manifesting a threat to integrity is of initial concern. To assist in setting priorities relative to the behavior of concern, the nurse, in collaboration with the person, identifies the focal, contextual, and residual stimuli influencing these responses. Specific contextual stimuli have been suggested by Roy and her colleagues as having an effect on behavior in each adaptive mode. These common stimuli are identified in Table 2–1.

Identifying Focal, Contextual, and Residual Stimuli

A stimulus has been defined as that which provokes a response. Stimuli can be internal or external and include all conditions, circumstances, and influences surrounding and/or affecting the development and behavior of the person. A collective term for all internal and external stimuli is *environment.*

Stimuli are assessed relative to behavior identified in the first level of assessment. Behaviors of disrupted integrity or the ineffective responses would be of initial concern. Ineffective behaviors are of concern since it is the goal of nursing to promote adaptation; the nurse assists the person to change ineffective behaviors to adaptive ones. Adaptive behaviors are also important; they are to be maintained and enhanced. The stimuli hold the key to the accomplishment of this goal. Changes in stimuli challenge the person's coping abilities. In many instances, stimuli can be altered by the person or the nurse, thereby enabling the person to cope more effectively. This idea will be discussed further in subsequent steps of the nursing process.

The skills used in assessment of stimuli are the same as those used to

TABLE 2–1.   COMMON STIMULI AFFECTING ADAPTATION

Culture—Socioeconomic status, ethnicity, belief system
Family—Structure, tasks
Developmental stage—Age, sex, tasks, hereditary, and genetic factors
Integrity of adaptive modes—Physiological (including disease pathology), self-concept, role function, interdependence
Cognator effectiveness—Perception, knowledge, skill
Environmental considerations—Change in internal or external environment, medical management, use of drugs, alcohol, tobacco

---

assess behaviors—perceptive observation, measurement, and interview. As the stimuli affecting each priority behavior or set of behaviors are identified, they are classified as focal, contextual, and residual. As with step 1, and with each step of the nursing process, consultation with the person and validation of observations are important.

The *focal stimulus* has been defined as the internal or external stimulus most immediately confronting the person. In assessing the focal stimulus, the nurse is looking for the most immediate cause of the identified behavior. Consider an example of a person experiencing a toothache. The focal stimulus in this situation is the fact that the person has just lost a filling from a rather deep cavity. This loss of filling and subsequent exposure of the nerve is the stimulus or change in environment with which the person is having difficulty coping.

Possible focal stimuli have been identified for given behaviors relative to each adaptive mode. These are identified in the chapters in which specific discussion of each adaptive mode is presented.

It is important to note that behavior in one adaptive mode may act as a focal stimulus in another. For example, as a manifestation of anxiety regarding her final exams, a teenage girl begins eating while she is studying and subsequently gains weight. This weight gain (physiological behavior) may become a stimulus to the self-concept mode causing low self-esteem when she does not meet her own and other's expectations that she remain slim.

Also, one focal stimulus can affect more than one adaptive mode. The loss of a limb not only affects the physiologic mode but it may disrupt the self-concept, role function, and interdependence modes. Not only is the person's mobility affected, self image, ability to perform roles, and interrelationships with others may be disrupted as well.

Contextual stimuli have been defined as all other internal or external stimuli evident in the situation. They contribute to the behavior triggered by the focal stimulus. For example, consider again the person with the toothache. One contextual stimulus may be that he or she has just been chewing on a very sticky piece of candy. The candy contributed to the loss of the filling but in the current situation the sugar on the exposed nerve is aggravating the pain. Contextual stimuli are important because they often are tied to the meaning a person attaches to the situation. A person with a toothache who has a family member with cancer of the jaw may react entirely differently than one who does not.

Residual stimuli are the third category of stimuli influencing behavior to be assessed. These stimuli have been defined as those having an indeterminate effect on the person's behavior; their effect has not or cannot be validated. Roy has identified two ways in which validation of a stimulus can occur: (1) The person confirms that the stimulus is affecting him; (2) the nurse has theoretical or experiential knowledge to establish confirmation. Residual stimuli become contextual or focal once they have been validated. When residual stimuli are identified as affecting the situation, they are no longer *possible* influencing stimuli; their effect on the person's behavior has been confirmed.

Residual stimuli affecting the person with the toothache could be the type of toothpaste being used or dental hygiene habits. If one is able to confirm that conscientious care of the teeth has not been taken, the stimulus then becomes contextual. Probable influencing factors can be identified through research and understanding of the human person. Still, based on philosophical assumptions Roy maintains that parts of the human person may remain a mystery.

It is important to note that changing circumstances can change the significance of the stimuli. What is contextual at one point in time might be focal at another. For example, at the point in time when the filling was actually dislodged, the most immediate cause was the chewing of the piece of candy; this focal stimulus later becomes a contextual factor.

Common Influencing Stimuli

As discussed in Chapter 1, the environment is considered to be all the internal and external stimuli affecting the development and behavior of the person. Certain contextual stimuli have been identified as having an effect on behavior in all of the adaptive modes. Table 2–1 presented an overview of these common influencing stimuli as initially identified by Martinez (1976) and selectively elaborated upon by Sato (1984).

Sato (1984) discussed culture, family, and developmental stage as of primary consideration for stimuli affecting human adaptation. **Culture** is described as involving socioeconomic status, ethnicity, and belief systems. Socioeconomic status provides an indication of the person's style of living and the material resources upon which the person has to draw. Different stimuli are evident in situations of different socioeconomic status. For example, an impoverished person suffering from malnutrition is affected by entirely different stimuli than those affecting a malnourished teenager from an upper middle-class family.

Ethnicity is viewed as including language, practices, philosophies, and associated values. Ethnic background may influence health practices and responses to illness. It is recognized that ethnicity is a stimulus in a person's response to pain. For example, some cultures are generally considered to be more stoic when compared to the expressiveness of persons of other cultural groups.

Belief system, as a component of culture, involves spiritual beliefs, practices, and philosophies and may influence all aspects of a person's life. As well as being a major support system for the person, one's belief system may have a specific influence on health practices and adaptation. For example, a person's attitude toward death is affected to a great extent by the person's belief system and the extent to which these beliefs are carried into practice. Often it is important for a Catholic, even one who has not been an active church member, to see a priest when death is imminent.

Another common influencing stimulus pertains to the **family** and its associated structure and tasks. Consider the different stimuli associated with a single-parent family as opposed to a nuclear or extended family. As well, a family in the beginning stages of child rearing has different duties and responsibilities than a family whose children are grown and have left home.

Consideration of factors related to the **developmental stage** of the person is important in assessment of contextual stimuli affecting adaptation. Based primarily on the developmental stages and tasks identified by Erikson (1963), it is known that factors such as age, sex, and heredity influence the person's behavior, especially relating to the role function mode.

The interrelationships among the aspects of the whole person as an adaptive system cannot be overemphasized. As noted earlier, it is important to recognize that behavior in one adaptive mode may function as a stimulus in another. Thus, **lack of integrity** in any area of a person's functioning (physiological, self-concept, role function, interdependence) would, in turn, act as a stimulus affecting behavior in another area. Since the nurse often encounters persons during treatment for disease, an important consideration relative to adaptation in the physiological mode is the presence of disease pathology. This lack of integrity in the physiological mode would act as a stimulus for behavior in each of the other modes.

Another stimulus demonstrating the interrelated aspects of the person relates directly to the **cognator subsystem** of the coping mechanisms and involves the effectiveness with which the system is functioning. Inherent in this stimulus are the knowledge, perception, and skill possessed by the person to assist in coping with environmental stimuli. Consider an example of a malnourished individual. If the person does not recognize what nutrients constitute a balanced diet, the knowledge necessary to provide for adaptive behavior relative to nutritional health is not present. Therefore, the cognator subsystem cannot perform effectively. Lack of knowledge is a stimulus affecting adaptation level.

The last stimulus to be mentioned here relates to the **environmental**

setting. Changes in environmental setting can have a pronounced effect on the person's state of adaptation. These changes tend to affect the individual's senses and include such stimuli as temperature changes, different noise levels, or unusual diet. The presence of unfamiliar people or absence of familiar ones may be a part of environmental change. Also related to the environmental setting are drugs, alcohol, and tobacco, the use of which has a distinct effect on the person's internal environment.

The effect on adaptation of each of the common stimuli identified is a study in itself, as would be the person's effect upon the environment. The discussion in this chapter is an attempt to identify common stimuli affecting a person's adaptation. It is not meant to be exhaustive. Many other stimuli will be evident as each individual is assessed. The stimuli that have been described, however, include those that have been found important for primary consideration in the assessment of the stimuli affecting the individual's behavior relative to each mode. Such assessment also contributes to the nurse's general understanding of the context and meaningfulness of the individual's world.

NURSING DIAGNOSIS

Since the nursing process is a problem-solving process, behavioral data, once gathered, must be interpreted. This interpretation is accomplished by considering the behaviors of the person (as assessed in the first level of assessment) together with the factors (stimuli) affecting those behaviors (as assessed in the second level of assessment) in establishing a nursing diagnosis.

Nursing diagnosis is defined in the Roy Adaptation Model as a judgment process resulting in a statement conveying the person's adaptation status. Based on the goal of nursing described in the model, that is, to enhance positive life processes and to promote adaptation, Roy (1988) has identified the utility of a typology of indicators of positive adaptation associated with each of the four modes. This typology is presented in Table 2–2. Adaptation problems, defined as broad areas of concern related to adaptation, also have been derived to describe deviations from the indicators of positive adaptation. These are presented in Table 2–3.

In establishing nursing diagnoses within the framework provided by the model (behavior related to stimuli), three alternatives have been suggested: (1) a statement of the behaviors within one mode with their most relevant influencing stimuli, (2) a summary label for behaviors in one mode with relevant stimuli, or (3) a label that summarizes a behavioral pattern when more than one mode is being affected by the same stimuli. Each alternative has particular utility in certain situations. For example, the first alternative is useful in teaching situations where learners are beginning to grasp the concept of nursing diagnosis whereas the third

TABLE 2–2. TYPOLOGY OF INDICATORS OF POSITIVE ADAPTATION

Physiological Mode

1. Oxygenation
   stable processes of ventilation
   stable pattern of gas exchange
   adequate transport of gases
   adequate processes of
       compensation
2. Nutrition
   stable digestive processes
   adequate nutritional pattern for body
       requirements
   metabolic and other nutritive needs
       met during altered means of
       ingestion
3. Elimination
   effective homeostatic bowel processes
   stable pattern of bowel elimination
   effective processes of urine formation
   stable pattern of urine elimination
   effective coping strategies for altered
       elimination
4. Activity and Rest
   integrated processes of mobility
   adequate recruitment of
       compensatory movement processes
       during inactivity
   effective pattern of activity and rest
   effective sleep pattern
   effective environmental changes for
       altered sleep conditions
5. Protection
   intact skin
   effective processes of immunity
   effective healing response
   adequate secondary protection for
       changes in skin integrity and
       immune status

6. Senses
   effective processes of sensation
   effective integration of sensory input
       into information
   stable patterns of perception, ie,
       interpretation and appreciation of
       input
   effective coping strategies for altered
       sensation
7. Fluid and Electrolytes
   stable processes of water balance
   stability of salts in body fluids
   balance of acid/base status
   effective chemical buffer regulation
8. Neurological Function
   effective processes of arousal/attention;
       sensation/perception; coding,
       concept formation, memory,
       language; planning, motor response
   integrated thinking and feeling
       processes
   plasticity and functional effectiveness
       of developing, aging, and altered
       nervous system
9. Endocrine Function
   effective hormonal regulation of
       metabolic and body processes
   effective hormonal regulation of
       reproductive development
   stable patterns of closed loop negative
       feedback hormone systems
   stable patterns of cyclical hormone
       rhythms
   effective coping strategies for stress

Self-Concept Mode

1. Physical Self
   positive body image
   effective sexual function
   psychic integrity with physical growth
   adequate compensation for bodily
       changes
   effective coping strategies for loss
   effective process of life closure

2. Personal Self
   stable pattern of self consistency
   effective integration of self ideal
   effective processes of moral-ethical-
       spiritual growth
   functional self esteem
   effective coping strategies for threats
       to self

continued

TABLE 2–2. TYPOLOGY OF INDICATORS OF POSITIVE ADAPTATION (*CONTINUED*)

Role Function Mode
effective processes of role transition
integration of instrumental and
expressive role behaviors
integration of primary, secondary, and
tertiary roles
stable pattern of role mastery
effective processes for coping with role
changes

Interdependence Mode
stable pattern of giving and receiving
nurturing
affectional adequacy
effective pattern of aloneness and
relating
effective coping strategies for
separation and loneliness

alternative is more relevant in situations of more advanced nursing practice. Throughout this text, alternatives one and two have been selected as the methods most appropriately illustrating the typology of positive adaptation and the related adaptation problems in each of the modes. Examples of the third method are provided since this approach is consistent with efforts in the profession to develop a language of diagnosis whereby nurses can communicate regarding the unique services they provide.

Alternatives for Stating Nursing Diagnoses

Data collected thus far in the nursing process take the form of statements about the person's behavior that has been observed, measured, or subjectively reported. Also, data include statements about the focal, contextual, and residual stimuli that are or may be influencing these behaviors. The third step of the nursing process involves the formulation of statements that interpret these data. Such a statement is the nursing diagnoses and is depicted in the diagrammatic representation of the Roy Adaptation Model in Fig. 2–1. The nursing diagnosis is a statement about the person. Roy has described three ways of establishing a nursing diagnosis from the data gathered in the first and second levels of assessment.

The first method described by Roy (1984) for making a nursing diagnosis involves stating the behavior together with the most relevant stimuli. Consider the assessment data associated with this physiologic adaptation problem. An individual's pulse is rapid and thready, breathing is rapid and shallow, blood pressure tends to rise at first and then fall. The person feels clammy, looks pale and may be agitated or confused. All these behaviors are indicative of inadequate circulation and thus insufficient oxygenation of body tissue. They result from a variety of causes (stimuli): loss of blood volume, an infectious process in the body, or a stressful physical or emotional event, to name but a few.

Using the first method for deriving a nursing diagnosis, the nurse may state, "blood pressure of 90/60 due to hemorrhage from incision." This would represent one nursing diagnosis related to the problem described. Advantages of this method are twofold: (1) It provides specific indication for nursing intervention since, as will be seen later in this chapter, nursing interventions relate directly to stimuli; and (2) it allows for the incompleteness of typologies of nursing problems.

In the second method, assessment information (behavior and stimuli) associated with one mode is clustered and labeled according to the suggested typology related to each of the four adaptive modes. This typology of commonly recurring adaptation problems that has evolved throughout the development and refinement of the Roy Adaptation Model was presented in Table 2–3.

The above-mentioned behavioral assessment information can be clustered and labeled "shock." Shock is a common adaptation problem of the physiologic mode and the person's need for oxygenation. A nursing diagnosis illustrating this second method could be "shock due to incisional hemorrhage."

The third method of making a nursing diagnosis provides for the fact that one stimulus may cause behaviors in more than one mode. An example is that of a person suffering the loss of a limb. Assessment data could include behaviors indicative of lowered self-esteem resulting from changes in body image, difficulties in role performance, changes in dependence requirement, in addition to the associated physiologic adaptation problems such as loss of appetite and disturbed sleep patterns. A nursing diagnosis that recognizes the interrelatedness of these data and crosses modes would be "depression related to the loss of limb." The advantage of the third approach to nursing diagnosis, that of summarizing behaviors in more than one mode being affected by the same stimulus, is that the holistic functioning of the person and the interrelatedness of the modes are recognized. This method of stating nursing diagnoses is very useful in the complex situations encountered in advanced nursing practice.

Nursing diagnoses may pertain to both adaptive and ineffective situations. Recall that the goal of nursing is to enhance positive life processes and to promote adaptation. An example of a positive diagnosis for the person suffering the amputation would be "effective coping strategies to grieve the loss of a limb."

Complex Adaptation Problems

In situations of advanced nursing practice such as that of the person suffering the loss of the limb, nurses encounter individuals with complex

TABLE 2–3. TYPOLOGY OF COMMONLY RECURRING ADAPTATION PROBLEMS

Physiological Mode

1. Oxygenation

   hypoxia/shock
   ventilatory impairment
   inadequate gas exchange
   inadequate gas transport
   altered tissue perfusion
   poor recruitment of compensatory
      processes for changing oxygen
      need

2. Nutrition

   weight 20/25% above/below average
   nutrition more/less than body
      requirements
   anorexia
   nausea and vomiting
   ineffective coping strategies for altered
      means of ingestion

3. Elimination

   diarrhea
   bowel/bladder incontinence
   constipation
   urinary retention
   flatulence
   ineffective coping strategies for altered
      elimination

4. Activity and Rest

   inadequate pattern of activity and rest
   restricted mobility, gait, and/or
      coordination
   activity intolerance
   immobility
   disuse consequences
   potential for sleep pattern disturbance
   fatigue
   sleep deprivation

5. Protection

   disrupted skin integrity
   pressure sores
   itching
   delayed wound healing
   infection
   potential for ineffective coping with
      allergic reaction
   ineffective coping with changes in
      immune status

6. Senses

   impairment of a primary sense
   potential for injury/loss of self care
      abilities
   potential for distorted communication
   stigma
   sensory monotony/distortion
   sensory overload/deprivation
   acute pain
   chronic pain
   perceptual impairment
   ineffective coping strategies for sensory
      impairment

7. Fluid and Electrolytes

   dehydration
   edema
   intracellular water retention
   shock
   hyper or hypo calcemia, kalemia, or
      natremia
   acid/base imbalance
   ineffective buffer regulation for
      changing pH

8. Neurological Function

   decreased level of consciousness
   defective cognitive processing
   memory deficits
   instability of behavior and mood
   ineffective compensation for cognitive
      deficit
   potential for secondary brain damage

9. Endocrine Function

   ineffective hormone regulation,
      reflected in fatigue, irritability, heat
      intolerance
   ineffective reproductive development
   instability of hormone system loops
   instability of internal cyclical rhythms
   stress

continued

TABLE 2–3. TYPOLOGY OF COMMONLY RECURRING ADAPTATION PROBLEMS (*CONTINUED*)

Self-Concept Mode	
1. Physical Self	2. Personal Self
body image disturbance	anxiety
sexual dysfunction	powerlessness
rape trauma syndrome	guilt
loss	low self esteem

Role Function Mode
role transition
role distance
role conflict
role failure

Interdependence Mode
ineffective pattern of giving and receiving nurturing
ineffective pattern of aloneness and relating
separation anxiety
loneliness

and interrelated problems. Behaviors in one mode may be acting as a stimulus for another mode. One stimulus may be affecting more than one mode. Such complex interrelationships among modes further demonstrate the holistic nature of the person.

In-depth exploration of complex adaptation problems is not within the scope of this introductory text. This topic can be dealt with in a future text addressing advanced nursing practice and the Roy Adaptation Model.

GOAL SETTING

Once the nurse has assessed the person's behavior and the stimuli influencing that behavior and has formulated nursing diagnoses from the assessment information, goals are established. Goal setting has been defined as the establishment of clear statements of the behavioral outcomes of nursing care for the person (Roy 1984).

The general goal of nursing intervention has been defined previously: to maintain and enhance adaptive behavior and to change ineffective behavior to adaptive. The person's behavior is the focus of this general statement and similarly, when establishing specific goals, the person's behavior is the focus.

Throughout the first and second levels of assessment, the person's behavior and the stimuli influencing it have been identified and recorded. This information was formulated into nursing diagnoses. Step 4 of the nursing process, goal setting, involves the statement of behavioral outcomes of nursing care that will promote adaptation. Figure 2–1 illustrated goal setting as it relates to the other steps of the nursing process.

Recall from previous discussion the person who, following surgery, was demonstrating a progressive drop in blood pressure caused by hemorrhage from his incision. A nursing diagnosis could be worded, "Blood pressure 90/40 related to hemorrhage." A goal for this person could be stated as follows: "The patient's blood pressure measurement will stabilize in a range of 110/70 to 130/80 within 30 minutes." This is a short-term goal that identifies a behavioral outcome promoting adaptation.

Goals may also be long term. A long-term goal pertaining to the example may be, "The patient will be able to return to his job on a part-time basis within six weeks."

The designation of goals as long or short term is relative to the situation involved. For some problems, especially those that are life threatening, short-term goals may be formulated on a minute-to-minute basis, and long-term goals on a day-to-day basis. In other situations, in the psychosocial realm, for example, short-term goals may involve the time frame of a week, and long-term goals, months.

A goal statement should designate not only the behavior to be observed but the manner in which the behavior will change (as observed, measured, or subjectively reported), and the time frame in which the goal is to be attained. Consider the following:

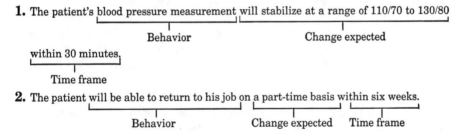

1. The patient's blood pressure measurement will stabilize at a range of 110/70 to 130/80
     Behavior   Change expected
within 30 minutes.
     Time frame

2. The patient will be able to return to his job on a part-time basis within six weeks.
     Behavior   Change expected   Time frame

Notice how each of the goals demonstrates the three elements identified above. These elements are important in the evaluation of goal attainment.

In these examples, the goals focus on ineffective behaviors in an attempt to change them to adaptive behaviors. However, it may be just as important to focus on adaptive behaviors in an effort to maintain and enhance them. Consider the following situation: A five-year-old boy, newly admitted to hospital for surgery, was interacting readily with his new roommate until it was time for his mother to leave, at which point he began to cry and cling to her hand. In this situation, the goal might focus on the adaptive behavior of interaction with roommate. The goal might be, "Within five minutes of mother's departure, child will be playing happily with roommate as evidenced by participation in mutual activity."

The person is actively involved in the formulation of behavioral goals whenever possible. This involvement provides the nurse with the opportunity to explore the rationale behind certain goals and gives the person the chance to suggest goals and evaluate whether others are realistic. A person who is actively involved in the formulation of goals is more likely to be committed to attainment of the goal. Consider the following goal: "Within 6 hours after surgery, the patient will stand unsupported by the bed for five minutes." Generally, it is considered important for persons undergoing surgery to be mobile as soon as possible following return from the operating room. The person involved in the formulation of this goal and who understands the underlying rationale is more likely to strive to achieve it, than someone who hears, "It's time to get you out of bed," for the first time while in pain and still drowsy. It can be noted that individual behavioral goals are aimed at the goals of adaptation, that is, survival, growth, reproduction, and mastery. Thus, the nurse helps the person strive for full human potential.

INTERVENTION

Once the goals have been established relative to behaviors that will promote adaptation, the nurse must determine how to intervene to assist the person in attaining these goals. This is the fifth step in the nursing process.

Intervention as the Management of Stimuli

In Roy's description of the person as an adaptive system, stimuli from the internal and external environment activate the coping mechanisms to produce behaviors. When ineffective behavior is identified, there is evidence that the coping mechanisms are not able to adapt effectively to the stimuli affecting them. The first three steps of the nursing process involve the assessment of these behaviors and the related stimuli and the synthesis of this information into the nursing diagnosis. Subsequent goal setting is the statement of the desired behavioral outcomes of nursing care relative to the problem areas identified. Intervention focuses on the manner in which these goals are to be attained. Just as the focus of goal setting is the person's behavior, the focus of intervention is the stimuli influencing the behavior. Figure 2–1 illustrated this in terms of the Roy Adaptation Model.

As was identified in Chapter 1, the person's ability to adapt or respond positively to a change taking place depends on the focal stimulus and adaptation level. The focal stimulus is the degree of change taking place. The adaptation level is a changing point determined by the pooled effect of the three classes of stimuli and represents the person's ability to respond positively in a situation. In order to promote adaptation, it may be necessary to manage other stimuli present. Management of stimuli involves altering, increasing, decreasing, removing, or maintaining them. Altering the stimuli enhances the ability of the person's coping mechanisms to respond positively, and the result is adaptive behavior.

Identification and Analysis of Possible Approaches

The identification of possible approaches to nursing intervention involves the selection of which stimuli to change. Roy incorporates the nursing judgment method as presented by McDonald and Harms (1966) in her description of this fifth step of the nursing process. In this method, possible approaches are listed and the approach with the highest probability of attaining the goal is selected. In applying this method to the Roy model, the stimuli affecting specific behavior are listed. Next the consequences of changing each stimulus are identified together with the probability of their occurrence. The value of the consequence is judged as *desirable* or *undesirable*. This is accomplished in collaboration with the person, when possible and appropriate.

Consider an example of the person who is unable to sleep in the hospital environment. The second level of assessment yielded the following stimuli as contributing to this sleeplessness.

- Noise level (focal)
- Uncomfortable bed (contextual)
- Person is hungry (contextual)

Application of the Nursing Judgment Method to these factors is illustrated in Table 2–4.

The first approach, that of altering the stimulus of noise level, has the best probability of accomplishing the desired goal with undesirable consequences having a low probability. On the other hand, the third approach has a moderate probability of achieving the desired result, but the undesirable consequence of disrupting plans for surgery is highly probable.

Whenever possible, the focal stimulus should be the focus of nursing interventions. However, when this is not possible, contextual stimuli must be managed in an effort to broaden adaptation level. It also may be appropriate to use several approaches in combination. For example, a person

TABLE 2–4. THE NURSING JUDGMENT METHOD AS APPLIED TO SELECTION OF APPROACHES

Alternative Approach	Consequence	Probability	Value
Alter noise level	Enhance sleep	High	Desirable
	Not enhance sleep	Low	Undesirable
Alter comfort of bed	Enhance sleep	High	Desirable
	Not enhance sleep	Low	Undesirable
	Disrupt intravenous	Low	Undesirable
Alter hunger	Enhance sleep	Moderate	Desirable
	Not enhance sleep	Moderate	Undesirable
	Disrupt plans for surgery in morning	High	Undesirable

may be suffering severe pain caused by the focal stimulus of a terminal disease process. In this case, it is not possible to deal with the disease itself, and efforts must be directed towards contextual factors enabling the person to handle the pain and be more comfortable. A personal support system may be one of the stimuli that must be increased or maintained. Other factors related to pain management are discussed in Chapter 9.

Implementation of Selected Approach

Once the most appropriate approach to nursing intervention has been selected, the nurse must determine and initiate the steps that will serve to alter the stimulus appropriately. Having decided that altering the noise level is the best approach to the patient's sleeplessness, the nurse must determine how to do it. Shutting the door to the person's room might help; it may be possible to reduce the volume of the paging system. It may be necessary to move the person away from a disruptive roommate.

Having accomplished the nursing intervention, the nurse then proceeds to evaluate its effectiveness.

EVALUATION

The last step of the nursing process as described by the Roy Adaptation Model is evaluation. *Evaluation* involves judging the effectiveness of the nursing intervention in relation to the person's behavior. Was the goal that was set in the fourth step of the nursing process attained? To make this decision, the nurse assesses the behavior of the person after the interventions have been implemented. As in the initial assessment steps, the skills of sensitive observation, measurement, and interview are used. The nursing intervention would be judged effective if the person's behavior aligns with the initial goals.

Evaluation as a Reflection of Goals

As has been discussed before, it is behavior that demonstrates the effectiveness with which the coping mechanisms are able to adapt to the stimuli affecting the person. Nursing interventions are directed towards altering stimuli in an effort to enhance the ability of the mechanisms to cope. When goals are established in step 4 of the nursing process, they are set in terms of the person's behavior and they aim to maintain and enhance the adaptive behavior and to change ineffective behavior to adaptive. To evaluate the effectiveness of nursing interventions in terms of these goals, the nurse, in collaboration with the individual, must look again at the person's behavior. Have the behavioral goals been achieved? This evaluation is the sixth and final step of the nursing process. Its relationship to the previous steps and to Roy's description of the person was illustrated in Fig. 2–1.

Skills Used in Evaluation

As in the first assessment steps of the nursing process, the nurse uses the skills of observation, measurement, and interview to evaluate the effectiveness of nursing interventions. Consider the earlier example of the person who was hemorrhaging following surgery. Some of the ineffective behaviors identified were falling of blood pressure (measured), large amount of blood on dressing (observed), and decreasing level of consciousness (observed through purposeful questioning). Goals relative to these behaviors would relate to stabilizing blood pressure, cessation of bleeding, and regaining of consciousness, respectively. To evaluate the effectiveness of nursing interventions relative to these goals, the nurse would measure the person's blood pressure, observe the amount of blood on a fresh dressing, and use an established format (see chapter 11) for determining the level of consciousness—all skills used in making the initial assessment.

Continuity of the Nursing Process

For the nursing intervention to be judged effective, the person's behavior will reflect the mutually set goals. If the goals are not achieved, the nurse must proceed to discover what went wrong. The goals may have been unrealistic or unacceptable to the person, the assessment data may have been inaccurate or incomplete, or the selected approaches may not have been carried out properly. The nurse returns to the first step of the nursing process to look closely at behaviors that continue to be ineffective and to try to further understand the situation.

In the example, the nurse may evaluate that the person's blood pressure has stabilized and that bleeding has stopped, but there may not be a change in the level of consciousness. Although it is still important to ensure that the stable blood pressure and cessation of bleeding are maintained, the nurse would begin to focus on the person's level of consciousness and proceed through the steps of the nursing process again in order to identify an alternative approach to the ineffective behavior of decreasing level of consciousness.

Although the steps of the nursing process have been separated and specified for clarity of discussion, it is important to recognize that the nursing process is ongoing. In fact, many of the steps occur simultaneously. The nurse may be assessing behavior in one area while proceeding with a nursing intervention in another area. She may be assessing behavior and stimuli at the same time and discussing goals in another area.

SUMMARY

The six-step nursing process described in the Roy Adaptation Model has been presented in this chapter. The nurse assesses the person's behavior and the stimuli influencing that behavior and proceeds to formulate nursing diagnoses. Goals establishing behavioral outcomes for the patient are formulated and interventions designed to manage stimuli are planned and implemented. Evaluation involves judging the effectiveness of the nursing intervention in relation to the person's behavior.

Roy's nursing process is closely aligned with the assumptions and concepts associated with the description of the person according to the Roy Adaptation Model. The importance of collaboration with the person throughout the nursing process steps has been pointed out and is emphasized. The effectiveness with which the nurse can assist the person in the promotion of adaptation depends on the nurse's understanding of the situation and collaboration with the person.

EXERCISES FOR APPLICATION

1. Situation: Two hours following surgery, a large amount of blood was noticed seeping through a patient's dressing. The nurse, on taking a pulse and blood pressure, noticed that both had dropped markedly (40 and 90/60, respectively) from the readings taken the previous time. The patient who had been waking normally from his anesthetic, was now impossible to rouse. In this situation, identify the behaviors being demonstrated and the skill used in their assessment. Label the behaviors as adaptive (A) or ineffective (I) and provide rationale for your decision.

2. Formulate a nursing diagnosis relative to the following situation: A child is complaining of severe stomach cramps and has had six loose bowel movements within two hours. It is discovered on investigating that he had eaten three green apples from the neighbor's crabapple tree.

3. Suggest a behavioral goal that could apply to you, as the reader of this text on your completion of this chapter. It should apply to the knowledge gained from reading this chapter.

4. Imagine yourself as a student who has just received a failing grade on an examination. Suggest several stimuli (focal, contextual), that may have influenced the poor performance. Identify and analyze possible approaches to the problem relative to the stimuli. Use the following table as a guideline. Select the approach with the highest possibility of success.

Alternative Approach	Consequence	Probability	Value

5. Assume that, as of last week, you have applied the nursing process to yourself relative to your daily diet and have set the goal that you will eat a nutritionally balanced diet containing all the recommended daily allowances for nutrients. In light of this goal, evaluate your intake of food in the past 24 hours and suggest whether your observations align with the preset goal or are ineffective in moving towards it. You may proceed through all the steps of the nursing process relative to your own situation.

ASSESSMENT OF UNDERSTANDING

Questions

1. Underline the behaviors demonstrated by the child in the following situation.

    A mother noticed that her five-year-old son was not actively participating in play with other children. When she questioned him, he stated that he did not feel well and had a sore throat. The mother noticed that he appeared flushed and felt warm to her touch. Looking at his throat, she noticed that it was very reddened and two rather large masses of tissue were protruding from either side.

2. Using the criteria presented in this chapter, label the following underlined behaviors as adaptive (A) or ineffective (I) and provide rationale for your decision.

    (a) _____ A woman of five feet weighs 60 pounds.

    (b) _____ The nurse measured her patient's blood pressure at 125/75.

    (c) _____ The patient asked the nurse three times to explain a simple procedure.

    (d) _____ A person whose pulse is 60 beats per minute states that his heart rate has been that low since he was a teenager.

    (e) _____ A person has not eaten nor had any fluid intake for two days.

3. In the following situation suggest stimuli that might be influencing the person's behavior of refusing to taste the food.

    An 80-year-old patient who had been placed on a salt-restricted diet received her first saltless meal. She announced to her nurse that she would rather go hungry than eat such tasteless food. The entire meal was left untouched.

4. In the following situation identify the stimuli that contributed to the student's performance and classify them as being focal, contextual, and residual.

    In preparation for an important exam, an anxious student who was having persistent problems in a course, studied all night before the day of the test. During the writing of the exam she found that she was having trouble concentrating on the questions and remembering what she had studied. Handing in her paper, she commented to the instructor, "That exam was really hard; I know I didn't make it." She was right.

5. Using each of the three methods of making a nursing diagnosis as presented in this chapter, formulate a nursing diagnosis statement relative to the behaviors and stimuli underlined in the situation below. Your statements need not include all behaviors and stimuli.

   A 55-year-old woman has lost the use of the right side of her body as a result of a stroke. She is presently in a program of rehabilitation which is aimed at helping her achieve a degree of independence relative to her activities of daily living. She appears to lack enthusiasm for the program and states that she can see no reason to make an effort to become active again as she has lost her position as an executive secretary. Since she lives alone, she feels she could not manage on her own anyway. She states she is just not motivated to participate.

6. Formulate several goal statements for each of the following segments of assessment information and nursing diagnoses.

Behavior	Stimuli	Nursing Diagnosis
(a) Sixteen-year-old girl. Weighs 85 pounds. Height 5 feet 7 inches. States she does not eat breakfast and only has candy bars for lunch. Feels tired. Appears drawn and pale.	Inadequate caloric and nutritive intake. Always short of time in morning. Peer group does not eat lunch. Parents work; must prepare meals herself. Does not understand principles of good nutrition.	Malnutrition due to inadequate intake of food and lack of knowledge.
(b) Elderly male patient. Withdrawn. Uncommunicative. Refuses to do anything for himself. States "No one cares whether I'm dead or alive." States "I'll never leave this place."	Long-term hospitalization. Hospital is long distance from home and family. Has one close relative (a son) who can visit only occasionally.	Loneliness due to absence of support systems.

7. The following table represents a segment of information obtained from steps 1 to 4 of the nursing process relative to an 80-year-old patient hospitalized for a fractured hip. Following surgical insertion of a pin and plate, there is a need to increase his mobility. Continue with step 5 of the nursing process and select interventions that would assist in the achievement of the specified goals.

Behavior	Stimuli	Nursing Diagnosis	Goals
Appears apprehensive. States "I'm afraid. I can't possibly support myself; I'm too weak."	Pain increases when he tries to move (focal). Has not been eating well (contextual). Lack of understanding of postoperative routine.	Apprehensive due to lack of understanding and pain.	Patient will demonstrate increased confidence in his ability to move by attempting to get out of bed with assistance in 1/2 hour.
States he is having pain.	Trauma from fracture and subsequent surgery.	Pain due to injury.	Patient will experience relief from pain in 15 minutes as evidenced by statement of same.
Appears uncooperative. Asks "Why do I have to move anyway?"	Lack of understanding of importance of mobility.	Uncooperative due to lack of understanding.	Patient will cooperate with attempts to increase his mobility by following instructions the next time he is asked to try to get up.

8. For the following goal statements, identify what one would look for in the person's behavior that would indicate that nursing interventions had been effective.

   (a) Within one week, the patient will have regained full use of his hand as evidenced by his ability to perform a full range of motion.

   (b) By tomorrow, the patient will demonstrate increased acceptance of her role as a new mother as evidenced by her assuming responsibility for feeding and bathing of the baby.

   (c) The patient will demonstrate an understanding of the importance of the postoperative exercise regime as evidenced by performance of voluntary exercise every two hours following surgery.

Feedback

1. five-year-old
   not actively participating in play
   stated that he did not feel well and had a sore throat
   appeared flushed
   felt warm
   (throat) very reddened
   large masses of tissue protruding

2. (a) I: Normally people of five feet weigh much more.
   (b) A: A blood pressure reading of 125/75 is within normal limits.
   (c) I: The patient appears to be demonstrating ineffective learning.
   (d) A: The person confirms the behavior is normal and adaptive for him.
   (e) I: Normal body requirements for fluids and nutrients are not being met.

3. Stimuli contribution to persons refusal to eat:

   • tastelessness of food,
   • inadequate explanation of reason for salt-free diet,
   • diminished acuity of taste sensation associated with aging.

4. Had trouble concentrating and remembering—focal
   Studied all night—contextual
   Had persistent problems—contextual
   Was anxious—contextual
   The exam was important—contextual

5. Method 1: "Appears to lack enthusiasm for rehabilitation and states she sees no reason to make an effort since she has lost her job and feels she will be dependent."—A statement of behavior is connected to the relevant stimulus.

Method 2: "Loss of body function due to stroke"—The woman has lost the use of the right side of her body as a result of a stroke. She can no longer physically perform her job nor can she care for herself. "Loss" is a common problem associated with the physical self-concept.

Method 3: "Depression as a result of a stroke"—Both the self-concept and interdependence modes are affected. "Depression" provides a summary label for the behaviors evident in each mode.

6. (a) Patient will begin to gain weight as evidenced by a measured gain of five pounds in one month.

   Patient will eat regular nutritious meals within one week as evidenced by a daily diary of food intake.

   Patient's appearance will improve within six months as evidenced by weight gain and improved coloring.

   Patient will have more energy within one week as evidenced by her statements that she feels less tired and has more energy.

   (b) The patient will begin to interact with other patients and staff by becoming involved actively in an occupational therapy session on a daily basis beginning tomorrow.

   Within two days, the patient will begin to assume responsibility for several self-care tasks as demonstrated by shaving himself and cleaning his own teeth.

   Within two weeks, the patient will begin to demonstrate optimism for the future by inquiring about potential for discharge to alternative care agency.

7. (a) ensure that there are two individuals to assist the patient out of bed,

   (b) pursue the patient's need for analgesic prior to getting him out of bed,

   (c) assess the patient's understanding of the importance of early mobility, carefully explain the procedure to be followed in helping patient out of bed, involve patient in establishing the best way to help him out of bed.

8. In each case, nursing interventions would be judged effective if the person was doing what was stated in the goal and in the time frame specified.

REFERENCES

Benner, P., and J. Wrubel. *The Primacy of Caring: Stress and Coping in Health and Illness.* Menlo Park, Calif.: Addison-Wesley, 1989.

Erikson, E.M. *Childhood and Society.* New York: W. W. Norton and Co. Inc., 1963.

Martinez, C. Nursing assessment based on Roy Adaptation Model, in *Introduction to Nursing: An Adaptation Model* (1st ed.), Sr. C. Roy, pp. 379–385. Englewood Cliffs, N.J.: Prentice-Hall, 1976.

McDonald, F.J., and M. Harms. Theoretical model for an experimental curriculum, *Nursing Outlook*, 14, no. 8 (August 1966): 48–51.

Roy, Sr. C. The Roy Model Nursing Process, in *Introduction to Nursing: An Adaptation Model* (2nd ed.), Sr. C. Roy, pp. 42–63. Englewood Cliffs, N.J.: Prentice-Hall, 1984.

Roy, Sr. C. The Roy Adaptation Model for nursing practice: Theorist's input for publications. Enclosure with correspondence to contributing authors dated November 4, 1988.

Sato, M.K. Major factors influencing adaptation, in *Introduction to Nursing: An Adaptation Model* (2nd ed.), Sr. C. Roy, pp. 64–87. Englewood Cliffs, N.J.: Prentice-Hall, 1984.

Additional References

Roy, Sr. C. The Roy model nursing process, in *Introduction to Nursing: An Adaptation Model* (2nd ed.), Sr. C. Roy, pp. 42–63. Englewood Cliffs, N.J.: Prentice-Hall, 1984.

Watson, J. *Nursing: Human Science and Human Care*. Norwalk, Conn.: Appleton-Century-Crofts, 1985.

Part II
The Physiological Mode

Inherent in Roy's description of the person as an adaptive system are four adaptive modes that manifest regulator and cognator activity: the physiological mode, the self-concept mode, the role function mode, and the interdependence mode. It is through these four major categories that responses are carried out and that adaptation level can be observed. The next four parts of this text are devoted to an exploration of these modes and the essential concepts associated with each.

Part II focuses on the physiological mode. Chapter 3 provides an overview of the mode while the subsequent nine chapters deal individually with the five needs and four complex processes that are the components of the mode. As a conclusion to Part II, a case study situation is presented to illustrate selected concepts associated with the physiological mode. The same situation is developed at intervals throughout the text to demonstrate application of the Roy Adaptation in a patient care situation.

Chapter Three —————————

Overview of the Physiological Mode

Heather A. Andrews and
Sister Callista Roy

The physiological mode as described in the Roy Adaptation Model is associated with the way the person responds physically to stimuli from the environment. Behavior in this mode is a manifestation of the physiological activity of all the cells, tissues, organs, and systems which comprise the human body. As with each of the adaptive modes, stimuli activate the coping mechanisms producing adaptive and ineffective behavior. In this case, the coping mechanisms are those associated with physiological functioning (primarily the regulator subsystem) and the responses produced are mainly physiological behaviors. However, the person functions as a whole with each mode affecting the other. In the physiological mode, it is the person's physiological behavior that indicates whether the coping mechanisms are able to adapt to the stimuli affecting them.

Five needs are identified in the physiological mode relative to the basic need of physiological integrity: oxygenation, nutrition, elimination, activity and rest, and protection. Also inherent in a discussion of physiological adaptation are the four complex processes involving the senses, fluids and electrolytes, neurological function, and endocrine function. These processes can be viewed as mediating regulator activity, integrating many physiological functions of the person and affecting the integrity of the other modes.

This chapter provides the reader with an overview of the physiological mode including a description of the components of the mode and the basis for nursing assessment relative to physiological functioning.

OBJECTIVES

After studying this chapter, the reader will be able to do the following:

1. Describe the physiological mode.
2. Identify the five needs inherent in physiological integrity.
3. Identify the four physiological processes that serve to mediate regulator activity and integrate physiological functions.

KEY CONCEPTS DEFINED

- *Physiological integrity:* the underlying need of the physiological mode; physiological wholeness achieved by adapting to changes in physiological needs.
- *Physiology:* a science dealing with knowledge about the physical and chemical phenomena involved in the function and activities of a living organism.
- *Physiological mode:* the manner in which a person manifests physiological activity.

DESCRIPTION OF THE PHYSIOLOGICAL MODE

Physiology has been described as a science that deals with knowledge about the physical and chemical phenomena involved in the function and activities of a living organism. The physiological mode is the manner in which a person manifests this physiological activity. An understanding of physiological behavior necessitates a knowledge of the anatomy and physiology of the human body as well as the pathophysiology underlying disease processes. The nurse must be knowledgeable about normal body function in order to recognize (1) variations from the norm based on the person's own adaptation level, and (2) behaviors that indicate problems with physiological functioning.

Earlier writers have used human needs as the basis for nursing knowledge. Abdellah et al (1960) focused on the problem-solving method and developed a typology of twenty-one nursing problems and skills to constitute the body of nursing knowledge. These were stated in terms such as: "to maintain good hygiene and physical comfort." Orlando (1961) used the person's "need-for-help" as the central concept of the nursing process. In this approach, nurses' efforts were to ascertain this need and help the person meet it. In an influential text, Henderson (1966) identified fourteen basic needs of the person, such as "breathe normally" and "eat and drink adequately," that were the components of nursing care. With developing knowledge in nursing and the related disciplines, the processes underlying human needs are increasingly the focus for structuring knowledge (Donaldson and Crowley 1977, Roy 1988). Since the Roy model focuses on adaptation, within the model, emphasis is placed on the life processes to meet human needs.

The underlying need of the physiological mode is *physiological integrity*. Integrity has been defined as the degree of wholeness achieved by adapting to changes in needs. When a person's physiological needs are met, physiological integrity is achieved. The Roy Adaptation Model suggests five basic needs inherent in physiological integrity: oxygenation, nutrition, elimination, activity and rest, and protection. These needs and the associated processes are briefly described here and addressed individually in following chapters.

1. *Oxygenation:* This need involves the body's need for oxygen and the processes of ventilation, gas exchange, and gas transport (Vairo 1984).
2. *Nutrition:* This need involves a series of processes associated with the ingestion and assimilation of food for maintenance of functioning, promotion of growth, and the replacement of worn or injured tissue (Servonsky 1984b).
3. *Elimination:* The need for elimination includes the physiological processes involved in the excretion of metabolic wastes primarily through the intestines and kidneys (Servonsky 1984a).
4. *Activity and rest:* The need for balance in physical activity and rest provides optimal physiological functioning of all body components and periods of restoration and repair (Cho 1984).
5. *Protection:* The body's basic defenses include processes of immunity and of the structures of integument (skin, hair, and nails) which serve an important protective function against infection, trauma, and temperature changes (Sato 1984).

In addition to the five basic needs listed, four complex processes have been identified as important areas of consideration when assessing physiological adaptation. These processes involve the senses, fluids and electrolytes, neurological function, and endocrine function. They are viewed in the model as mediating regulator activity and integrate many physiological functions of the person.

1. *The senses:* Sight, hearing, touch, taste, and smell enable persons to interact with their environment. The sensation of pain is an important consideration in assessment of the senses (Driscoll 1984).
2. *Fluids and electrolytes:* A delicate balance of fluids and electrolytes in terms of water, electrolytes, and acid/base is necessary for cellular, extracellular, and systemic function. Conversely, ineffective functioning of physiologic systems can produce electrolyte imbalance (Perley 1984).
3. *Neurological function:* Neurological channels are an integral part of a person's regulator coping mechanisms. They function to control and coordinate bodily movements, consciousness, and cognitive-emotional processes as well as to regulate activity of body organs (Robertson 1984).

4. *Endocrine function:* Endocrine action through hormone secretion serves, along with neurological function, to integrate and coordinate body functioning. Endocrine activity plays a significant role in the stress response and is also part of the regulator coping mechanism (Howard and Valentine 1984).

These complex components of physiological adaptation together with the five basic needs and their processes, as described previously, form the basis for physiological behavioral assessment in the Roy Adaptation Model.

THEORETICAL BASIS FOR THE PHYSIOLOGICAL MODE

The theoretical background for the physiological mode lies in basic life sciences, particularly anatomy, physiology, pathophysiology, and chemistry. In addition, the meeting of human needs is influenced by psychological processes such as motivation and concepts from sociology and anthropology, for example, social class and customs. Insights for all of the adaptive modes also can be gained from disciplines within the humanities. For example, literature provides understanding of how fictional characters have been drawn to deal with basic themes of life. These fields can be described briefly as follows:

1. *Anatomy:* As the study of the structure of the human body, human anatomy provides the structural basis for the physiological mode.
2. *Physiology:* Physiology provides the nurse with knowledge of the processes involved in the functioning and activities of the human body. This knowledge is the basis for judgment of adaptive and ineffective physiological behavior.
3. *Pathophysiology:* As the study of abnormal physiological changes accompanying illness, pathophysiology provides the nurse with rationale for identification of ineffective behavioral responses and the stimuli influencing them.
4. *Chemistry:* Knowledge from chemistry, dealing with the composition, properties, and reactions of substances, provides the basis for an understanding of body processes such as those involved in fluid and electrolyte activity.
5. *Psychology:* The study of the mind and behavior provides a basis for the understanding of psychosocial processes and how they relate to illness and ineffective behavior.
6. *Sociology:* The study of the development, structure, interaction, and collective behavior of organized groups of people provides a foundation for the nurse's assessment of the sociological modes and their influence on physiological function in situations of effective and ineffective adaptation.

7. *Anthropology:* The study of people in relation to their distribution, origin, classification, and the relationship of races including physical character, environmental and social relationships, and culture contributes to nurse's ability to identify the impact of psychological and sociological factors on the integrity of the person's physiological mode.
8. *Humanities:* Knowledge from other disciplines focusing on the attributes or qualities of the human person enables the nurse to more effectively consider the person's situation and intervene appropriately in situations of physiological as well as psychosocial need.

These disciplines provide direction for some of the knowledge needed to support the study of nursing itself. At the same time, the view of nursing indicates what knowledge is relevant and what knowledge needs to be developed. From their experience with persons who are healthy or unhealthy, nurses can determine what knowledge is relevant for nursing care. As with each of the modes, consideration of the physiological mode involves knowledge from a variety of related disciplines. This knowledge is viewed in the light of nursing's view of the person as a whole system and of the goal of promoting adaptation. The balance of physiological and psychosocial concepts in studying nursing is increasingly recognized.

APPLICATION OF THE NURSING PROCESS

Application of the nursing process in the physiological mode is illustrated in a general manner in the diagrammatic conceptualization of the model in Fig. 3–1. As the following chapters address the five physiological needs and the four complex processes, specific information about the application of the nursing process is presented. The following section takes a general look at how the six steps of the nursing process are applied within the physiological mode.

Assessment of Behavior. Behavioral assessment of the physiological mode provides the nurse with an indication of how the person is managing to cope with environmental changes affecting the physiological coping mechanisms. Nurses are taught specific ways to conduct physical assessment of the person under their care. These methods must be thorough and yet efficient. In the Roy Adaptation Model, the approach to assessment of physiological behavior lies in the five basic needs and the four complex processes of physiological adaptation. In the study of each of these areas, the nurse learns what behaviors reveal adaptive status in the person. The nurse's background in anatomy, physiology, pathophysiology, and nutrition provides the basis for the decision as to whether the observed behavior in each of the categories is adaptive or ineffective.

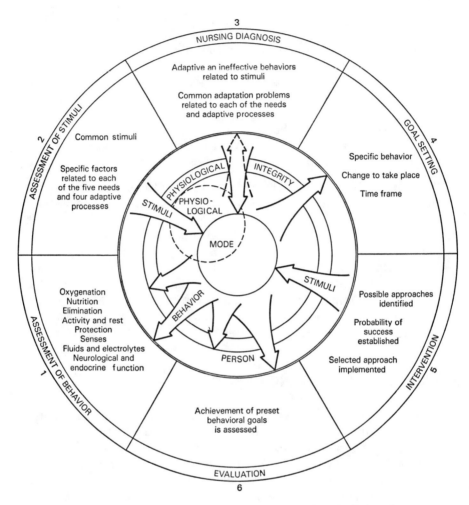

Figure 3–1. The nursing process applied to the physiological mode

For each of the behaviors applying to the needs and process components, there are both general and individual norms against which to judge the person's behavior. The nurse's theoretical background in the previously identified disciplines provides the knowledge necessary for this assessment step and for the assessment of stimuli influencing the observed physiological behaviors. The nursing model helps to focus that knowledge and provides a lens for looking at the person's physiological mode.

Assessment of Stimuli. The second level of assessment involves the assessment of the internal and external stimuli influencing the identified physiological behaviors. In Chapter 2, common stimuli were identified as affecting adaptation in all four modes and important for primary consideration in the assessment of the stimuli affecting the person's behavior relative to each mode. In addition, stimuli of particular relevance to each of the needs and components have been suggested. These are specified in the subsequent chapters dealing with the five physiological needs and four complex processes. Many of these stimuli relate directly to the common stimuli. Again, the nurse's background knowledge from the supporting disciplines provides the insight required for the assessment. The use of a nursing model provides the perspective for integrating and making nursing judgments based on that knowledge.

Stimuli are identified, in consultation with the person, as being focal, contextual, or residual. At this point, it is also possible to determine whether their effect on the person is positive or negative.

Nursing Diagnosis. Three methods of stating a nursing diagnosis were presented in Chapter 2. These were (1) the stating of behavior within one mode with most relevant stimuli, (2) the clustering of behavioral information and labeling according to indicators of positive adaptation and a typology of common adaptation problems related to each mode with the relevant stimuli, and (3) the summarizing of behaviors crossing modes and being affected by the same stimuli.

A typology of indicators of positive adaptation and common adaptation problems were presented in Tables 2–1 and 2–3. Specifically, indicators and problems were identified as related to the five needs and four complex processes. Each of these problems represents a cluster of assessment information. To compensate for the incompleteness of the typology, and to provide specific direction for nursing intervention, the nurse may prefer to identify individual behaviors and their relevant stimuli. Examples of nursing diagnoses stated in these ways are provided in the following chapters.

Goal Setting. The goal of nursing when applied to behavior in the physiological mode is to maintain and enhance adaptive physiological behavior and to change ineffective physiological behavior to adaptive behavior. Thus, the focus of goal setting in the physiological mode, as with any other mode, is the person's behavior.

The goal statement consists of three entities identified in Chapter 2: the behavior to be observed, the change expected, and the time frame for achievement of the goal. Examples of physiological goal statements are provided throughout the following nine chapters.

Intervention. In order to promote adaptation, it is necessary to manage the stimuli influencing the behavior under specific consideration. It may be necessary to change the focal stimulus or to broaden the adaptation level by managing other stimuli present. In selecting approaches, the nurse considers possible alternatives and then selects the approach with the highest probability of achieving the agreed upon goal.

Evaluation. The final step of the nursing process, evaluation, involves assessment of the person's behavior in relation to the established behavioral goal. If the goal has been achieved, the intervention was effective; if not, further assessment and reconsideration of goals and intervention is required.

SUMMARY

The physiological mode represents the manifestation of the person's ability to cope with changes in the environment affecting his or her physical being. Five basic needs and four adaptive processes were identified as the basis for physiological assessment. The major disciplines adding to a knowledge base for nursing activities relative to the physiological mode were listed. Figure 3–1 provided a diagrammatic representation of the nursing process as applied to the physiological mode.

EXERCISES FOR APPLICATION

1. Select one of the areas for assessment in the physiological mode and suggest behaviors that would be important to consider. Check your list with those suggested in the relevant following chapter.
2. Compare another framework for physical assessment to that suggested in the Roy Adaptation Model. Look particularly for commonalities. An example of another framework is "Head-to-toe assessment."

ASSESSMENT OF UNDERSTANDING

Questions

1. Which of the following statements describe the *physiological mode*?
   (a) It is the manner in which the person responds to changes affecting him or her physically.
   (b) It is associated with nine basic needs.
   (c) It incorporates functioning of cells, tissues, organs, and systems.
   (d) It affects functioning in each of the modes.
   (e) It is based on knowledge from psychology and sociology.
   (f) It is the most important mode at all times.

2. Which of the following are needs associated with the basic need of physiological integrity?
   (a) Fluids and electrolytes
   (b) Oxygenation
   (c) Endocrine functioning
   (d) Protection
   (e) Elimination
   (f) Nutrition
   (g) Neurological functioning
3. Four complex adaptive components were identified as important in the consideration of physiological functioning. List these four components.
   (a) _____
   (b) _____
   (c) _____
   (d) _____

Feedback

1. a, c, d
2. b, d, e, f
3. (a) The senses
   (b) Fluids and electrolytes
   (c) Neurological function
   (d) Endocrine function

REFERENCES

Abdellah, F., I. Beland, A. Martin, R. Matheney. *Patient-Centered Approaches to Nursing.* New York: Macmillan, 1960.

Cho, J.S. Activity and rest, in *Introduction to Nursing: An Adaptation Model* (2nd ed.), Sr. C. Roy, pp. 138–158. Englewood Cliffs, N.J.: Prentice-Hall, 1984.

Donaldson, S.K., and D. Crowley. Discipline of nursing: Structure and relationship to practice, in *Communicating Nursing Research,* vol. 10, ed. M. Batey. Boulder, Colo.: Western Interstate Commission on Higher Education, 1977.

Driscoll, S. The senses, in *Introduction to Nursing: An Adaptation Model* (2nd ed.), Sr. C. Roy, pp. 168–188. Englewood Cliffs, N.J.: Prentice-Hall, 1984.

Henderson, V. *The Nature of Nursing: A Definition and Its Implications for Practice, Education, and Research.* New York: Macmillan, 1966.

Howard, M., and S. Valentine. Endocrine function, in *Introduction to Nursing: An Adaptation Model* (2nd ed.), Sr. C. Roy, pp. 238–252. Englewood Cliffs, N.J.: Prentice-Hall, 1984.

Orlando, I. *The Dynamic Nurse-Patient Relationship.* New York: Putnam's, 1961.

Perley, N.Z. Fluid and electrolytes, in *Introduction to Nursing: An Adaptation Model* (2nd ed.), Sr. C. Roy, pp. 189–210. Englewood Cliffs, N.J.: Prentice-Hall, 1984.

Robertson, M.M. Neurological function, in *Introduction to Nursing: An Adaptation Model* (2nd ed.), Sr. C. Roy, pp. 211–237. Englewood Cliffs, N.J.: Prentice-Hall, 1984.

Roy, Sr. C. *Introduction to Nursing: An Adaptation Model* (2nd ed.). Englewood Cliffs, N.J.: Prentice-Hall, 1984.

Roy, Sr. C. An explication of the philosophical assumptions of the Roy Adaptation Model. *Nursing Science Quarterly.* 1 (1), 1988: 26–34.

Sato, M.K. Skin integrity, in *Introduction to Nursing: An Adaptation Model* (2nd ed.), pp. 159–167. Englewood Cliffs, N.J.: Prentice-Hall, 1984.

Servonsky, J. Elimination, in *Introduction to Nursing: An Adaptation Model* (2nd ed.), Sr. C. Roy, pp. 125–137. Englewood Cliffs, N.J.: Prentice-Hall, 1984a.

––––. Nutrition, in *Introduction to Nursing: An Adaptation Model* (2nd ed.), Sr. C. Roy, pp. 110–124. Englewood Cliffs, N.J.: Prentice-Hall, 1984b.

Vairo, S. Oxygenation, in *Introduction to Nursing: An Adaptation Model* (2nd ed.), Sr. C. Roy, pp. 91–109. Englewood Cliffs, N.J.: Prentice-Hall, 1984.

Chapter Four

Oxygenation*

Catherine Thompson

Oxygenation is identified in the Roy Adaptation Model as one of five physiological needs. Concepts from respiratory and cardiovascular physiology provide the framework for determining adaptation relative to oxygenation. Concepts from pathophysiology provide the basis for understanding ineffective behaviors.

In this chapter, ventilation, gas exchange, and gas transport are addressed along with the parameters for assessment of behaviors and stimuli related to oxygenation. Guidelines for formulating nursing diagnoses, establishing goals, planning interventions, and evaluating nursing care are described.

OBJECTIVES

After studying this chapter, the reader will be able to do the following:

1. Describe the physiological structures and functions regulating ventilation, gas exchange, and gas transport.
2. Describe adaptive and selected ineffective behaviors related to oxygenation.
3. List common stimuli that affect oxygenation.
4. State the common adaptation problems and nursing diagnoses related to oxygenation.
5. Derive goals for a patient with ineffective oxygenation in a given situation.

*This chapter is a revision of the chapter, "Oxygen and Circulation," Sharon Vairo in the first edition of *Introduction to Nursing: An Adaptation Model,* Sister Callista Roy, Englewood Cliffs, N.J.: Prentice-Hall, 1976, pp. 109–123 and the chapter "Oxygenation," Sharon A. Vairo in the second edition (1984) pp. 91–109.

6. Describe common nursing interventions used for oxygenation problems.
7. Propose approaches to determine the effectiveness of nursing interventions.

KEY CONCEPTS DEFINED

- *Gas exchange:* the movement of oxygen through the alveolar and capillary membranes into the blood and the reverse movement of carbon dioxide from the blood through the capillary and alveolar membranes into the alveoli.
- *Hypoxia:* oxygenation deficiency anywhere in the body tissue.
- *Pulmonary ventilation:* the movement of air into the alveoli of the lungs and back out into the atmosphere.
- *Respiration:* a combination of cardiovascular and pulmonary processes whereby oxygen is supplied to all body cells and carbon dioxide is removed.
- *Tidal volume:* the amount of air inhaled or exhaled with each breath under resting conditions.

STRUCTURES AND FUNCTIONS RELATED TO OXYGENATION

Oxygenation refers to the processes by which cellular oxygen supply is maintained in the body. The major mechanisms responsible for cellular oxygenation are ventilation, alveolar/capillary gas exchange, and transport of gases to and from the tissues. If all of these mechanisms are functioning properly and sufficient environmental oxygen is available, there will be adequate oxygenation of the body tissues.

Ventilation

For ventilation to take place, numerous complex activities must occur in the body. These activities are coordinated by the respiratory center. This center is composed of groups of neurons located in the medulla oblongata and lower pons of the brain stem. Various afferent and efferent neural pathways transmit signals to the respiratory center to regulate ventilation based on the body's current need. Further, the peripheral chemoreceptor system, including carotid and aortic bodies, are responsive to changes in oxygen, carbon dioxide, and hydrogen ion concentrations and transmit signals to the main center. Functioning respiratory muscles and rib cage serve as respiratory bellows which move air into and out of the lungs through a patent airway. Lung tissue compliance (stretchability) contributes to the respiratory process. In effective ventilation, the intrapleural and intrapulmonic pressure volumes are within normal range.

Exchange of Gases

Once atmospheric air reaches the alveoli, oxygen diffuses across the alveolar capillary membranes and carbon dioxide diffuses in the reverse manner for normal gas exchange to occur. The diffusion capabilities of these gases are influenced by the concentration gradient of the gases. That is, there will be a larger amount of oxygen in the alveoli than in the blood and a smaller amount of carbon dioxide in the alveoli than in the blood. In addition, exchange of gases requires that the alveolar membrane be intact and perfusion of the alveoli be adequate.

Transport of Gases

After its diffusion across the alveolar and capillary membranes, oxygen is transported to the tissues for uptake. This transport process depends on functional myocardial contractility and a patent vasular tree that is capable of transporting an adequate blood volume. A second physiologic basis for this vital stage of oxygenation is a sufficient red blood cell population and quantity of hemoglobin to combine with oxygen in the circulation. Of the oxygen, 99 percent is attached to the hemoglobin to form oxyhemoglobin, and the remaining 1 percent is dissolved in the plasma (Po_2). Under normal conditions, hemoglobin has a high affinity for oxygen which means it readily absorbs the oxygen transported from the lungs and releases it at the tissue level.

At the tissue level, carbon dioxide is picked up and returned to the lungs for disposal. Carbon dioxide is 20 times more soluble than oxygen, however, hemoglobin still plays a major role in its conversion to bicarbonate. Once formed, bicarbonate diffuses out of the red blood cells into the plasma where it combines with sodium to form sodium bicarbonate. Of carbon dioxide, 70 percent is carried back to the lungs by the circulation in the form of sodium bicarbonate, 23 percent is attached to hemoglobin, and the remaining 7 percent is dissolved in the plasma (Pco_2).

APPLICATION OF THE NURSING PROCESS

Oxygenation of body tissues is a priority requirement for the person's physiological adaptation. The nurse caring for the patient must have an understanding of behavioral norms associated with oxygenation and the indicators of ineffective and inadequate oxygenation. The effectiveness with which the nurse intervenes in disruptions of oxygenation may be crucial to the person's survival. The mechanisms for oxygenation—ventilation, gas exchange, and transport of gases—serve as a framework for the assessment of oxygenation.

Assessment of Behavior

Behavioral assessment of oxygenation involves physical assessment skills, observation and measurements, as well as interviewing techniques.

Ventilation. In assessment of ventilation, the characteristics of respirations—rate, rhythm, and depth—are observed. Normal respiratory rate in adults is 12 to 18 breaths per minute when awake. Rates above 24 per minute are termed tachypnea, and below 10 per minute, bradypnea. Apnea means the periodic absence of respirations. Respiratory arrest is the term used for prolonged periods of apnea, an ineffective behavior incompatible with life.

Normal respiratory rhythm consists of equal intervals between respiratory cycles with the inspiratory phase shorter than the expiratory phase. Cheyne-Stokes respiration involves a decrescendo–crescendo type of breathing with a period of apnea between. This type of breathing may be seen in patients prior to death or in severe cases of heart failure and drug overdose.

Depth of respirations in terms of tidal volume, the amount of air moved in and out of the lungs during normal respiration, is estimated by observing chest movements during inspiration and expiration. Direct measurement of tidal volume is possible using a spirometer. Hyperpnea involves breathing an abnormally large amount of tidal volume, and hypopnea is the reverse. Kussmaul's respirations is a term used to describe an abnormal increase in rate and depth of respirations.

The patient should perceive breathing as effortless and without conscious thought. Shortness of breath is a term indicating observable difficulty with respirations. Dyspnea is a subjective sensation of difficult or painful breathing. In cases of difficult respirations caused by obstruction, respiratory sounds are audible without the use of a stethoscope. For example, obstruction of the trachea produces a harsh crowing sound (stridor) on inspiration. Severe constriction of the bronchioles as in asthma produces a sound called wheezing.

Breath sounds are produced by air flow through the airway and are audible through a stethoscope. Normal breath sounds are low pitched with a swishy, breezy quality. Abnormal breath sounds are commonly described as crackles, rhonchi, and wheezes. Those nurses experienced in assessment of the lungs are able to distinguish the different abnormal breath sounds.

The cough reflex and the sneeze reflex are protective mechanisms that help rid the airways of debris and inhaled foreign substances. Hypo- or hyperactivity of these reflexes can constitute ineffective behavior for the patient. In addition to the cough reflex, the secretions of the airways must also be assessed for volume, consistency, odor, and color.

Gas Exchange. Assessment of actual gas exchange is not possible using the skills of sight, hearing, or touch. Adequate gas exchange can be inferred from arterial blood gas levels in laboratory testing. If there is a normal concentration of oxygen and carbon dioxide in the blood, it is assumed that there is adequate gas exchange across the alveolar and capillary membranes.

Transport of Gases. Pulses, blood pressure, and heart sounds provide an indication of adaptation relative to the transport of gases as do indicators in the other components of the physiological mode. Normal adult pulse rates are considered to range from 60 to 100 beats per minute. A rate below 60 is called bradycardia and above 100 is called tachycardia. Both are considered out of the normal range but may not necessarily indicate a pathological condition. Persons who are frightened or anxious may temporarily have tachycardia caused by the stimulation of the sympathetic nervous system. Any condition which causes a decrease in tissue oxygenation will automatically increase the heart rate.

Pulse rhythm is normally regular, that is, the time intervals between beats are of equal duration. An irregular rhythm is referred to as an arrhythmia or dysrhythmia. Pulse rhythm is recorded as either "regular" or "irregular." A pulse deficit exists if the apical rate, on auscultation, is higher than the radial pulse rate, indicating some ventricular contractions are weaker.

Peripheral pulses are assessed for their presence and strength and these are important indicators of the oxygenation status of distal tissues. Patients with heart problems or peripheral vascular disorders may have absent or diminished strength in the peripheral pulses.

Blood pressure consists of two readings: systole (the upper reading) and diastole (the lower reading). Normal blood pressure readings in adults average about 120/80 mm Hg. It may be necessary to take blood pressure reading in a supine, sitting, and standing positions. Normally, from the supine to the standing position, the systolic pressure should not drop more than 15 mm Hg and the diastolic pressure not more than 5 mm Hg. When assessing blood pressure, it is imperative that the patient's blood pressure range is known so that a sound interpretation of adaptive or ineffective can be made relative to the readings obtained. For example, if a patient's normal range is 150/86 to 138/80, then a sudden change to 106/60 must alert the nurse to possible problems and be reported to the physician. The most common abnormality seen in relation to high systolic and diastolic pressure is hypertension.

Increasingly, nurses, in their assessment of oxygenation, are becoming skilled with the auscultations of heart sounds. Discussion of the procedures associated with auscultation of heart sounds can be found in physical assessment resources such as Seidel, Ball, Dains, and Benedict (1987).

Other components of the physiological mode may manifest behavioral indicators of oxygenation. The skin, mucous membranes, and nail beds are considered later for their protective functions, however, the pallor and cyanosis of these are abnormalities seen in situations of decreased tissue perfusion. Decreased body oxygenation stimulates the sympathetic nervous system response which causes the skin to be cool and clammy. A decrease in the level of consciousness may be an early indicator of cerebral hypoxia. With respect to elimination, decreased urinary output may be indicative of a decrease in cardiac output. Monitoring hourly output of urine and detection of production of less than 30 ml per hour signifies ineffective behavior and must be reported to the physician.

There are numerous diagnostic studies used specifically to evaluate the respiratory and cardiovascular systems. A detailed discussion of these can be found in medical-surgical or laboratory studies texts. The most common of these are hematocrit, hemoglobin, red blood cell count, arterial blood gases, chest x-ray, and electrocardiogram. The hematocrit, hemoglobin, and red cell count provide information about the oxygen-carrying capabilities of the red blood cells. Arterial blood gas studies indicate the actual amount of oxygen and carbon dioxide in the blood. These findings provide an indication of the effectiveness of ventilation and gas exchange. Chest x-ray provides information about the gross structure of the lungs and pleural cavity, indicating abnormal growths, inflammation, and fluid within the lungs, for example. The electrocardiogram shows the electrical activity of the heart. Significant results from diagnostic studies may be important in the nursing assessment as they may reflect oxygenation problems.

Once the nurse has completed the behavioral assessment of oxygenation, a tentative nursing judgment is made as to whether the behaviors are adaptive or ineffective. As has been presented previously, normal values are available to guide this judgment, as are general expectations relative to the identified behaviors. In other situations, pronounced regulator activity with cognator ineffectiveness may provide the key to the identification of ineffective adaptation. By obtaining the behavioral indication of whether the person is receiving adequate oxygenation, priorities can be established with respect to the next level of the nursing process—assessment of stimuli.

Assessment of Stimuli

After assessing the individual's oxygenation behaviors, stimuli that influence and activate the regulator and cognator subsystems to produce either adaptive or ineffective behaviors are assessed. Assessment of stimuli requires data gathering focused on the patient's physiological status and environmental factors affecting the individual. Possible stimuli are identified from the patient's records, health care workers, and significant others. These are validated with the patient, when appropriate.

Ventilation. Impairment of structure or function can lead to compromise of the basic processes that meet oxygen needs, that is, ventilation, gas exchange, and transport of gases. A great demand to compensate for the impairment results. Of the other common stimuli affecting oxygenation adaptation, lack of integrity of the physiological mode is an important source of oxygenation disruption. Airway patency, musculoskeletal structure of the rib cage, functioning of the respiratory center in the medulla and pons, and the neural pathways are important factors in the mechanism of ventilation. Assessment of the patency of the patient's airway is one of the primary responsibilities of the nurse. Foreign bodies in the airway; inflammatory reactions from infections, irritants, and allergens; and aspiration of fluids or emesis are all factors which can cause airway problems.

Pathological processes may lead to deformity or atrophy of the musculoskeletal structures of the rib cage. Barrel chest, as seen in emphysema, is an abnormal condition where the anterior diameter is increased because of chronic over use of the expiratory muscles. Muscular dystrophies and conditions interfering with the neuromuscular junctions can affect the respiratory muscles. Poliomyelitis, Guillain-Barre syndrome, and myasthenia gravis are disorders which can interfere with the neuromuscular function of the respiratory muscles. Distention or pain in the abdomen decreases the movement of the diaphragm. Skeletal problems of the thoracic cage such as scoliosis and rib fractures affect ventilation by decreasing thoracic expansion.

Trauma or bleeding in the central nervous system can cause increased intracranial pressure which, in turn, can affect the respiratory center in the brain. Depression of the respiratory center can occur with the use of narcotics and anesthetics. Alterations in the oxygen or carbon dioxide center of the blood will also cause a change in the respiratory center. Pneumothorax is a critical condition in which intrapulmonic and intrapleural pressures are disrupted. This can lead to severe problems with inspiration or collapse of the lung tissue.

Exchange of Gases. Pathogenesis causing an alteration in the expandability and elastic recoil of the lung tissue compromises ventilation. Examples of diseases causing this pathophysiology are pneumonia, tuberculosis, chronic bronchitis, and emphysema.

Stimuli influencing the exchange of gases include the concentration of oxygen in the air, adequacy of blood supply to the alveoli, and integrity of the alveolar membrane. Pulmonary emboli or thrombi are examples of situations that decrease perfusion to the alveoli. If the alveolar membrane is thick and fibrotic or if the alveoli are filled with exudate or fluid, there will be minimal or no gas exchange.

Transport of Gases. Stimuli that influence the transport of gases relate to cardiac function and the circulating blood volume. Any condition which decreases the pumping ability of the heart will cause oxygenation problems because there will be a deficiency in the number of red blood cells reaching the tissue. Inflammatory conditions of the heart such as bacterial endocarditis, myocardial infarction, and congestive heart failure are disorders which can interfere with the pumping ability of the heart. Hemorrhage and dehydration are common causes of a decrease in cardiac output and circulating blood volume.

A decrease in the number of red blood cells or a lack of hemoglobin will decrease the oxygen-carrying capabilities of the blood. Under certain circumstances, the ability of hemoglobin to carry oxygen is compromised. Situations which decrease the uptake of oxygen at the alveolar level are acidosis and increase in body temperature. On the other hand, oxygen release at the tissue level is depressed by alkalosis and decreased body temperature.

Exercise, stress, changes in altitude, and temperature changes are all stimuli that alter the oxygen demands of the body. Changes of these stimuli are a normal part of the person's external environment. The body, if healthy, adapts to these stimuli by changing behaviors related to ventilation and gas transport. In a state of illness, these stimuli can have an overwhelming effect on the individual's ability to adapt. The demands are greater than one can meet and assistance is needed.

Noxious environmental stimuli such as tobacco smoke, allergens, and irritating fumes can be considered individually and are also part of the pathogenesis of many of the various diseases previously mentioned. These stimuli and other risk factors can be considered contextual stimuli.

Once the stimuli influencing oxygenation have been identified, the nurse proceeds to suggest whether they are focal, contextual, or residual in their effect on the person's physiological integrity. As was described in Chapter 1, the focal stimulus is the one most immediately confronting the person. Contextual stimuli are all other internal or external stimuli evident in the situation and contributing to the behavior precipitated by the focal stimulus. Residual stimuli represent those stimuli whose effect on the person has not or cannot be validated.

The nurse's knowledge from many related disciplines may suggest residual stimuli that should be pursued as contributing to the person's adaptation relative to oxygenation. The information generated in the assessment of behavior and stimuli is then interpreted. The interpretive statement forms the nursing diagnosis.

Nursing Diagnosis

As was described in Chapter 2, Roy has suggested three alternatives for stating nursing diagnoses: (1) a statement of the behaviors within one mode with their most relevant influencing stimuli, (2) a summary label for behaviors in one mode with relevant stimuli, or (3) a label that summarizes a behavioral pattern when more than one mode is being affected by the same stimuli. It is possible to derive nursing diagnoses that reflect positive adaptation as related to oxygenation. A nursing diagnosis illustrating adaptation could be, "Adequate oxygenation of toes of left foot due to good circulation in leg with cast." In situations of disruption of oxygenation, it is important that the nursing diagnosis convey the essence of the problem such that direction is provided for subsequent steps of the nursing process.

In situations of ineffective adaptation, terminology must be identified to communicate the adaptive problem. *Hypoxia* is an encompassing term referring to oxygen deficiency anywhere in the body tissue. However, one can be more specific and use the terms "ventilatory impairment," "inadequate gas exchange," and "inadequate gas transport" to specify the nature of the hypoxia. Using these labels to assist with conveying the essence of the problem constitutes an appropriate method of stating the nursing diagnosis. An example of such a nursing diagnosis would be, "Ventilatory impairment related to copious secretions in the airways." Both the ineffective behavior and the focal stimulus are identified in this statement.

Using a label that summarizes a behavioral pattern when more than one mode is being affected by the same stimuli normally involves a very complex concept and assumes that the nurse is an experienced practitioner. The concept of hypoxia provides an example of this method of stating a nursing diagnosis. The diagnostic statement could be "hypoxia due to compromised cardiac output." Much information is contained in the terms of "hypoxia" and "compromised cardiac output" that would provide meaningful direction for the experienced nurse but may be less meaningful and provide less direction for the beginning nurse.

The statement of nursing diagnoses provides concrete direction for the next step of the nursing process. Based on the nursing diagnosis, the nurse proceeds to the fourth step—goal setting.

Goal Setting

Goal setting, according to the Roy Adaptation Model, involves the establishment of clear statements of behavioral outcomes for the person as the result of the nursing care provided. A complete goal statement contains the behavior of focus, the change expected, and the time frame in which the goal should be achieved. Goals may be short term or long term and these time frames are relative to the situation.

Consider the example of a patient with a newly applied leg cast. Although the nursing diagnosis indicated that, at that point, there was adequate circulation to the toes, swelling that often occurs after the application of a new cast would be something that the nurse would be aware of and need to monitor. A short-term goal pertaining to this situation could be, "Circulation to toes will remain adequate within the next hour." The behavior in this goal would be "circulation to toes," the change expected is no change, that is, circulation would remain adequate, and the time frame is "within the next hour."

In the case of the patient whose diagnosis was "ventilatory impairment related to copious secretions in the airways," the behavior on which the goal should focus is the ventilatory impairment. A goal could be, "Within 10 minutes, the patient will be breathing effortlessly." The patient's breathing is the behavior of focus, the criterion is "effortless," and the time frame is "within 10 minutes."

Generally, the goal of the nurse relative to oxygenation is to ensure an adequate level of oxygen supply to all parts of the body. This goal is operationalized by the identification of the specific goals that address ventilation, gas exchange, and transport of gases. The importance of anticipating potential problems associated with oxygenation is evident. Much of the nurse's role in relation to oxygenation involves monitoring the person's condition to detect oxygenation problems before they become serious. Thus, many goals established for the patient may be preventive in nature rather than focusing on an already ineffective situation.

In order to assist the patient in the achievement of the established goals, the nurse proceeds to planning of nursing interventions.

Intervention

The four previous steps of the nursing process provide specific direction for the identification of nursing interventions to assist the patient. Whereas the goal focused on specified patient behaviors, the interventions address the stimuli that are causing these behaviors. This management of stimuli involves either altering, increasing, decreasing, removing, or maintaining them.

Nursing measures used to facilitate ventilation and gas exchange include deep breathing and coughing, positioning to encourage maximal breathing capacity, using lung inflation devices, providing oxygen therapy, promoting drainage and removal of tracheobronchial secretion, providing hydration, and providing pulmonary resuscitation in situations of respiratory arrest. Nursing interventions to enhance gas transport include maintaining adequate circulation through proper positioning and nonrestrictive clothing, providing adequate nutritional intake of iron, and providing cardiopulmonary resuscitation in situations of cardiac arrest.

In the previous situation involving the patient with the new cast, the stimulus that could interfere with oxygenation of the toes is swelling within the cast and the subsequent interruption of blood flow to the toes. In considering interventions to prevent such an occurrence, the nurse would identify and analyze possible approaches and then select the approach with the highest probability of achieving the goal. Possible interventions could be splitting the cast, elevating the leg on a pillow, or packing the leg in ice to prevent swelling. The last alternative may have a detrimental effect on the plaster cast; the first is not something that would be tried as a preventive measure. Thus the nurse would select the intervention of elevating the leg on a pillow in an attempt to minimize swelling before it becomes a problem. Nursing intervention in situations of oxygenation disruptions involves facilitating the processes of ventilation, gas exchange, and gas transport.

In the situation of the patient with ventilatory impairment due to bronchial secretions, the nursing intervention would focus on clearing the secretions from the person's airway. Possible interventions include positioning of the patient, postural drainage, encouraging the person to cough, and suctioning of the patient's airway. The approach selected would depend on the circumstances. A person with an altered level of consciousness may require suctioning while a patient who is aware and can follow instructions may benefit by assistance and encouragement with effective coughing.

Whatever the nursing interventions selected, their effectiveness in attainment of the goals is addressed through evaluation.

Evaluation

The key to evaluation of the effectiveness of nursing interventions lies in determining if the behavior changed within the time frame stated in the goal. Consider the previously identified goal: "Within 10 minutes, the patient will be breathing effortlessly." The behavior of interest in evaluating success in achieving the goal is the person's breathing. If it is effortless within the 10-minute time frame, the goal has been achieved.

Suppose that within one hour, the nurse identified that the patient with the cast was demonstrating decreased circulation to his toes in that they were dusky in color and the patient was reporting numbness. This situation would necessitate immediate action on the part of the nurse and prompt, continued reassessment, and further intervention.

Such a situation demonstrates the simultaneous and continuous nature of the nursing process. Although the steps are addressed separately for purposes of teaching and learning, the experienced nurse assesses behavior and stimuli simultaneously, perhaps while setting goals with the patient and carrying out an intervention. The interrelatedness of the steps of the process, based on Roy's conceptualization of the person as a whole, becomes increasingly evident as the nurse becomes more experienced in its application.

SUMMARY

This chapter has focused on the application of the Roy Adaptation Model to the physiological need of oxygenation. A brief overview of the structures and functions associated with ventilation, gas exchange, and gas transport was provided. These were used to provide a framework for the application of the nursing process to the physiological component of oxygenation.

EXERCISES FOR APPLICATION

1. Develop a tool to assist you with the assessment of oxygenation. Address in the tool important behavioral indicators and stimuli that affect ventilation, gas exchange, and gas transport.
2. Using the tool developed in item 1, assess a patient's status relative to oxygenation. Assess the adequacy of your tool by comparing it to an oxygenation assessment guideline in a physical assessment resource.

ASSESSMENT OF UNDERSTANDING

1. Identify the three major mechanisms associated with cellular oxygenation.
   a. _____
   b. _____
   c. _____
2. Which of the following are important behaviors associated primarily with the assessment of the adequacy of transport of gases?
   a. breath sounds
   b. respiratory rate
   c. blood pressure
   d. rhythm of respirations
   e. tidal volume
   f. peripheral pulses
3. Which of the following stimuli influence exchange of gases?
   a. adequacy of blood supply to alveoli
   b. integrity of alveolar membrane
   c. concentration of oxygen in the air
4. State a nursing diagnosis reflecting effective adaptation relative to oxygenation.

Situation:

A patient has been admitted in the emergency department with carbon monoxide poisoning. The nursing diagnosis as formulated reads: Skin cyanotic, respirations shallow and slow, and nonresponsive to stimuli due to depression of respiratory center from carbon monoxide poisoning.

5. Derive a goal statement for this patient that contains the behavior of focus, the change expected, and the time frame involved.
6. Identify three common nursing interventions to facilitate gas exchange. Specify the approach* with the highest probability of achieving the goal you derived in item 5.
   a. _____
   b. _____
   c. _____

7. If the goal developed in item 5 was, "Within 8 hours, the patient will evidence a stable pattern of gas exchange by regaining consciousness and normal coloration," on what behavior(s) would the nurse focus in evaluating the effectiveness of the intervention?

Feedback

1. a. ventilation
   b. gas exchange
   c. gas transport
2. c and f
3. a, b, and c
4. Example: Stable processes of ventilation due to appropriate positioning of head to prevent blockage by tongue.
5. Example: Within 8 hours, the patient will evidence stable pattern of gas exchange by regaining consciousness and normal coloration.
6. a. positioning to encourage maximal breathing capacity and prevention of aspiration
   b. providing oxygen therapy*
   c. utilizing lung inflation devices
7. Level of consciousness, coloration.

REFERENCE

Seidel, H.M., J.W. Ball, J.E. Dains, and G.W. Benedict. *Mosby's Guide to Physical Examination*. St. Louis: The C.V. Mosby, 1987.

Additional References
Bates, B. *A Guide to Physical Examination and History Taking* (4th ed.). Philadelphia: J.B. Lippincott Company, 1987.
Bullock, B., and P. Rosendahl. *Pathophysiology: Adaptation and Albertations in Function* (2nd ed.). Boston: Scott, Foresman and Co., 1988.
Lehrer, S. *Understanding Lung Sounds*. Philadelphia: W. B. Saunders, 1984.
Long, B., and W. Phipps. *Medical-Surgical Nursing: A Nursing Process Approach* (2nd ed.). St. Louis: The C. V. Mosby, 1989.
Marieb, E.N. *Human Anatomy and Physiology*. Redwood City, Calif.: Benjamin/Cummings Publishing Co., 1989.
Miller, M. *Pathophysiology: Principles of Diseases*. Philadelphia: W. B. Saunders, 1983.
Porth, C.M. *Pathophysiology: Concepts of Altered Health States*. (3rd ed.) Philadelphia: J.B. Lippincott Company, 1990.
Rambo, B. *Adaptation Nursing: Assessment and Interventions*. Philadelphia: W. B. Saunders, 1984.
Tilkian, A., and M. Conover. *Understanding Heart Sounds and Murmurs*. Philadelphia: W. B. Saunders, 1984.

Chapter Five —————————————

Nutrition

Jane Servonsky

Nutrition, identified in the Roy Adaptation Model as one of five physiological needs, relates to the series of processes by which the person takes in and assimilates food necessary for maintenance of human functioning, promotion of growth, and replacement of injured tissues. Marieb (1989:851) described nutrition as "one of the most overlooked areas in clinical medicine." This observation has important implications for the role of nursing in promoting health since one's level of nutrition influences every phase of metabolism and plays a major role in each person's overall health. Consideration of the individual's state of nutrition and promotion of an optimal nutritional level are important nursing activities in the holistic role that nurses occupy in the promotion of adaptation and health.

Basic concepts related to digestion and metabolism provide the framework for determining adaptation relative to nutrition. In this chapter, an overview of these basic concepts is provided. In addition, the application of the nursing process in terms of the assessment of behaviors and stimuli, nursing diagnoses related to nutrition, goal setting, intervention, and evaluation is explored.

OBJECTIVES

After studying this chapter, the reader will be able to do the following:

1. Describe the person's need for nutrition in terms of the processes related to digestion and metabolism.
2. Assess behaviors related to nutrition.
3. Identify common stimuli related to nutrition.
4. Define common adaptation problems of the need for nutrition.
5. Develop a nutritional goal in a given situation.

6. Identify nursing interventions to assist in the achievement of a nutritional goal.

7. Suggest ways to evaluate the person's achievement of nutritional goals.

KEY CONCEPTS DEFINED

- *Absorption:* the process by which the products of digestion pass through the alimentary canal mucosa into the blood or lymph.
- *Anorexia:* the loss or lack of appetite for food.
- *Digestion:* the chemical and mechanical processes of breaking down food into substances that can be absorbed (Marieb 1989:752).
- *Metabolism:* the sum total of all chemical reactions occurring in the body cells (Marieb, 1989:804).
- *Nutrients:* substances that provide nourishment to the body. These include proteins, fats, carbohydrates, vitamins, and minerals.
- *Nutrition:* the processes by which the person takes in and assimilates food necessary for maintaining human functioning, promoting growth, and replacing worn or injured tissues.
- *Satiety:* a condition of satisfaction or a lack of desire for food after its ingestion.

STRUCTURES AND FUNCTIONS RELATED TO NUTRITION

Nutrition is a basic need second only to the need for oxygen. The term nutrition refers to the series of processes by which the person takes in and assimilates food necessary for maintaining human functioning, promoting growth, and replacing injured tissues. For purposes of this overview of the need for nutrition, two major processes are identified: digestion and metabolism. The food that the person ingests influences every phase of metabolism and plays a major role in the overall health of the individual.

Digestion

Digestion can be described in general terms as a series of processes by which food is taken into the body and prepared for absorption into the blood and lymph for transport to body cells. The organs of the digestive system function to keep the body supplied with the nutrients required by the body tissues and organs. Digestive organs can be categorized into two main groups. (1) The **gastrointestinal tract** or **alimentary canal** consists of the mouth, pharynx, esophagus, stomach, small and large intestines, and the anus—the terminal opening. Within the alimentary canal, food is digested and digested fragments are absorbed. (2) The **accessory digestive organs** include the teeth, tongue, gallbladder, salivary glands, liver, and pancreas. These assist in the process of digestive breakdown of foods.

Marieb (1989:754) described digestion in terms of the following six major processes:

1. *Ingestion:* the process of taking food into the digestive tract,
2. *Propulsion:* the peristaltic movement of food through the alimentary canal,
3. *Mechanical digestion:* the preparation of food for chemical digestion by chewing, mixing, and churning.
4. *Chemical digestion:* the breaking down of food into molecules small enough to be absorbed.
5. *Absorption:* the movement of digested substances into the blood or lymph for transport to body cells.
6. *Defecation:* the elimination of undigested substances.

The physiology of these processes is introduced in the following chapter, however, the reader is referred to a physiology text for a more thorough explanation.

Metabolism

Marieb (1989:804) described *metabolism* as the sum total of all chemical reactions occurring in the body cells. Metabolism is the process by which digested nutrients are used within body cells as metabolic fuels and to build cells, to replace worn structures or to synthesize functional molecules.

Nutrients are described as substances that provide nourishment to the body and are used by the body to promote normal growth, maintenance, and repair. Three major and two minor nutrients have been categorized by Marieb (1989:805). The major nutrients include carbohydrates, fats, and proteins while the minor nutrients, required in smaller amounts, are vitamins and minerals. Each is essential for normal body functioning.

The role of nursing in the person's need for nutrition relates to the ensuring that the individual's diet is meeting body requirements. The factors to be considered when evaluating a diet for optimal nutrition are described by Williams (1986:341–343). To promote health, the diet should provide all essential nutrients in adequate amounts for the daily needs of the body. Accepted standards for recommended daily allowances of nutrients have been developed. An example is that developed by the National Academy of Sciences (1989). The optimal diet provides a caloric level that will meet the energy needs of the body. Foods containing fiber should be ingested since the fiber provides bulk which stimulates intestinal elimination. The food eaten should promote health and provide a measure of prevention in protecting the person from illness throughout all stages of the life cycle.

The established dietary pattern must be acceptable to the person or family. Acceptability includes establishing a diet that includes culturally defined differences such as those noted later in this chapter. Taking account of such differences can be accomplished with ease since there are many kinds and combinations of foods that constitute a well-balanced diet. Finally, the diet chosen should promote a good supply of energy for optimum performance of the person's activities of daily living and total human functioning.

The Department of Agriculture in the United States and National Health and Welfare Canada (1983) have developed a daily food guide for the purpose of promoting good nutrition. This guide provides a flexible framework to help a person achieve the nutrient needs as outlined in the Recommended Daily Dietary Allowances. The daily food guide combines foods with similar nutritional values into four main groups—milk, meat, vegetable and fruit, and grain—commonly referred to as the Basic Four. In planning a diet, the person should choose from each group a variety of foods that they like and can afford. (Refer to nutritional text books for further information about nutritional requirements and dietary planning.)

APPLICATION OF THE NURSING PROCESS

A nursing role relative to the need for nutrition is that of counselor, wherein the nurse collaborates with the person regarding nutritional needs and provides for education when required. In recent years, there have been increased awareness of and interest in nutrition on the part of the general public. To respond to this interest effectively, the nurse requires a basic knowledge related to nutrition and a framework within which to assess a person's dietary patterns and identify the health implications and to initiate referrals to other health professionals when required.

Assessment of Behavior

When assessing the need for nutrition as described in the Roy Adaptation Model, the nurse observes several categories of behavior. These include appetite and thirst, height and weight, eating patterns, food allergies, and condition of the oral cavity.

Appetite and Thirst. *Appetite* is a pleasant sensation involving the person's desire for and anticipation of food or drink. Frequently, the appetite is affected by such specific stimuli as the sight, smell, and thought of food. It is psychological and is dependent on memory and associations. *Hunger*, however, is physiologically aroused by the body's need for food. The hypothalamus is the principal organ involved in the physiological regulation of eating. A functioning hypothalamus is responsible for sending internal cues that signal the person to eat in order to supply the body with needed energy. This process is one example of the regulator activity outlined in

Chapter 1. The hypothalamus again signals through the *satiety* center, telling the person to stop eating. A healthy individual who responds to these internal cues that regulate energy balance is able to maintain a normal weight and control their appetite. An example of an adaptive appetite behavior would be the statement: "I have a good appetite in the morning and eat a well-balanced breakfast," whereas an ineffective appetite behavior would be: "Although I had eaten a large lunch, the smell of a freshly baked cake tempted me into eating a big slice. I now feel very uncomfortable."

Thirst is a desire for fluid or the dry sensation resulting from a lack of, or need for, water. Often this sensation of dryness is felt in the mouth and back part of the throat. The hypothalamus contains the mechanism for stimulating thirst and is activated by an increase in the solute concentration in body fluids. Thirst is usually a reliable guide to the body's need for water. The normal adult should consume an average of 1 to 1½ litres of water or other liquids daily in order to provide a sufficient amount of water needed for all physiological processes. Water is available to the body through other sources, such as beverages, solid foods, and a small amount through the oxidation of essential nutrients. The maintenance of water balance is explored further in Chapter 10.

Height and Weight. In a behavioral assessment of nutrition as a need, the nurse measures and records the height and the weight of the person. Height measurements are taken without shoes and the weight preferably is taken without clothing.

A daily weight is also useful when assessing a person's fluid balance. In this case it is particularly important that the weight be taken at the same time of day and on the same scale. When a person is underweight or overweight, measurements taken over a period of time are more useful than a single measurement. Tables specifying appropriate height and weight for male and female adults have been established and serve as a guideline when making judgments regarding adaptive weight according to a person's height, sex, and body build. These tables are found in textbooks on nutrition. In general, the nurse may use the following criterion: the person should weigh 100 pounds for 5 feet, with 5 pounds added for each additional inch of height. For males, an extra 5 pounds per inch is suggested. Standard and reference growth charts for infants, children, and youth also have been established, and these guidelines are found in any growth and development or pediatric textbook.

Eating Patterns. The nurse obtains a diet history listing the quantities of all food and fluids ingested during a 24-hour period. The recommended dietary allowances and daily food guide can be used as standards in determining if the quantity and quality of the nutrients ingested are adaptive or ineffective.

Food Allergies. The nurse assesses whether the person has a known food allergy or sensitivity. An allergic reaction to a certain food or food group is the result of an inappropriate antibody-antigen reaction in the body. Foods causing problems are identified and behaviors (such as skin rash, swelling of the face or mouth, or gastrointestinal reaction) occurring if the food is ingested are noted.

Condition of the Oral Cavity. Appraisal of the oral cavity, that is, the lips, teeth, gums, and tongue, is useful in determining the person's nutritional health and in identifying deficiencies. The lips of the healthy adult are smooth and free from lesions. The skin is thin with many vascular structures which give the lips their reddish appearance. The oral mucosa is normally smooth, moist, and pinkish red in color, with expected variations based on ethnic differences. The adult has 32 permanent teeth. They are examined for conditions that decrease their grinding action, such as loose or missing teeth, cavities or wear. If dentures are used, they are removed to allow complete inspection of the mouth. Normal gums are solid in turgor and free of inflammation or bleeding. The tongue is pinkish in color. The dorsal surface is rough and the ventral surface is smooth.

Pain. The nurse assesses for any pain related to the ingestion of food or fluids. Pain may be noted as a behavior by listing the person's statements regarding discomfort and pain following ingestion of food. For example, persons may state that they experience a burning sensation which they refer to as heartburn after the ingestion of foods such as onions. All verbal and nonverbal behaviors are recorded as are severity, duration, and onset of the pain.

Altered Ingestion. If the person is unable to eat and drink normally, the altered means of nutritional intake should be assessed. For example, a person may be nourished through a nasogastric or gastrostomy tube. The amount and substance ingested should be noted. If the person is receiving intravenous fluids and electrolytes or a hyperalimentation solution, the solutions and rate of delivery are assessed. The knowledge and skills related to these particular altered means of ingestion are continually developing. The nurse is challenged to maintain the knowledge and skill necessary to provide nursing care in these situations through reading, clinical practice, and continuing education.

Sense of Taste and Smell. The normal person determines taste on the anterior two-thirds of the tongue. Four basic substances are experienced: sweet, sour, bitter, and salt. The sensory receptors for taste are the glossopharyngeal nerve (cranial nerve IX) and the facial nerve (cranial nerve I). Nasal passages should be patent. Testing each nostril separately, the person should be able to identify such odors as coffee or tobacco.

Once behaviors pertaining to nutrition have been identified, the nurse makes an initial judgment as to whether they are adaptive or ineffective. This assists in establishing priorities for the following steps of the nursing process. That is, ineffective behaviors would be of initial concern.

Assessment of Stimuli

The nurse assesses stimuli related to the ingestion and assimilation of nutrients by identifying the factors influencing the stated behaviors. This assessment of stimuli includes the body's adaptive ability to maintain structure, function, and regulation of the digestive system, as well as coping strategies the person uses to maintain or change the behaviors.

Integrity of the Physiological Mode. The nurse knows the normal homeostatic responses of the digestive system that function to receive and transfer nutrients from the external to the internal environment of the body. Through these responses, the body maintains a constancy of the internal environment. The alimentary canal consists of the upper, middle, and lower regions and is responsible for the digestion and absorption of nutrients. When food is ingested, a series of physical and chemical changes occurs which prepare the nutrients for absorption and utilization by the cells. The alimentary canal is regulated by the neural-chemical-endocrine processes that Roy describes as the regulator subsystem (presented in Chapter 1). Residue remaining after digestion and absorption is then excreted from the body.

The nurse identifies whether or not a disease state is present that affects the normal structure, function, and regulation of the digestive system. Examples would include such conditions as obstructive lesions of the esophagus and malabsorption, which are explained in general textbooks of pathology. Also, the nurse assesses if a condition exists that prohibits the person from eating, such as recent surgery, or if the person is on a restricted or special diet, such as that for a person with a medical diagnosis of diabetes.

Cognator Effectiveness. The person's level of knowledge regarding nutrition and perception of what constitutes a diet that promotes a healthy state and that fulfills nutritional needs is a major stimulus. The nurse assesses this knowledge and perception since it greatly influences what the person is presently ingesting or what the person desires to eat and thus results in either adaptive or ineffective patterns of nutrition. Based on the patient's level of knowledge about sound nutrition, diet counseling may be required. The nurse is also aware of the person's beliefs regarding the types of food eaten. Many people, for religious, economic, health, and ethical ecological reasons, are vegetarians. Such beliefs are taken into account in diet counseling.

Medication. The nurse identifies whether or not the person takes any medication that may influence the intake of food or the digestive process. For example, drugs that may decrease the appetite may be taken if the person is attempting to lose weight. It is important to ascertain whether supplemental vitamins and minerals are used.

Caloric Requirements. Factors affecting caloric requirements to consider are age, sex, size, activity, temperature, diet, race, climate, pregnancy, and endocrine hormones (Williams, 1986:18). For example, an infant, because of a high rate of metabolism and relatively large body surface area, requires more calories per kilogram of body weight than an adult. A person exposed to severely cold weather expends additional calories to maintain body temperature. In periods of rapid growth during infancy, adolescence, and pregnancy, there is an increased caloric need. Males, who usually have a greater body size and greater proportion of lean body tissue, have a greater caloric requirement than do females. There is a steady decline in caloric need starting with the early adulthood years. Inactive people require fewer calories than those with greater levels of activity (Phipps, Long, and Woods 1987). Exercise patterns of the person are assessed, as they will influence caloric requirements.

Condition of the Oral Cavity. In addition to behaviorally manifesting nutritional status, the condition of the oral cavity influences the ingestion of food. Any mouth lesions, gum disease, teeth in need of dental repair, or improperly fitted dentures are noted. The nurse identifies whether or not there is dental pain and if it affects the ability of the person to chew or swallow food, or to ingest hot or cold foods. The coping strategies which the person uses to deal with difficulties are important to determine including whether they are effective or ineffective.

Availability of Food. The nurse considers the availability of food to the person including monetary and other resources. For example, an elderly person may find it difficult to travel to the store and may have limited funds or fixed income to purchase food.

Conditions of Eating. The nurse identifies who purchases and prepares the food the person eats. In the family setting, the health beliefs of this person regarding nutrition will influence greatly the ingestion behaviors of all members. One looks at whether or not the family meal planning provides a well-balanced diet and notes what social and moral values are placed on eating. For example, is eating a highly social event, and is food used as a punishment or reward? The nurse further identifies the level of family or peer group influences regarding eating. The nurse considers if the person or family sets aside a special time for mealtime. Are the meals taken alone, with a group, at home, at fast-food services, or in a restaurant? Another important consideration is the person's familiarity with different types of food.

Culture. The nurse determines the person's cultural, social, and religious patterns that influence eating and drinking. The person's food habits and preferences based on cultural experience begin early in life. Some general examples provided by Williams (1986) are cited here. *Seventh Day Adventists* do not eat meat, fish, or poultry, but allow cheese, milk, and eggs as a source of animal protein, with nuts and legumes as other sources of protein. *Orthodox Jewish* dietary habits prohibit pork in any form. They do allow goats, sheep, deer, and cows, which are classified as quadrupeds that have a cloven hoof and chew a cud. The poultry allowed includes chicken, duck, goose, pheasant, and turkey. All meats and poultry must be prepared by the process known as "koshering" or "clean." This is the prescribed ritual of soaking the meat in salted water to remove all traces of blood. All fish eaten must have fins and scales; therefore, shellfish are not allowed. Combining milk and meat in the same meal is prohibited. The Jewish Sabbath and religious holidays also have dietary laws. On the Sabbath no food is to be cooked. No leavened bread may be taken during Passover week. Yom Kippur is a fast day, and no food or drink is taken for a 24-hour period. The *Roman Catholic* dietary restrictions and fast days have been liberalized in recent years. Therefore, customs, days of abstaining from meat, and fasting may vary in different locations.

The *American* living in the South consumes a diet that is described as "soul food." This term conveys special feelings of happiness and enjoyment. Their diet consists of the use of hot breads, not made with yeast, such as cornbread and biscuits. They use a wide variety of greens (turnip, collard) cooked in liquid using some form of pork. Grits, corn, and rice are popular sources of carbohydrates, with dried beans as a source of protein. Meats that are high in bone and connective tissue, such as spareribs, pigsfeet, and chitterlings (intestines) are favored. Meats are frequently prepared by stewing, barbecuing, and frying. Sweets are eaten in large quantities and milk products and cheese are used less frequently.

In the diet of the *Mexican American,* the use of a variety of dried beans, especially the pinto bean, chili peppers, rice, corn, and some vegetables is favored. Little meat is used in the diet. Corn tortillas are eaten as bread. Popular dishes include chili con carne, tamales, tacos, and enchiladas. Coffee is consumed in large amounts and is sometimes given to children.

The dietary habits of the *Chinese* include the use of meat, fish, eggs, cereals, and a variety of vegetables. Rice is used instead of bread. Meat is eaten in small amounts and is usually served with vegetables. Food is cut or chopped into small pieces and cooked quickly in small amounts of liquids or fats.

The *Japanese* diet has changed during the past decades because of the influence of Western culture. Their diet had consisted primarily of the use of rice, beans, curd, vegetables, fruit, raw or cooked fish, and pickles, but now includes eggs, meat, milk, and cheese. A whole meal may consist of noodles cooked in broth seasoned with bits of vegetables and fish. Tea has been the traditional favored drink.

With *Italian Americans,* bread and pasta served with a variety of sauces and cheeses are eaten. Foods are highly seasoned with spices and many dishes use a lot of eggs, tomatoes, green vegetables, and fruit. Italian foods are usually cooked or simmered in oil or in liquids such as broth or tomato sauce.

Starchy vegetables and tropical fruits are common in the *Puerto Rican* diet. Rice and beans are other staples. The favorite meats include beef, pork, and chicken. A typical dish would include dried beans cooked with tomatoes, onions, peppers, salt pork, and seasonings. Milk is used on a limited basis.

People with *Middle East* cultures, such as the Lebanese, Armenians, and Greeks, receive their major source of energy from the use of grains. The favored meat is lamb. Bread is the center of every meal, and they favor cheeses and yogurt. Vegetables are generally the main dish. Their food is rich in fat and not highly spiced.

North American Hutterites have special diets for mothers in the post-partum period. As Hostetler and Huntington (1980) reported, "During the first five weeks, in addition to the zwieback and the regular colony meals, the new mother is served omelets, rich chicken soups, milk puddings and chicken roasted in butter which are prepared especially for her by the diet cook."

Cues for Eating. When assessing factors influencing the person's amount of food intake, it is important to identify the internal and external cues to which the individual responds. As mentioned earlier, a healthy, functioning hypothalamus sends the person internal cues to signal that enough food has been ingested. In cases of overeating, the nurse helps the person identify what external cues they are responding to when eating if the person is failing to respond to internal cues relating to appetite and hunger control. For example, some people might over eat as a means of coping with the stresses of daily living. The nurse identifies if the person's eating and drinking behaviors are influenced by emotions, social pressures, habits, or the good taste and palatability of food rather than the internal cues that control appetite. Cues from the external environment, such as a pleasant environment and freedom from pain and stress, also influence ingestion.

Weight Consciousness. Finally, the nurse identifies the person's desire to gain, lose, or maintain body weight. This weight consciousness influences the person's present and future eating patterns.

Nursing Diagnosis

As has been described previously in this text, the assessment information related to behaviors and stimuli are interpreted in the form of a nursing diagnosis. The three alternatives suggested by Roy for structuring a nursing diagnosis include: (1) a statement of behaviors within one mode with their most relevant influencing stimuli, (2) a summary label for behaviors in one mode with relevant stimuli, or (3) a label that summarizes a behavioral pattern when more than one mode is being affected by the same stimuli. It is possible to derive nursing diagnoses that reflect positive adaptation related to nutrition. A nursing diagnosis illustrating adaptive nutrition could be, "evidence of adequate nutritional pattern related to a balanced diet for body requirements containing appropriate foods from all four food groups."

In situations where problems exist relative to the need for adequate nutrition, it is important that the nursing diagnosis convey the essence of the problem such that direction is provided for the subsequent steps of the nursing process. This is facilitated by the use of the first method for stating nursing diagnoses. For example, the nurse may determine that, in relation to the individual's height, the person is overweight and that this appears to be related to an excessive intake of high caloric foods. The nursing diagnosis in such a situation may be "weight 40 percent above average related to diet exceeding body requirements and high in fat content."

The North American Nursing Diagnosis Association (Gordon 1987) identified two nursing diagnoses pertaining to altered nutrition, one identifying alterations (actual or potential) resulting in more nutrients than required by the body, and the second, less than body requirements. Such diagnoses would constitute summary label diagnoses for behaviors in the one mode, the physiological. Using the second method of structuring a nursing diagnosis, the statement might read, "Altered nutrition: more than body requirements due to excessive intake of food during stressful situations."

Labels that summarize a behavioral pattern when more than one mode is being affected by the same stimuli are often very meaningful to experienced nurses. They convey much information in a single term. An example of such a label would be the term *anorexia*, that is, the loss or lack of appetite for food. Stimuli contributing to anorexia are often very complex and are associated with modes in addition to the physiological mode. For example, the self concept and interdependence modes may be involved. The person may feel attractive only when their weight is less than one hundred pounds. Significant others may reinforce this belief by commenting adversely whenever additional weight becomes evident. A nursing diagnosis illustrating this third method of structuring could be, "Anorexia related to peer pressure and low-self-esteem."

Considering further nursing diagnoses related to altered nutrition, "more or potentially more than body requirements," defines the state in which a person experiences or is at risk of experiencing an intake of nutrients which exceeds metabolic needs. This is one of the most common adaptation problems related to nutritional need in contemporary North America. Excessive accumulation of fat in the body increases the weight beyond the recommended measures with regard to bone structure, height, and age. The male is termed as having an intake exceeding metabolic needs when his weight exceeds 20 percent of the average weight found in standard height/weight tables. For the female, excess weight is 25 percent above the listed standard.

The behaviors and stimuli related to these diagnoses are individual and may include such assessment factors as sedentary activity level or responding inappropriately to internal and external cues for eating. It is important to consider metabolic and endocrine factors that may be contributing to the problem. If these physiologically based factors do not exist, other stimuli should be explored.

A diagnosis of "altered nutrition, less than body requirements" is defined as the state in which a person experiences an intake of nutrients insufficient to meet metabolic needs. Stimuli related to this diagnosis may include the person's inability to ingest or digest food or absorb nutrients because of psychological, biological, or economic factors. The person is termed as having an intake of nutrients insufficient to meet metabolic needs when the body weight is 20 percent or more under the ideal weight for bone structure, height, and age. The behaviors and stimuli related to this diagnosis are varied and may include such assessment factors as lack of interest in food, decreased availability of food, or sore, inflamed condition of the oral cavity.

Nausea and vomiting are other common adaptation problems related to nutritional needs. These problems frequently are associated but may be experienced separately. *Nausea* is an unpleasant sensation reported as a feeling of sickness with the urge to vomit. *Vomiting* is the forceful ejection of stomach contents through the mouth. The vomiting reflex can be stimulated by a number of intrinsic and extrinsic factors, for example, unpleasant odors, tastes, sights; sensations such as severe pain; chemical agents used in the treatment of disease; and radiation therapy. Identification of the stimuli contributing to the problem are important factors in its solution.

Once the nursing diagnosis related to nutrition has been established, the nurse proceeds to formulate goals that address each of the identified problems or support areas in which adaptation has been observed.

Goal Setting

In the fourth step of the nursing process as described in the Roy Adaptation Model, the nurse, in collaboration with the person receiving care, establishes goals, that is, statements of clear behavioral outcomes of nursing care for the person. The goal should address the behavior, the change expected, and the time frame in which the goal is to be achieved. Goals may be long term or short term and these time frames are relative to the situation involved.

When setting a goal for the person experiencing an intake of nutrients exceeding metabolic needs, it is realistic and healthy to establish a goal providing for gradual weight loss of 1 to 2 pounds per week while eating a well-balanced diet. An appropriately worded goal for this could be, "The patient will lose 2 pounds each week for the next 4 weeks." In this objective, the person's weight is the behavior of focus, the change expected is the loss of 2 pounds each week and the time frame is 4 weeks.

An appropriate goal for the person experiencing altered nutrition with less than body requirements may be for the individual to ingest a well-balanced, high-caloric diet so as to initially stabilize the weight and then increase the weight gradually. A short-term goal may relate to the daily intake: "Today the person will ingest multiple small feedings high in caloric content and rich in nutrients." A longer term goal could relate to the person's status in one month: "By this date next month, the person will have gained 5 pounds and documented a balanced intake containing all recommended nutrients."

For the person experiencing the adaptation problems of nausea and vomiting, the goal should directly reflect a decrease in the stated assessed behavior or an increased ability to cope with it. As has been identified before, goals pertain directly to the person's behavior are stated in behavioral terms from the patient's perspective.

The focus for the next step of the nursing process, intervention, is change of the stimuli identified as contributing to the observed behaviors.

Intervention

Once the goals have been established relative to behaviors that will promote adaptation, the nurse determines the interventions that will assist the person in attaining the stated goals. Nursing interventions for the promotion of nutritional needs depend on the stimuli identified. The nurse manages the stimuli by either promoting or reinforcing them or by taking action to change or eliminate the stimuli. For example, if the stimulus related to over eating in response to internal cues of feeling stressed has been identified, the nurse may assist the person in establishing coping strategies to adapt to the stresses of daily living. Additionally, if a decreased exercise pattern is identified as a stimulus, the nurse may assist the individual with measures to increase activity level.

If a person decides that he or she is overweight and wants to do something about it, it is important to establish the motivation for the desired weight losing regimen. Some reasons for wanting to lose weight may include an improved health status in order to avoid many of the chronic disorders linked to obesity. Other motivations may be a desire for improvement in personal appearance and avoidance of pressures from family and friends to lose weight.

An intervention that has been used successfully for changing a person's response pattern of eating because of external cues is behavior modification (Stuart and Davis 1972). It is often helpful for the person to write down specific feelings before eating in order to identify if the eating is in response to emotions such as anxiety, boredom, or loneliness. The person then is instructed to try to substitute other activities in place of eating at these times. Other techniques within this approach include slowing down and making the act of eating a conscious acknowledged action. A meal should last at least 20 minutes so that the hypothalamus can send out satiation signals. In the process of slowing down, doing only one activity at a time may be helpful, that is, preparing each bite of food separately, putting the utensils down between bites, taking a sip of beverage between bites, and using the napkin frequently while concentrating on slowing down all actions.

General interventions for nausea and vomiting should focus, where possible, on the stimuli causing the problem. For example, unpleasant, strong odors in the environment should be eliminated; or the person's environment should be kept quiet and sudden movements prevented. If pain is causing the problem, it may be that something can be done to alleviate it. Other conservative treatments for nausea and vomiting include limiting the person's food and fluid intake until the problem subsides. If fluids are tolerated, offering carbonated beverages may be comforting. Ice chips may be tolerated and oral hygiene is refreshing for the patient. Positioning the patient with head raised and turned to the side may assist and will be necessary if vomiting is occurring. If none of these interventions is successful, it may be necessary to administer an antiemetic medication as ordered by the physician. When the problem subsides and the diet is resumed, offering foods that are bland, such as dry toast or soda crackers, is often appropriate. If nausea and vomiting persist, the use of intravenous fluids to prevent fluid and electrolyte imbalance may be warranted.

The nurse's intervention in relation to nutritional planning may be to provide for referral to a health professional involved exclusively in dietetics and nutrition.

Evaluation

Evaluation involves judging the effectiveness of nursing interventions in relation to the person's behavior and in terms of the preset goals. The nursing interventions would be identified as effective if the person's behavior is in accordance with the stated goal. For example, in the previous illustration, the goal was, "The patient will lose 2 pounds each week for the next 4 weeks." Achievement of this goal could be measured by weekly assessment of weight. The goal would be achieved if the person loses 2 pounds each week for 4 weeks. If the goal has not been achieved, the nurse identifies alternative interventions or approaches by reassessing the behavior and stimuli and continuing with the other steps of the nursing process.

SUMMARY

This chapter has provided basic guidelines for the nurse to use in helping a person maintain physiological integrity by meeting nutritional needs. The steps of the Roy Adaptation Model nursing process were applied to the component of nutrition. Behaviors associated with nutrition were identified and described and stimuli that influence behaviors were presented. Nursing diagnoses and adaptation problems related to nutrition were discussed as were the steps of goal setting, intervention, and evaluation.

EXERCISES FOR APPLICATION

1. Assess your own eating patterns by recording a diet history for a 24-hour period. Determine if the quantity and quality of the nutrients ingested are adaptive or ineffective.
2. Identify a person with good eating habits and preferences based on cultural experience that is different from your own. Determine the cultural, social, and religious patterns that influence that person's ingestion of food and fluids.

ASSESSMENT OF UNDERSTANDING

Questions

1. List the six major processes associated with the digestion of food.
   a. _____
   b. _____
   c. _____
   d. _____
   e. _____
   f. _____
2. Label the following behaviors related to nutrition as adaptive (A) or ineffective (I).
   a. _____ body weight less than 20 percent of norm for height, gender, bone structure
   b. _____ lack of appetite for food
   c. _____ "I normally eat three meals a day."
   d. _____ average daily consumption of water: 2 cups
   e. _____ "My three-year-old won't touch anything but hot dogs."

3. Identify four stimuli that commonly influence adaptation relative to nutrition.

   a. _____

   b. _____

   c. _____

   d. _____

Situation:

Nancy James is a forty-year-old career person who works as an executive for a publishing company. She commutes 2 hours each day, leaving early and arriving home late. She rarely has time for breakfast and does not bother preparing supper for herself. She frequently has business luncheons and thus does not feel hungry until later in the evening. Whenever she does feel hungry, she snacks on pop, chocolate bars, and chips since the dispensing machine is located close to her office. Nancy is wanting to lose some weight. She is 5 feet 2 inches tall and weighs 160 pounds. "I can't understand why I keep putting on weight; I usually eat only one meal a day!"

4. Formulate a nursing diagnosis for the described situation.

   _____

5. State a goal to address weight loss in the described situation. Identify the behavior, the change expected, and the associated time frame.

   Goal: _____

   Behavior: _____

   Change expected: _____

   Time frame: _____

6. List two interventions that might assist Nancy in the achievement of the goal stated. What stimuli are being managed?

Interventions	Stimuli
a. _____	_____
b. _____	_____

7. What behavior would provide evidence that the identified goal had been achieved?

   _____

Feedback

1. a. ingestion
   b. propulsion
   c. mechanical digestion
   d. chemical digestion

    e. absorption
    f. defecation
2. a. I, b. I, c. A, d. I, e. I
3. a. condition of the oral cavity
    b. culture
    d. cognator effectiveness
    d. integrity of the physiological mode
4. Nursing Diagnosis: "Body weight greater than 20 percent above average due to diet in excess of body requirements."
5. Goal: "Within 4 weeks, Nancy will have lost 10 pounds."
   Behavior: weight
   Change expected: loss of 10 pounds
   Time frame: within 4 weeks

6. **Interventions**	**Stimuli**
a. Documentation of intake	cognator effectiveness: Nancy's perception of how much she eats is erroneous.
b. Adherence to 1000 calorie diet	Caloric requirements: Nancy's required intake for weight loss will relate to her needs.

7. Within 4 weeks, Nancy will have lost 10 pounds.

REFERENCES

Gordon, M. *Nursing Diagnosis: Process and Application*. New York: McGraw-Hill, 1987.

Health and Welfare Canada. *Canada's Food Guide Handbook* (Revised). Ottawa, Canada: Minister of National Health and Welfare, 1983.

Hostetler, J.A., and G.E. Huntington. *The Hutterites in North America*. New York: Holt, Rinehart and Winston, 1980.

Marieb, E.N. *Human Anatomy and Physiology*. Redwood City, Calif.: Benjamin/ Cummings, 1989.

National Academy of Sciences, *Recommended Dietary Allowances*. Washington, D.C.: National Academy Press, in *Understanding Nutrition* (5th ed.), Whitney, E.N., E.M.N. Hamilton, and S.R. Rolfes. St. Paul: West, 1990.

Phipps, W., B. Long, and N. Woods. *Medical-Surgical Nursing: Concepts and Clinical Practice* (3rd. ed.). St. Louis: The C. V. Mosby Company, 1987.

Stuart, R., and B. Davis. *Slim Chance in a Fat World: Behavioral Control of Obesity*. Champaign, Ill.: Research Press, 1972.

Williams, S.R. *Essentials of Nutrition and Diet Therapy* (4th ed.). St. Louis: Times Mirror/Mosby College, 1986.

Additional References

Atkinson, R.L. A comprehensive approach to outpatient obesity management, *Journal of the American Dietetic Association,* 84(4): 439–443, 1984.

Fuller, J., and J. Schaller-Ayers. *Health Assessment: A Nursing Approach.* Philadelphia: J. B. Lippincott, 1990.

Pipes, P.L. *Nutrition in Infancy and Childhood* (3rd. ed.). St. Louis: The C. V. Mosby Company, 1985.

Schneider, E.L. Recommended dietary allowances and health of the elderly, *New England Journal of Medicine,* 314: 157–160, 1986

Whitney, E.N., E.M.N. Hamilton, and S.R. Rolfes. *Understanding Nutrition* (5th. ed.). St. Paul: West, 1990.

Chapter Six

Elimination

Jane Servonsky

Elimination is a basic life process essential to adaptation. Just as by the processes of digestion, absorption, and metabolism, nutrients are provided for survival and to maintain physiological balance, so does the person need to eliminate metabolic waste products. These waste materials are expelled to maintain homeostasis. Wastes are excreted from the intestines, by the kidneys, and by the skin and lungs. Excretion of the lungs, through gas exchange with the environment, was dealt with in Chapter 4, and excretion by the skin through perspiration is included in Chapter 8. This chapter describes the structures and functions that comprise the process of elimination from the intestines and kidneys. The nursing process then is applied to the elimination component of the physiological adaptive mode. Essential knowledge is used as a guideline for describing assessment of behaviors and stimuli, nursing diagnosis related to elimination, goal setting, intervention, and evaluation.

OBJECTIVES

After studying this chapter, the reader will be able to do the following:

1. Outline the basic structures and functions that make up the processes of elimination.
2. Assess behaviors related to elimination of the intestines and the kidneys.
3. Identify common stimuli that affect elimination.
4. Define common adaptation problems of the elimination component.
5. State a goal for nursing care related to elimination.

6. Derive common nursing interventions for problems of elimination.

7. Propose plans to evaluate the effectiveness of nursing interventions and appropriate methods for revising the plan for nursing care.

KEY CONCEPTS DEFINED

- *Anal incontinence:* inability to control fecal excretory function.
- *Constipation:* a condition in which the fecal matter in the bowel is too hard to pass with ease, or a state in which the bowel movements are so infrequent that uncomfortable symptoms occur.
- *Diarrhea:* rapid movement of the fecal material through the intestines, resulting in poor absorption of water, essential nutrients, and electrolytes, and in an abnormally frequent passage of watery stool.
- *Flatus:* gas or air in the gastrointestinal tract which may result in pain or feelings of abdominal fullness.
- *Peristalsis:* movements of the intestinal tract that both mix and propel the mixture of food and enzymes that comes from the digestive process of the stomach.
- *Urinary incontinence:* inability to control the release of urine from the bladder.
- *Urinary retention:* the inability to void, with the resultant accumulation of urine within the bladder.

STRUCTURES AND FUNCTIONS RELATED TO ELIMINATION

Maintenance of adequate elimination requires a functioning gastrointestinal tract and urinary system. As noted in the previous chapter, it is the primary function the gastrointestinal, or alimentary tract, as a whole to provide water, electrolytes, and nutrients to sustain life. Basic structures of the upper **gastrointestinal tract** consist of the mouth, esophagus, stomach, and duodenum. The lower gastrointestinal tract is made up of the small intestines, jejunum and ileum, and the large intestine, which includes the ascending, transverse, descending, and sigmoid colon, rectum and the anus. This tract carries out three processes: (1) the movement of food through the tract, (2) secretion of digestive juices, and (3) absorption of the digested nutrients, as well as water and electrolytes. The upper gastrointestinal tract deals with ingestion and digestion of food. The small intestine involves both digestion and absorption of nutrients. The function of the large intestine is primarily the absorption of water and electrolytes, and the elimination of the waste products of digestion through the anus.

Movements of both the small and large intestine are key to the process of elimination. Such movements are divided into two types, mixing and propulsive movements. In the small intestine, rapid segmental contractions chop the solid food particles to promote mixing them with digestive secretions. The peristaltic waves are weak and die out quickly, thus chyme (mixture of food with stomach secretions as it passes on down the tract) moves slowly, taking 3 to 5 hours to pass from the stomach to the large intestine.

The proximal half of the colon is concerned primarily with absorption, and the distal half with storage. Less intense mixing movements are required for these functions. Thus in the colon, the fecal material is gradually turned over and exposed to the surface of the large intestine where fluid is progressively absorbed. In this way, about 1500 ml of chyme enters the large intestines each day, but only 80 to 150 ml are excreted as feces. The propulsive movements of small and large intestine also differ. In the latter case, instead of peristaltic waves, mass movements primarily occur in the large intestine. The movements include a constrictive ring occurring at a distended or irritated point, followed rapidly by a long segment, for example 20 cm or more, of colon contracting almost as a unit. This action forces the fecal material as a mass down the colon. These movements usually occur only a few times a day, most frequently for about 15 minutes during the first hour or so after eating breakfast. On the other hand, the peristaltic waves of the small intestine occur throughout the day, but are greatly increased after a meal.

Defecation is the action whereby feces is emptied from the rectum. A weak sphincter approximately 20 cm from the anus, at the juncture between the sigmoid colon and the rectum, keeps the rectum empty of feces most of the time. Normally, when a mass movement forces feces into the rectum, the process of defecation is initiated. This process includes the defecation reflex and conscious sphincter control. Control of fecal evacuation involves tonic constriction of two sphincters. The internal sphincter is a circular mass of smooth muscle that constricts immediately inside the anus. The external anal sphincter is composed of striated voluntary muscle and surrounds the internal sphincter, slightly distal to it.

The defecation reflex initiates the process that ordinarily results in defecation. Sensory nerve fibers in the rectum are stimulated by stretch and carry their signals to the spinal cord, then reflexly, back to the lower gastrointestinal tract by way of the parasympathetic system. These signals set up strong peristaltic waves that can effectively empty the entire large bowel. Other effects that are part of the reflex response are taking a deep breath, closing the glottis, and contracting the abdominal muscles and the pelvic floor muscles. In infants and persons without conscious control, this process proceeds naturally to defecation. However, in other persons, despite the defecation reflex, voluntary efforts are used in expel-ling feces. Through a conscious cognitive process, the person voluntarily controls the external sphincter. The person may inhibit its contraction and thereby allow defecation to occur, or may contract the sphincter if the time is not socially acceptable for defecation to occur. If the sphincter is kept contracted, the defecation reflex can die out after a few minutes. Usually it does not return until an additional amount of feces enters the rectum, possibly in several hours.

In addition to several other reflex systems, the gastrointestinal tract has an intrinsic nervous system of its own called the enteric nervous system (Guyton 1987). It begins at the esophagus and extends all the way to the anus. This system particularly controls gastrointestinal movements and secretions. However, the degree of activity of the enteric nervous system can be altered strongly by both parasympathetic and sympathetic nervous system signals from the brain. (See Chapter 11.) The influence of both branches of the autonomic nervous system, parasympathetic and sympathetic, are particularly active at the upper end of the gastrointestinal system, down to the stomach, and at the distal end, from the midcolon region to the anus. The neurons of the parasympathetic system generally enhance activity of most gastrointestinal functions; whereas, stimulation of the sympathetic branch inhibits activity of the tract. Strong stimulation of this branch can block totally movement of food. Understanding these connections, and the relationship of these processes within the thinking and feeling person, can be useful in assessing problems of elimination and in planning nursing care.

The structures of **urinary elimination** include the kidneys, ureters, bladder, and urethra. One function of this system, to balance body fluids and electrolytes, is discussed in Chapter 10. The second function of these structures is the excretion of most of the end-products of bodily metabolism. The intact operating of both of these functions contributes to internal homeostasis and to the regulation of body processes.

The functional nephron is the basis for understanding renal function. The two kidneys together contain more than two million nephrons, each of which is capable of forming urine by itself. The nephron cleans, or clears, the blood plasma of unwanted substances as it passes through the kidney. The nephron's filtering process is the clearing process that prevents waste substances from being reabsorbed. These unwanted substances are end-products of metabolism such as urea, creatinine, uric acid, and urates. Wanted substances such as water and electrolytes are reabsorbed into the plasma. In addition, the nephron clears the plasma of excesses of other substances, such as sodium ions, potassium ions, chloride ions, and hydrogen ions, that tend to accumulate in the body. The unwanted portions of the fluid from the nephron filtration process are passed into the urine. This system has two special feedback mechanisms that act together with the arterial blood pressure to bring about the necessary degree of filtration autoregulation. These principles of urine formation and the mechanisms of metabolism in the kidney are discussed further in basic physiology texts.

As urine collects in the kidneys, pressure increases and initiates a peristaltic contraction of the ureter. The *ureters* are small smooth muscle tubes that pass downward from the kidneys to the bladder. The ureters have both sympathetic and parasympathetic nerves, as well as other nerve fibers along their entire lengths. The urinary bladder is composed of smooth muscle and has two principal parts: the body, where the urine collects, and the neck, a funnel-shaped extension of the body. The muscle of the bladder neck is referred to as the internal sphincter. It acts to keep the bladder neck empty of urine. Beyond the bladder neck, the urethra passes through a layer of muscle called the external sphincter of the bladder. This is a voluntary skeletal muscle. As with the gastrointestinal track, this voluntary sphincter is under the control of the central nervous system and can be used consciously to prevent urination.

Micturition is the process by which the urinary bladder is emptied. A micturition reflex is a cycle involving three stages: (1) progressive and rapid increase in pressure in the bladder, (2) a period of sustained pressure, and (3) return of the pressure to a base-line level. After such a reflex cycle that has not ended in emptying the bladder, the nervous system structures remain inhibited for at least a few minutes to as long as an hour before another micturition reflex occurs. With an increasingly distended bladder, the micturition reflexes occur more frequently and powerfully. Eventually they will force the bladder neck to open, leading to further reflexes. The micturition reflex is a completely automatic spinal cord reflex. It is the basic initiator of urination, but the higher brain centers normally exert final control. According to Guyton (1987) these include strong facilitatory and inhibitory centers in the brain stem, probably located in the pons and several centers located in the cerebral cortex that are mainly inhibitory but can at times become excitatory. The higher centers keep the micturition reflex inhibited when micturition is not desired, facilitate it when desired, and can inhibit the closure of the external urinary sphincter so that urination can occur.

APPLICATION OF THE NURSING PROCESS

The formation of a positive nurse-client relationship is essential in order to collect data about a person's elimination patterns. Since the topic of bodily secretions is considered personal by many, the nurse is aware of the privacy needs of the person, and her own reaction when inquiring about another's elimination pattern. In addressing elimination, the nurse establishes privacy and an intrusion-free environment. The nurse's interaction with the patient considers the person's language level and communication skills as influenced by his or her cultural and educational background.

Assessment of Behavior

When assessing intestinal elimination, the nurse observes the following behaviors. **Stool** is described by stating the amount, color, consistency, frequency, odor, and effort. Normally, the stool that is evacuated is soft, formed, and brown in color for adults. The frequency of a bowel movement varies with each individual, although one bowel movement a day is average. In healthy persons, variations may range from a stool evacuated twice a day to a stool evacuated every 2 to 3 days. When making a judgment as to whether the frequency is adaptive or ineffective, the nurse assesses if the observed behavior represents a change from the person's normal pattern. Stool is to be passed with ease without straining or discomfort when the defecation reflex is first felt.

Stool containing any unusual matter such as the presence of blood, mucus, pus, or intestinal worms is also noted. A careful, exact description of the stool is essential when blood is present. Observe whether the blood appears on the surface of the stool, or if it is mixed throughout. If the client is menstruating, this may be the source of bright-red blood on the surface of stool. Normal stool has a characteristic odor caused by bacterial action on the foods that are eaten. Any unusual odor should be noted, for it may have clinical significance.

Bowel sounds indicate the movements within the small and large bowel. In assessing these, the nurse notes the presence, frequency, or absence of bowel sounds. The abdomen is auscultated in all four quadrants proceeding in a clockwise fashion. Using the diaphragm part of the stethoscope, listen in each quadrant, changing the auscultatory site 2 or 3 inches with each move. It is important to remove the stethoscope completely from the abdomen when changing locations, for pulling the stethoscope across the abdomen will produce interfering sound, may cause involuntary muscle spasms, and may be uncomfortable for the person.

Normal bowel sounds will be high-pitched, gurgling noises usually occurring five or more times a minute. Ineffective bowel sounds include extremely weak or infrequent sounds, or a complete absence of sounds, which may indicate bowel hypomobility or immobility. Before a determination of bowel sounds can be made, the abdomen is auscultated for at least 3 minutes. Bowel sounds indicating possible hypermotility of the bowel will be heard as frequent rushes of loud, high-pitched sounds. Passage of gas is a good indication that peristaltic movement is occurring.

Pain related to bowel elimination is included as assessment of behavior by listing the person's statements regarding discomfort and pain on evacuation of the bowel or the excessive accumulation of flatus or gas in the intestines. All verbal and nonverbal behaviors and the location, severity, duration, and onset of the pain are noted. In completing the behavioral assessment of the bowel elimination component of the physiological adaptive mode, **laboratory results** related to stool are checked, if available. Specimens of the feces may be tested for occult blood when intestinal bleeding is suspected, but gross blood is not visible on inspection. (Laboratory values and procedures for assisting with these tests are available from resource texts such as Cella and Watson 1989.)

When assessing urinary elimination the nurse observes the following behaviors. The amount of **urine** per voiding and the total for 24 hours is stated. The color and transparency, odor, frequency, urgency felt, and effort are noted as well.

Normally, the amount of urine voided by the average adult will vary from 1000 to 2000 cc in a 24-hour period. Urine is normally pale yellow or amber in color, because of the presence of the yellow pigment urochrome. In healthy individuals, urine that is pale and almost colorless is probably very dilute with a low specific gravity, while urine that is darker in color may have a higher specific gravity. Freshly voided urine has a clear transparency, and cloudy urine or urine containing a sediment may represent a disease state. This change in transparency could be caused by a reactional change of the urine if left standing for a period of time, as the pH changes from acidic to alkaline. The odor of fresh-voided urine is aromatic. When left standing, urine may develop an ammonia smell caused by decomposition of urea by bacteria.

The frequency of urination, urgency felt, and effort in starting and stopping the flow of urine may depend on many factors. In general, the musculature of the bladder is capable of distending to the approximate capacity of 300 cc before the urge to void is felt. This begins the process of the micturition reflex described earlier. The stretch receptors in the bladder being stimulated, together with involuntary and voluntary control of the sphincters located at the opening of the bladder into the urethra, permit the flow of urine.

The nurse assesses any **pain** related to urinary elimination. This includes pain or burning sensations prior to, during, or after urination. Normally, the person will void with ease, without pain or discomfort. Finally, **laboratory data** is useful, especially in comparing the findings in a routine urinalysis and findings of other specific tests with normal values.

Assessment of Stimuli

With the assessment of stimuli, the nurse gathers data about factors influencing the behaviors identified in the assessment phases of the adaptation nursing process. This includes the important factor of the body's adaptive ability to maintain the structure, function, and regulation of the eliminative component, as well as the coping strategies the person uses to maintain or change behaviors.

Homeostasis comprises the steady physiological states which enable persons to counteract changes both in external conditions and in internal bodily functions. The **intact homeostatic process** in the bowel is primarily responsible for adaptive stool behaviors. As noted earlier, the digestion of food is completed in the small intestine as it absorbs nutrients from the ingested substances. Peristaltic waves push the substance through the ileocecal valve into the large intestine, which absorbs a high percentage of the liquid from the wastes as well as salts. Intestinal contents are then propelled toward the rectum for evacuation.

A major stimulus disrupting intestinal elimination is the presence of a **disease state** which affects the normal structure, function, and regulation of the gastrointestinal system. Examples would include such conditions as ulcerative colitis and intestinal obstruction, which are explained in general textbooks on pathology.

The type and amount of **diet** are focal to bowel elimination. The nurse notes the person's present daily nutritional intake and evaluates whether or not these foods: (1) provide roughage and bulk, such as high-residue foods of fresh fruits and vegetables; (2) contain natural laxative effects that promote normal stool consistency, such as prunes and brans; (3) influence the production of excessive intestinal gas, such as cabbage and beans; and (4) influence the color or consistency of stool. For example, the high-milk intake of an infant may cause light-colored stool, and intolerance to certain foods may promote diarrhea.

Assessment of stimuli influencing bowel elimination includes **fluid intake**, including noting the amount of fluid the person is taking, both orally and intravenously. Decreased fluid intake may promote stool that is dry and hard.

The **immediate environment** contributes to adaptation in this mode component as it does in others. This would include whether or not the person has maintenance or lack of privacy for evacuation. The nurse assesses the availability of the toilet to the person, or if the use of a bedpan is required. The person immobilized in traction who uses a bedpan while in the reclining position may have difficulty adapting usual bowel evacuation to this changed environment. The temperature and comfort of the room is assessed since this also may influence the situation.

Other factors in the immediate situation that influence bowel elimination are medications, treatments or tests, and pain. The nurse notes specific **medications** that the person may be taking that influence stools. For example, iron may cause dark, hard stools; codeine may cause behavior indicative of constipation; and sensitivities to certain other drugs may cause behaviors of diarrhea. Any **treatments** or **tests** influencing bowel elimination behaviors, such as barium enemas, gastrointestinal x-ray series, or soapsuds enemas are identified, as well. Of specific significance is any altered means of elimination, such as an ileostomy or a colostomy.

Furthermore, the nurse validates with the person the cause of any **pain** related to bowel elimination. Possible causes would include the presence of disruptive processes, such as hemorrhoids, anal fissure, or abdominal cramping caused by excessive intestinal gas. The coping strategies the person uses for this pain are assessed. For example, with hemorrhoids, the person may use sitz baths, ointments, or special skin care for the irritated skin around the anus.

The nurse also assesses the **normal pattern of bowel habits** as influencing the current behavior observed. She notes factors that maintain or increase peristalsis, such as the person's daily activity level or pattern of exercise. Factors that decrease peristalsis include bed rest, immobility, or recent anesthesia. The coping strategies the person uses to maintain his or her pattern of elimination are identified. These could include drinking a hot liquid or fruit juice or the use of laxatives, mineral oil, enemas, or suppositories. The nurse assesses if the person has a routine schedule or time set aside each day for evacuation. Whether the person thinks the strategies used are effective or ineffective is important to note.

Because of the connectedness of bowel motility and the defecation reflex with the autonomic nervous system, **stress** may be an important factor influencing on-going habits and current behaviors noted by the nurse. Awareness of signs of physical and psychological stress, such as illness or anxiety is part of nursing assessment as these factors influence stool behaviors.

Family or **cultural beliefs** concerning elimination often begin early in childhood and may involve specific views about the need and schedule to eliminate wastes from the bowel. The expected schedule of elimination may be related to beliefs about health. These background factors are relevant information regarding assessment of bowel elimination. Similarly, **age** is a contextual stimulus that the person brings to the situation. The age of the person is noted, since this will influence intestinal elimination. For example, the older person may show a decline in the motility of the gastrointestinal tract which occurs with advancing years, or the young child may have difficulties with toilet training.

The adaptive response of the urinary system, as noted earlier, plays a major role in homeostasis or physiologically steady states by the removal of waste products from the bloodstream, and regulation of fluid and electrolyte balance, acid-base balance, and osmotic pressures within the body. Nursing assessment of factors influencing urinary elimination begins with an understanding of the **intact homeostatic processes** that result in the production and elimination of urine. (These processes are described earlier in this chapter and in other basic physiology and nursing science texts.) As these processes operate, bladder elimination is influenced by many of the same categories of stimuli that influence intestinal elimination. Specifically, the following are factors to be considered in the assessment of stimuli for urinary elimination.

The nurse identifies if a **disease process** or condition, a surgical procedure, or trauma has taken place which affects the normal structure, function, or regulation of the urinary system. Examples include urinary tract infections; disturbances of the central nervous system pathways, causing loss of voluntary control; tissue damage to the sphincters; relaxation of the perineal structures from childbirth; pressure on the bladder during pregnancy; poorly regulated diabetes mellitus; and chronic renal failure.

Of particular significance as a stimulus for urinary output is the amount of **fluid intake**. The nurse notes the amount of fluids taken in both orally and intravenously for the previous 24 hours and presently. This influences the amount of urine excreted. Insensible loss of water through the skin and lungs are considered in relation to urinary output. Basically, when evaluating intake and output per 24 hours, these values will be approximately equal, allowing for some margin of difference. In instances that are critical to the person's maintenance of health, a basic measurement of fluid loss or gain in daily weights is taken at the same time each day. Related to fluid balance, the person is assessed for conditions that may affect the **fluid and electrolyte balance** of the body, for example, losses of fluids via other routes, such as liquid stools, nasogastric tube drainage, emesis, or insensible loss occurring with high body temperature. Fluid and electrolytes are discussed further in Chapter 10.

In assessing the **immediate environmental** stimuli, the nurse observes for factors that may influence the person's ability to void, such as the maintenance or lack of privacy to void; temperature and comfort of the room; availability of the toilet, bedpan, or urinal; and the position the person is required to be in to void. For example, the male who is unable to stand to void may have difficulty adapting his usual pattern within this environmental change. Another immediate influence to consider is **medications** the person may be taking that can influence the color or amount of urine. For example, certain vitamins and Pyridium may cause dark orange urine, and diuretics increase the amount of urine excreted.

When the person has **pain** or discomfort with urination, the nurse assesses both the factors influencing the pain and the coping strategies the person uses to deal with the pain. For example, one stimulus influencing pain could be mucosal irritation caused by recent removal of a urinary catheter or by a cystoscopy examination. The presence of a urinary tract infection may also be the source of pain. The nurse also considers the person's **ability to cope** with ineffective behaviors such as burning or pain with urination. How these behaviors have affected the voiding pattern and how they are coped with are assessed. For example, the person may use sitz baths, or avoid voiding. For behaviors indicating retention, incontinence, difficulty starting or stopping the stream of urine, or dribbling, the effect of these alterations on the person's activities of daily living and social relations is assessed. Predisposing factors that make the urinary behaviors better or worse are noted. For example, urinary incontinence may be precipitated by laughing, coughing, stress, activity, and so forth. The nurse assesses what coping strategies are being used presently and if the person feels they are effective or ineffective.

A key assessment factor is the person's **usual daily urinary elimination pattern**. The usual pattern is noted and its effect on and comparison with the behaviors observed are assessed. A change in the present pattern from the person's normal patterns is particularly important. **Stress** may be present as a focal or contextual stimulus in the daily pattern or for a currently observed behavior. The nurse thus assesses for physical or psychological states that may stimulate or hinder urination. For example, frequently with anxiety or stressful situations, the person may notice a feeling or urgency to void, although he or she has just emptied the bladder. Or the person who has experienced a painful urination may develop muscular tension resulting in an inability to relax the perineal muscles that promote urination for fear of a repeat of the painful situation. Finally, in assessing usual patterns, the nurse is aware of any **altered means of elimination** that the person uses, such as a urinary catheter or ureterostomy.

As with bowel elimination, there may be **family and cultural beliefs** concerning the need, schedule, and particular circumstances for emptying the bladder. The nurse identifies these beliefs as contextual stimuli.

Similarly, the **age** of the person is an important contextual stimulus affecting urinary elimination. For example, the young child may lack sphincter control or not be toilet trained yet. With the natural aging process, there are generalized circulatory changes, and blood flow to the kidneys may be diminished due to a decrease in cardiac output. Therefore, renal function may decrease. With aging, the pelvic floor muscles become weakened and the supporting connective tissue alters, causing the bladder to become funnel shaped. This change may result in bladder wall irritability. There may also be decreased bladder capacity due to its inability to elongate. Therefore, the aging person may present behaviors of frequency, incontinence, retention, and dysuria (Phipps, Long, and Wood 1987). Another example would be an elderly male who has frequency of voiding accompanied by problems in initiating and ending the stream of urine. This may be due to prostatic enlargement with resultant urinary retention. Also, consider the elderly female with relaxation of the perineal muscles, who may present with behaviors of stress incontinence.

Nursing Diagnosis

Assessment factors of behaviors and related stimuli are interpreted and used in establishing a nursing diagnosis. The nurse prepared to use the Roy Adaptation Model of nursing can state diagnoses as specific behaviors with the stimuli that are most relevant. Some examples have already been given, for example, involuntary release of urine related to relaxed muscles in an elderly person.

A second way of stating nursing diagnoses according to the model is to identify a summary label that connotes the nature of the general adaptation problems. Such an approach can use the specific diagnoses accepted by the North American Nursing Diagnosis Association (Gordon 1987). The categories related to bowel and bladder elimination include the following.

Bowel elimination, altered: *constipation*. One of the most common adaptation problems of elimination is that of constipation. Simple constipation may present with the behaviors of excessive hardness of stool, without regard to the frequency of bowel movements, or an infrequent passage of dry, hard stools with accompanying excessive straining. The stimuli related to this diagnosis are individual for each person. Examples of stimuli that may affect stool behaviors which define the problem of constipation include decreased fluid intake or lack of high-residue foods in the diet.

Bowel elimination, altered: *diarrhea*. This nursing diagnosis may be defined as a state in which the person experiences a change in normal bowel habits characterized by the frequent passage of loose, fluid, unformed stools. When the person presents with behaviors of diarrhea, abdominal cramping and tenesmus (ineffectual and painful straining) may also occur. Frequently, diagnostic procedures or laboratory tests may be necessary to determine the exact cause and other related influencing factors for this problem.

Bowel elimination, altered: *incontinence*. This nursing diagnosis would apply when the person experiences a change in normal habits characterized by involuntary passage of stool.

Urinary retention. The inability to void, with resultant accumulation of urine within the bladder, is termed *urinary retention*. Possible causes include obstruction at or below the bladder outlet, spinal or general anesthesia, muscular tension, emotional anxiety, and medications such as sedatives, opiates, psychotropic drugs, and antispasmodics, which interfere with the normal neurologic function of the voiding reflex. Besides the absence of voided urine, in retention, the nurse may assess a distended bladder. As the bladder fills with urine, it rises above the level of the symphysis pubis, and may be displaced to either side of the midline. The absence of voided urine from retention is to be distinguished from *anuria*, complete suppression of urine formation by the kidneys, or *oliguria*, diminished urine secretion in relation to fluid intake.

Urinary incontinence. The inability of the urinary sphincters to control the release of urine from the bladder is *urinary incontinence*. Causes may be both psychological and physiological. Common causes of sphincter damage or loss of control include weak abdominal perineal musculature, obstetrical trauma, complications from pelvic surgery or radiation treatment, use of medications such as narcotics or sedatives, and use of alcohol.

According to the terminology of the North American Nursing Diagnosis Association (Gordon 1987), the occurrence of either of these two problems is given the nursing diagnosis of *urinary elimination, altered patterns*.

Excessive gas in the stomach and intestines is termed **flatulence** and may be accompanied by abdominal distension. Certain foods contribute to the formation of excessive gas and should be reduced or eliminated from the diet. These include beans, cabbage, cauliflower, onions, and highly seasoned foods. Milk products may produce excessive gas in some adults. If abdominal distention is present, the person should avoid those activities that might promote air swallowing such as using a drinking straw or chewing gum. Carbonated beverages are to be avoided. It may be helpful to eat more slowly and to increase the activity level to facilitate the passage of the gas.

The final way of stating a nursing diagnosis according to the Roy Adaptation Model is to use a label that summarizes a behavioral pattern when more than one mode is being affected by the same stimulus. Urinary incontinence related to spinal cord damage might be such a diagnosis because the nurse would be immediately aware that the person's physical self-concept, role function, and interdependence modes would also be involved. After extensive, successful rehabilitation, a person with such injuries might have the diagnosis of "effective coping strategies for altered elimination."

Goal Setting

Based on thorough assessment and understanding of adaptation problems related to elimination, the nurse sets goals in terms of outcomes for the person. A complete goal statement includes the behavior of focus, the change expected, and the time frame in which the goal is to be achieved. For example, for the person experiencing the adaptation problem of constipation related to poor normal bowel habits, the long-term goal may be: within two weeks, the person will establish a regular pattern of bowel movements. An initial short term could be that during the next week, the person would identify the best time of day for bowel elimination. This would take into consideration personal patterns of mass movements of the large bowel and the individual's life activities. Then the person would both try and evaluate the effectiveness of either hot liquid or fruit juice in facilitating normal evacuation on three days of the week.

Intervention

The intervention step of the nursing process according to the Roy Adaptation Model depends on the identified stimuli as the nurse either promotes or reinforces the stimuli or takes action to change or delete them. Interventions for the common adaptation problems related to elimination will be discussed.

For the problem of constipation, general interventions include: increasing fluid intake to ensure adequate hydration; exercise; providing a diet that is adequate in residue, including increasing the intake of fruits, juices, bulk-producing vegetables, and bran cereals; responding to the urge to defecate to prevent additional reabsorption of water from the stool, thus avoiding hard, dry stools. Setting time aside to evacuate the bowel (for example, 30 minutes after the morning meal), or drinking a warm beverage or water early in the morning, may help to initiate a movement for some people. In learning healthy habits, chronic laxative use is avoided, for this abuse may lead to atonic bowel syndrome. However, if other conservative measures fail, the occasional use of a laxative to stimulate peristalsis and bowel evacuation may be indicated.

Interventions should be directed toward those identified causes when intervening for the problem of diarrhea. Other interventions include avoidance or elimination of allergic dietary substances or drugs that promote loose, watery stools. Many persons are aware of the foods that cause diarrhea, for example, alcoholic beverages, highly caffeinated liquids such as coffee, or rich pastries high in sugar content.

With mild cases of diarrhea, nothing but clear liquids, such as water, tea, carbonated beverages, bouillon broth, and sweet fruit juices, is taken during the first 12 hours. Citrus juices are avoided. Cold liquids and concentrated sweets are tolerated poorly and thus are avoided.

During the next 12 hours, more foods, such as toast, soda crackers, and uncreamed soups may be added. After the stool begins to firm, other bland foods can be added, with gradual advancement to the person's regular diet.

With more severe cases of diarrhea, fluid and electrolyte replacement may be necessary, and/or the person may need administration of medication to decrease peristalsis and relieve abdominal cramping. Medical treatment of diarrhea is discussed in texts concerned with pathology.

The person with diarrhea is provided with an atmosphere conducive to relaxation and rest. The anal region is cleansed with mild soap and water after each movement to reduce local irritation and discomfort.

When anal incontinence (the inability of the anal sphincter to control the passage of feces) is present, a bowel training program may be initiated. It is important to set aside a consistent time for evacuation. Hot fluids may be given, followed by a glycerine suppository, or for some, the insertion of a gloved finger into the rectum will provide enough stimulation. The person should then attempt evacuation and allow adequate time.

In addition, the person should be encouraged to follow many of the interventions outlined in the section addressing constipation, such as adequate fluid intake, a diet high in roughage, and the intake of fruit juices.

Incontinent persons may be embarassed and have emotional distress. Special nursing care includes support and understanding, as well as measures to reduce possible skin irritation, odor, and the soiling of clothing and linen.

For urinary retention, interventions include early ambulation following surgery, acquiring a sitting position or a standing posture in the male, providing the person with privacy, listening to the sound of running water, dangling the hands in warm water, pouring warm water over the perineum or sitting in a warm bath to promote perineal muscle relaxation, or any other measure that might promote relaxation. If these measures fail, medications may be employed to promote the ease of voiding, or bladder catheterization may be used.

A complete diagnostic workup is done to identify the causative and contributing stimuli for the adaptation of incontinence. If stress incontinence is present, the person tries to avoid excessive straining or conditions such as chronic coughing. Weight reduction and pelvic exercises are helpful in regaining bladder control. Kegel exercises increase the tone of the perineal muscles. Instruct the person to contract the perineal muscles as though trying to stop the flow of urine. This should be done 10 to 15 times per session at least four times a day. Also, the person should try to start and stop the stream of urine when voiding.

A bladder training program may be required which includes an adequate intake of fluids, strengthening exercises for the perineal muscles, and a definite schedule set aside for voiding. The intake of fluids should be carefully spaced throughout the day and limited before sleep to promote adequate rest. The person is encouraged to void every 30 minutes to 2 hours, and as the program progresses, the urine is held for longer periods of time. As with anal incontinence, nursing care should include supportive measures to decrease emotional stress and possible skin irritation. (Additional information on nursing management of incontinence is found in basic nursing texts and in textbooks on neuroscience nursing and care of the elderly.)

Evaluation

Evaluation involves judging the effectiveness of the nursing interventions in relation to the person's adaptive behavior. Whether or not the patient has attained the behavior stated in the goal is identified. The nursing interventions would be identified as effective if the person's behavior is in accordance with the stated goal. If the goal has not been achieved, the nurse identifies alternative interventions or approaches by reassessing the behavior and stimuli and continuing with the other steps of the nursing process.

Consider the example given earlier of a short-term goal set with the person with constipation. In one week the person has identified before breakfast as the best time of day for bowel elimination and used a cup of hot-decaffeinated coffee on awakening, as well as prune juice with breakfast. During the week he had four bowel evacuations in the morning that were hard, but expelled without undue difficulty. At this point another short-term goal would be set. This would be to add other contextual factors to create good bowel habits, such as drinking more fluids, getting more exercise, and a diet higher in residue.

SUMMARY

In this chapter, the steps of the Roy adaptation nursing process were applied to the human need of elimination. Knowledge of the underlying processes related to intestinal and urinary elimination were highlighted as basic to planning nursing care. Behaviors and stimuli were identified and described. Nursing diagnoses and adaptation problems related to elimination were discussed as were the steps of goal setting, interventions, and evaluation.

EXERCISES FOR APPLICATION

1. Assess the bowel elimination behaviors of a young child, adolescent, adult, and elderly person. Relate the stimuli of age for each person to the assessed behaviors.
2. Develop a teaching plan to help a person utilize strategies to cope with the adaptation problem of urinary incontinence.

ASSESSMENT OF UNDERSTANDING

1. Recall three functions of the intestines.
   a. _____
   b. _____
   c. _____

2. List four behaviors to assess related to urinary elimination.
   a. _____
   b. _____
   c. _____
   d. _____

3. Discuss stimuli that can influence peristalsis and relate these to your understanding of the processes involved in movements of the intestines.
4. State a potential nursing diagnosis related to urinary elimination for a patient after surgery.
5. Identify two interventions that help the person cope with increased flatulence.
   a. _____
   b. _____

6. If a suggested nursing intervention has not been effective in meeting the goal established with the patient to meet elimination needs, discuss how the nurse will proceed based on the Adaptation Model nursing process.

Feedback

1. Any three of the following: digestion, absorption, and metabolism of nutrients; absorption of water and electrolytes; and elimination of waste products of digestion.
2. Any four of the following: Disease processes, fluid intake, fluid and electrolyte balance, environmental stimuli, medications, factors that influence and cope with pain and discomfort, usual daily urinary elimination pattern, stress, altered means of elimination, family and cultural beliefs, and age.
3. Factors that maintain or increase peristalsis, include the person's daily activity level or pattern of exercise. Factors that decrease peristalsis include bed rest, immobility, or recent anesthesia. Movements of the intestines are both mixing and propulsive types. Mixing movements aid in absorption functions and propulsive movements move waste products toward elimination. General increase of muscle activity and related neurological activity promotes such movement, thus facilitating bowel elimination.
4. Urinary retention related to recent anesthesia.
5. Any of the following: reduce or eliminate foods that contribute to flatus formation such as beans, cabbage, onions, cauliflower, and milk products; avoid carbonated beverages; avoid swallowing excessive air; and increase activity level.
6. The nurse will return to the earlier steps of the process to see if the assessment is accurate and complete, the diagnosis appropriate, the goal realistic, and the interventions adequate.

REFERENCES

Cella, J., and J. Watson. *Nurse's Manual of Laboratory Tests*. Philadelphia: F. A. Daves Company, 1989.

Gordon, M. *Nursing Diagnosis: Process and Application*. New York: McGraw-Hill, 1987.

Guyton, A. *Human Physiology and Mechanisms of Disease* (4th ed.). Philadelphia: W. B. Saunders Company, 1987.

Phipps, W., B. Long, and N. Woods. *Medical-Surgical Nursing: Concepts and Clinical Practice*, (3rd ed.). St. Louis: The C. V. Mosby Company, 1987.

Additional References
Ellickson, E. Bowel management plan for homebound elderly, *Gerontology Nursing*, 14(1): 16–19, 1988.

Luckmann, J., and K. Sorensen. *Medical-Surgical Nursing: A Psychophysiologic Approach,* (3rd ed.). Philadelphia: W. B. Saunders Company, 1987.

Maresca, T. Assessment and management of acute diarrhea illness in adults, *Nurse Practitioner,* 11(11): 15–16, 1986.

McShane, R., and A. McLane. Constipation: Impact of etiological factors, *Journal of Gerontology Nursing,* 14(4): 31–34, 1988.

Resnick, B. Constipation: Common but preventable, *Geriatric Nurse,* 6(4): 213–215, 1985.

Chapter Seven

Activity and Rest

Sister Callista Roy*

Activity and rest are basic needs in the physiological mode of adaptation. Activity is important because through activity one goes about one's daily living and presents who one is within the environment. Activity also provides the physical stresses on body structures that promote normal growth and development. Rest, on the other hand, provides the periods of restoration, repair, renewal of energies and effectiveness of life processes. Maintaining an appropriate balance in both rest and activity is one of the challenges of adaptation. In this chapter the theoretical bases for how activity and rest act to maintain health are discussed. The predictable consequences of inadequate activity and rest will be identified. The steps of the nursing process will be described: This includes the behaviors to be assessed, the common stimuli, nursing diagnoses, goals, and nursing interventions, particularly aimed at preventing problems of activity and rest and promoting health in this physiological mode component.

OBJECTIVES

After studying this chapter, the reader will be able to do the following:

1. Describe how activity and rest are important in maintaining health.
2. List the consequences of inadequate physical activity.
3. Describe how the major body functions are affected by inadequate physical activity.

*This chapter is a revision and expansion of the chapter "Activity and Rest" by Joan Seo Cho in the second edition of *Introduction to Nursing: An Adaptation Model* by Sister Callista Roy, Englewood Cliffs, N.J.: Prentice Hall, 1984, pp. 138–158.

4. Derive a preventive nursing intervention for a specific disuse consequence.
5. Discuss the effects of inadequate rest and sleep on integrity of the adaptive modes.
6. Propose approaches to promote adequate rest.

KEY CONCEPTS DEFINED

- *Body alignment:* natural or anatomically correct posture in which the body parts are arranged in their functional position.
- *Disuse consequences:* predictable physiological and psychological changes resulting from inadequate physical activity and affecting all four adaptive modes.
- *Gait:* manner of walking, thus providing the basic means of moving around from place to place.
- *Immobility:* relative inactivity beyond necessary rest periods.
- *Muscle conditioning:* maintenance of muscle tone by regular and deliberate use of muscles such as in isotonic, isometric, and resistive muscle exercises.
- *Range of motion (ROM) exercise:* movement of joints according to the range of motion of the particular joint; may be active, passive, or assisted.
- *Rest:* relative decrease or change of activity which renews more energy than is expended.
- *Sleep:* a form of rest in which there is diminished ability to respond to environmental stimuli; physiologically defined by polygraph criteria.
- *Sleep stages:* five separate periods of rhythmic changes that occur during one night, each having its own characteristics and time frame.

STRUCTURES AND FUNCTIONS RELATED TO ACTIVITY AND REST

Activity and rest are both key to one's survival. Activity refers to body movement and serves various purposes such as carrying out daily living chores and protecting self or others from bodily injuries. Recreation is a change in activity in which one becomes renewed for other activities. Rest involves changes in activity in which energy requirements are minimal. During rest energy is conserved and restored, and during sleep most of the physiological processes slow down to allow renewal of energy for future activity. As more of the institutionalized patient population, as well as persons receiving health care at home, is made up of elderly or seriously ill persons, the concept of immobility and its effect becomes an important focus for nursing care. At the same time there are increasing numbers of persons in society whose daily activity leads to stresses that interfere with getting adequate rest. Because of increasing difficulties in meeting the needs for activity and rest in today's society, the nurse is concerned with assisting persons in meeting these needs.

Activity

Activity involves the structures of normal movement, that is, the voluntary and autonomic neuromuscular and skeletal systems. Nurses note that in addition to intact body systems, activity involves also the motivation to move and a free nonrestrictive environment in which to move (Hodges and Callihan 1988). In terms of brain function, limbic and nonlimbic structures of the brain are involved. (See Fig. 7–1.) The limbic system governs basic biological drives and emotional behavior by control-

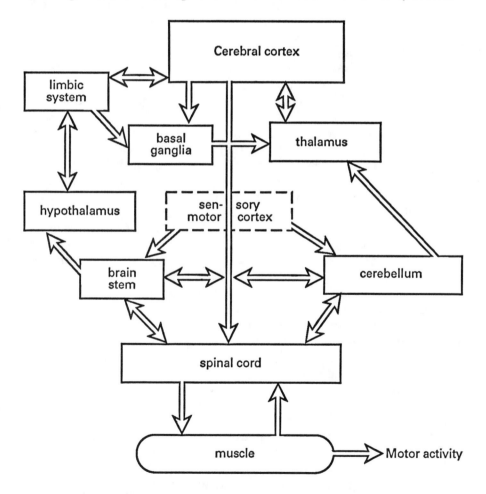

Figure 7–1 Central nervous system structures involved in motor activity

ling the neuroendocrine and autonomic systems through the hypothalmus. A need for action is generated that influences, and is influenced by,
the sensorimotor part of the brain. The nonlimbic structures consist of
sensory and motor cortex and their associative systems.

Brooks (1986) describes a command hierarchy for the control of pos-
tures and movements. The highest level operates in the association areas
of the cerebral cortex and elaborates perceptions and overall motor plans
or strategies. As part of this process, the limbic system denotes what is
relevant to the perceived needs of the body. The middle level of the command hierarchy is where strategies are converted into motor programs or
tactics. This level consists of sensorimotor cortex, the cerebellum, the
basal ganglia, and the brain stem. These programs correlate body equilibrium, movement directions, force, and speed, as well as mechanical stiff-
ness of the joints, that is, whether the joint moves or is held in one
position. Natural movements of everyday life involve several joints and
are composed of simple movements that affect only one joint. This lowest
level of control is the spinal cord which translates commands into muscular activity. The spinal cord also regulates such activity through stretch
reflexes. (Chapters 9 and 11 further describe related neurologic processes
and relevant reviews are found in basic anatomy and physiology texts.)

All of these processes are integrated so intricately that human activity
has not yet been duplicated in efforts to built robots. An article in a
popular science journal (Dworezky 1987) noted: "It's no wonder movie-
makers still use people dressed up in robot suits instead of using the real
thing. Today's commercial robots don't walk like men (sic people), actually balancing their bulk, but stay on their feet statically, like tables on
wheels. They're incapable of counter-balancing, of shifting their center of
gravity to make lifting or pushing more efficient, so they must be over-
engineered into glorified forklifts in order to work without toppling over."

The stress caused by physical activity is essential in maintaining all
major body functions. Physical activity promotes the normal oxygenation
process by stimulating cardiovascular circulation, and proper lung expansion with mobilization of its secretions. The musculoskeletal system maintains its muscle tone and bone strength only if adequate stresses are
imposed on them regularly. Physical activity promotes the normal urinary flow through its tract and stimulates the gastric mobility that is
essential for proper digestion of foods. It also has an effect on bowel
elimination. Maintenance of normal metabolic rate requires adequate
physical stresses in order to maintain proper equilibrium between the
catabolic and anabolic activities.

The human dimensions of what it means to a person to plan and carry
out activity is noted in a neurologist's account of witnessing his patients
become suddenly mobile, after years of virtual immobility (after receiving
a new treatment for parkinsonian symptoms induced by encephalitis).
Sacks (1983) called what he saw in patients "awakenings" and he com-

mented that we are critically dependent on a continual flow of impulses and information to and from all the sensory and motor organs of the body. More poignantly he states: "We must be active or we cease to exist: activity and actuality are one and the same" (p. 302).

Rest
Rest cannot be defined as mere physical inactivity. Rest includes the quality of relaxation that comes with freedom from physical discomfort and psychological stresses such as anxiety. Most especially, rest is an individualized matter. What leads to relaxation and restoration of energy will vary from person to person. Napping or sleeping are forms of rest. Other forms of rest may be changing activity such as taking a walk during lunch break at work. Vacation and other kinds of recreation function to provide rest. For some persons rest is best attained by doing nothing, for example, sitting outside watching the ocean or beside a fireplace indoors in winter or watching raindrops on the window in spring.

During rest physiological processes slow down to allow renewal of energy. Physiologically, heart rate recovery is greatest at the beginning of a rest period. Thus it is suggested that several short rest periods rather than one long, extended period is more effective. Industrial studies suggest that 15 percent of work time be given to rest, with increases of 20 to 30 percent in evenly distributed times for strenuous work loads.

Sleep
Most rest is done through sleep with human beings spending an average of one-third of their lives in sleeping. Behaviorally, rest becomes sleep when one's ability to respond to minute environmental stimuli is diminished. Sleep is a rhythmic and active process. Physiologically, sleep is defined by polygraph criteria that include: cortical activity scored from electroencephalogram (EEG) waveforms, muscle activity noted on the electromyogram (EMG), and eye movements recorded by electro-oculogram (EOG). Standardized terminology, techniques, and a scoring system are used to define the stages of sleep in the adult (Rechtschaffen and Kales 1973) and in the child (Anders and Parmelee 1971.) During a typical night of 7 to 8 hours of sleep, the person goes through several cycles of sleep in an orderly sequence of stages approximately every 60 to 90 minutes. Stages 1 through 4 are called the NREM (non-rapid eye movement) phase, and Stage 5 is called the REM phase because of the rapid eye movements characteristic of this stage. This pattern of sleep, including occurrence, timing, and duration of stages, is called the architecture of sleep.

Generally, the night's sleep begins with lights out and less than 20 minutes of awake time. A period of drowsiness, Stage 1, follows and will reoccur at intervals throughout the night, especially to begin a new sleep cycle. Stage 1 makes up less than 1 to 5 percent of the night. A person is easily aroused during this stage. In stage 2 there is increased muscular relaxation and several cortical changes, including low-voltage activity and bursts of sleep spindles. The person's ability to respond spontaneously to stimuli is further diminished. Stages 3 and 4 are the deeper levels of sleep, also known as delta sleep, or slow wave sleep (SWS). The percent of particular waveforms differentiates the two stages. The fourth stage is actually deep sleep in which one may be able to respond only to strong stimuli. Bedwetting in children usually takes place during this stage because of inability to respond to internal stimuli as well as external stimuli.

Following the fourth stage, the cycle usually reverses, returning to Stage 2 before entering Stage 5, the REM phase of sleep. On the EEG, REM sleep looks much the same as the awake state. However, the characteristic eye movements are both phasic and tonic (high number of movements and periods of fewer movements). These movements can be observed through the closed eyelids as well as on the EOG.

During sleep, the person's physiology differs significantly from that of a waking person (Robinson 1986). The cardiovascular, respiratory, and gastrointestinal systems are most affected. Other alterations include cerebral blood flow and metabolism, temperature regulation, and endocrine and renal function. These effects differ in the various stages of sleep and are based on the characteristics of sleep. For example, with the loss of wakefulness, neural control of respiration changes as the cortical component is lost and metabolic control predominates. The result may be normal variations such as rapid or irregular breathing or abnormal responses such as snoring or obstructive apnea.

Beginning in Stage 1 there is decreased activity in vital bodily functions such as heart rate, temperature, respiration, and basal metabolic rate. During the deep sleep that starts with Stage 3, one's basic metabolic rate is decreased by 10 to 20 percent, and this is demonstrated by a drop of body temperature, heart rate, and blood pressure. Muscle tone becomes atonic. The skin may become flushed and warm, with mild diaphoresis. Blood pressure decreases during Stages 3 and 4. It is believed that during Stage 4, growth hormone is released and there is a decreased concentration of corticosteroids. These changes seem to promote protein synthesis, which assists in restoration and repair of biological structures and functions (Oswald 1976). Thus sleep researchers postulate that NREM sleep is an anabolic state and responsible primarily for one's physiological restoration. This possibilitiy is supported by the fact that NREM sleep takes precedence over REM sleep when one is recovering from sleep deprivation. Still, more is known about the description and mechanisms of sleep than about its functions, or how it acts to renew the person for another day's activities.

Variability of both blood pressure and heart rate are increased during REM sleep, possibly due to other changes such as decreased cardiac output. During this stage there is an overall, but transient increase in physiological activities in the body. This may result from a marked, but brief cutaneous vasoconstrictions, a reduction in urine volume, and possibly, an increased level of plasma catacholamines. The body temperature, heart rate, and blood pressure are all increased, sometimes even to above the level of the person's waking state. An increase in cerebal activity is indicated by increased cerebral flow. When awakened during this stage, many persons report vivid dreams. Nocturnal attacks of such conditions as anginal pain, gastric pain, and asthma may be triggered during this stage. Although REM sleep is included within each cycle, the cycles occurring later in the sleep period, that is, closer to normal awakening, have more REM sleep, thus there is greater vulnerability to these attacks around 5 or 6 A.M.

In relation to the mechanisms whereby sleep occurs, researchers have worked out the neurotransmitter-active neurons and the anatomical sites they act upon for each stage of sleep (Robinson 1986). One model attempts to provide a global view of the action and interaction of three neurochemical systems of the brain that are the mechanisms for the cycles of waking and sleeping (Hobson 1974). As the processes continue to be understood better, then the functions can be identified more clearly. This knowledge, what causes sleep and what sleep does for people is important to nursing practice in helping persons meet the need for rest.

APPLICATION OF THE NURSING PROCESS

Activity and rest are important to the person's physical and psychological integrity. The nurse will look at specific assessment factors to determine the adequacy of activity level and to identify any existing adverse consequences of inactivity. These observations and the nursing care plan derived are based on an understanding of structures and functions related to these needs. Similarly, behavioral observations of adequacy of meeting rest and sleep needs, and background knowledge in this area, provide the basis for planning nursing care.

Assessment of Behavior

Two major categories of assessment factors for activity are considered: (1) the type and amount of physical activity carried out by the person, and (2) the person's motor function status which depends on muscle and joint mobility, posture and gait, and coordination. For rest and sleep, the following are assessed: (1) quantity and quality of daily rest, (2) sleep pattern, and (3) signs of sleep deprivation. The behavioral assessment factors are summarized in column one of Table 7–1.

The benefits of physical activity for fitness have been widely recog-

TABLE 7–1. NURSING PROCESS FOR ACTIVITY AND REST[1]

Behavior	Stimuli	Nursing Diagnoses	Goals
Acvitivity Need			
1. Type and amount of daily physical activity.	A. Neuromuscular and skeletal systems disruptions.	1. Inadequate physical activity due to: Stimuli C or D.	1. To increase physical activity.
2. Motor function - Muscle masses, tone, and strength - Joint mobility, size, function - Posture - Gait - Motor coordination - Abnormal or involuntary movement	B. Disease or illness requiring imposed restriction of activity, including mechanical constraints and medical protocols. C. Reluctance to perform activity. D. Immediate environmental factors.	2. Development of disuse consequences due to Stimuli A or B.	2. To prevent the effects of immobility on various bodily functions.
Rest and Sleep Need			
1. Quantity and quality of daily rest.	A. Physical condition - Heavy physical activity - Discomfort and pain of illness and disease. - Jet travel - Rotating work shifts.	1. Inadequate rest due to Stimuli A, B, or C.	1. To increase quantity and quality of rest.
2. Sleep pattern - Frequency and duration of sleep period - Number of arousals during sleep	B. Psychological condition - Heavy mental work - Psychological stresses such as anxiety, depression or loneliness.	2. Difficulty initiating or maintaining sleep due to Stimuli A, B, C, or D.	2. To improve normal sleep-wake cycle.
3. Past sleep history related to current pattern.	C. Change in sleep habits and environment.	3. Sleep deprivation due to Stimuli A, B, C, or D.	3. To increase the quantity and quality of sleep.
4. Signs of sleep deprivation - Psychological - Physical	D. Drug or alcohol use.		
5. Subjective feelings related to rest/sleep.			

[1]Developed by Joan Seo Cho

nized since the 1950s when President Eisenhower of the United States called attention to this need. Regular exercise by adults has increased in this country since that time. Federal programs and policy on health promotion have continued to emphasize physical exercise. However, current studies show that the majority of people, particulary women, children, low-income populations, and minorities, still do not get enough regular exercise. Obtaining information on the person's patterns of physical activity is important in planning nursing care to avoid the consequences of inadequate activity and to promote health, fitness, and well being. By observing, discussing, and recording the type and frequency of *physical activity,* the nurse can judge the adequacy of activity level in relation to the person's total physical condition.

Through assessment of *motor function,* the nurse determines the type of physical activity the person is capable of performing, and identifies consequences of inactivity. Types of physical activity the person can perform are evaluated by functional assessments. Specific instruments developed for functional assessment are divided into three basic categories: (1) global instruments for comprehensive assessments, (2) activites of daily living scales, and (3) functional profiles which enable one to assess limitations of a specific condition, or to evaluate a single function, such as use of one's hand or climbing stairs (Hollerbach 1988). Of particular significance is whether or not one is capable of performing self-care activities.

Assessment of muscle and joint mobility is made by active or passive demonstration of the range of motion. All active movements, such as lifting, pushing, and pulling, require muscle contractions. *Muscle mass* (size) and *tone* (firmness) are assessed by grasping the center of the muscle and feeling that it is firm, supple, and full-bellied. In the older person it is expected that there is less shape and contour of major muscles. In the child, muscles are softer and have less mass. Muscle *strength* varies widely according to age and training. Strength is tested by asking the person to move, using certain muscles, against resistance, or to hold the part still while the examiner tries to move it. An example is testing flexion and extension at the elbow by having the patient pull and push against the examiner's hand. Levels of strength are commonly scaled from 0, no muscular contraction either seen or felt, to 5, normal muscle strength. Table 7–2 describes commonly used levels of strength. Generally a muscle strength rated below 3 is considered indicative of disability.

Joint mobility is assessed by an active or passive demonstration of each joint's range of motion. The range of motion is the direction and degree a joint is capable of moving. This varies for different joints, for example, the ankle moves by flexing about 50 degrees and extending about 20 degrees, whereas, the hip can flex as much as 135 degrees, extend 28 degrees, abduct 50 degrees, and adduct about 30 degrees as well as rotate. (See Fig. 7–2). Some expected limitation of joint mobility occurs

TABLE 7–2. LEVELS OF MUSCLE STRENGTH

Grade	Strength
5	Free range of motion against normal resistance and gravity
4	Full range of motion against moderate resistance and gravity
3	Full range of motion against gravity only
2	Full range of motion with gravity eliminated
1	Slight muscle contraction palpable, but no movement noted
0	No visible or palpable contraction; paralysis of limb

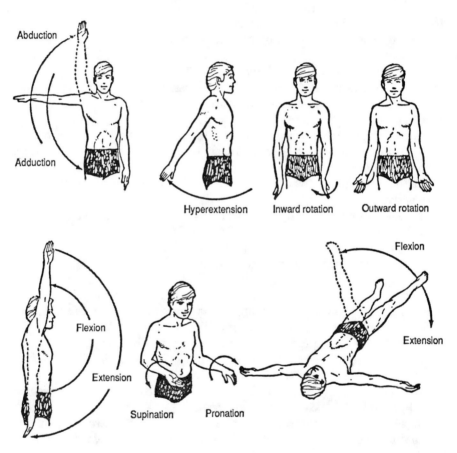

Figure 7-2 Range of Motion Movements

with aging. When there is good mobility, bones move freely and smoothly, without pain (Mourad 1986).

The anatomical arrangement of body parts in a given position is called *posture.* Correct posture is a factor in physical saftey since not appropriately alligning muscles and joints during activity can result in injury or deformity. Good posture is body alignment that permits optimal weight balance and operation of the motor function. In the upright standing position, the head, shoulders, and pelvis are aligned; the arms hang freely from the shoulders; and the feet are aligned with toes pointing straight ahead. (See Figure 7–3.) Observation of the person's preferred posture is significant as a possible sign of some dysfunction, for example, a person with obstructive lung disease tends to lean forward with arms braced.

Gait is the manner of walking and provides the basic means of moving around from place to place. One assesses whether or not the person walks easily, comfortably, with self-assurance, good balance and symetry of movement or has a limp, pain or discomfort, fear of falling, loss of balance, difference in movement from one side to the other, or unusual movements. An improper gait may impose undue stress on certain musculoskeletal parts and in time can lead to deformity. For example, when a patient is using a "swing through" gait on crutches, the movement is not the same as normal walking and will eventually result in weakening of the lower extremities. A proper gait with good posture will allow a safe and optimal level of mobility.

Good motor *coordination* requires both intact neurological and mus-

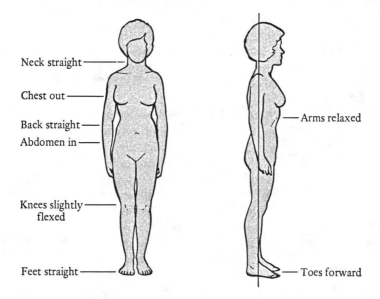

Neck straight

Chest out

Back straight

Abdomen in

Knees slightly flexed

Feet straight

Arms relaxed

Toes forward

Figure 7–3 Correct standing position.

culoskeletal function and will have an effect on the person's activity status, particularly self-care activities. Coordination is easily tested by having the person do rapidly alternating movements such as placing one foot on the opposite knee and sliding it down that shin to the big toe or a finger from the examiner's finger to his or her own nose. A child as young as 6 years can easily do these tasks. (Further details on assessing each of these aspects of motor functions can be found in texts on physical assessment.)

Behavior related to *rest* can be assessed simply by observing and recording rest periods throughout the day. The need for daily rest periods other than nightly sleep depends on one's physical and psychological condition in a given situation. However, for most hospitalized patients, deliberately planned rest periods may be a necessary part of total care. Continuous tossing and turning while resting in bed or fidgeting of hands may indicate restlessness. The mere absence of physical activity may not provide effective rest for a person who is under mental stress. For persons with activity intolerance, they may show one or more of the following behaviors: exertional discomfort, difficulty completing activities, and verbal report of being easily fatigued (American Nurses' Association and American Association of Neuroscience Nurses 1985). The person's feelings of being well rested are the most important behavior to be assessed.

A person's *sleep pattern* is assessed by recording observations or reports of how long it takes to fall asleep, restlessness during sleep, number of arousals during each sleep period, early awakening and sleepiness during the day. Behavioral cues of sleep deprivation include reddened eyes, puffy eyelids, dark circles around the eyes, and frequent yawning. Understanding the person's usual pattern of sleep in relation to any recent changes is important in the assessment. Characteristics of a sleep pattern disturbance include the following additional behaviors: reduction in one's role performance (work, school, or home), increasing irritability, restlessness, disorientation (progressive), listlessness, slight hand tremors, expressionless face, and thick speech with mispronounced and wrong choice of words (Schreier 1986).

The effects of sleep on physiological and psychological integrity have been studied by observing and recording behavioral changes that occur following a period of *sleep deprivation* (Pasnau et al 1986, Sassin 1970, Opstad et al 1978). These studies indicate that loss of sleep brings changes in brain function and causes alteration in biochemical processes in the body. Sleep loss causes not only physical fatigue and poor neuromuscular coordination, but also signs of psychological dysfunction which manifests itself as general irritability, inability to concentrate, disorientation, and confusion. The severity of these effects depends on the degree and length of deprivation and the individual's predeprivation condition.

More extensive assessment tools for clinically evaluating sleep and rest have been developed, for example, *Sleep Questionnaire and Assessment of Wakefulness (SQAW)*, from the Stanford Sleep Disorders Clinic

(Miles 1979). These tools are useful because they depend on self report and subjective feelings of being well rested. The person's sense of having enough sleep is the important behavior to assess regardless of additional data from observation.

Assessment of Stimuli

After the behavioral assessment of activity and rest needs, the nurse assesses the stimuli affecting these needs and how they are being met. Some of the categories of possible focal, contexutal, and residual stimuli are: (1) physical condition, (2) current psychological condition, (3) the environment particularly at bedtime, (4) personal habits related to activity and rest, and (5) drug and alcohol consumption. (See listing in column 2 of Table 7–1.)

These factors act together and will be assessed as the pattern of stimuli affecting the person. For activity needs, disruptions in the structure and function of the musculosketal system are *physical condition* factors that act as key focal stimuli affecting the person. Such disruptions can occur by either direct physical injuries to muscles and bones or by central nervous system disorders. Regardless of the underlying causative factor, a dysfunctioning musculoskeletal system will cause a direct and immediate effect on one's motor function. A fractured bone will inevitably necessitate a limitation of one's physical activity due not only to the loss of function, but also to the discomfort and pain one may experience.

A person with an illness, depending on the nature and severity of the condition, will limit physical activity either voluntarily or because of medically imposed restrictions. Bed rest is often an integral part of therapeutic treatment because rest provides a period of restoration and repair. Particular concerns for planning nursing care when the person is on bed rest will be addressed later in this chapter.

One's rest and sleep also are influenced by the physical stresses one experiences at a given time. The extent of illness is assessed as affecting rest and sleep. The more serious one's illness, the more time one will need to spend in rest and sleep. Levels of daily physical activity also are assessed. Whereas vigorous physical activity tends to lengthen the deep sleep cycle, a lack of physical activity will cause a feeling of unsatisfied sleep caused by lack of deep sleep. Physical discomfort and pain are other common causes that reduce the level of satisfactory rest and sleep. Travel by jet airplane across time zones or working shifts that rotate can alter the body's rhymic sleep-wake cycle.

Another contextual stimuli for sleep is age. Generally, the younger one is, the longer the time spent for sleep, until the individual reaches young adulthood. The average time spent for sleep in different age groups can be summarized as follows: 22 hours for the neonate, 14 to 16 hours for infants, 10 to 12 hours for toddlers and preschoolers, and 8 to 10 hours for school children. Young adults and elderly individuals spend an average of

7 to 8 hours daily for sleep. Recent studies have demonstrated that elderly men and women have multiple miniature arousals to stage 1 or awake during the normal night's sleep for that age group.

One's *psychological condition* in a given situation and at a given time has an effect on both activity and rest. Besides intact body systems, it was noted earlier that activity involves the motivation to move. Such motivation includes knowledge about activity and its beneficial effects for health. An example, of misinformation being a focal stimulus for inactivity is a mother on a postpartum unit who does not get out of bed to take a shower. With further assessment, the nurse might learn that the mother's cultural upbringing taught her not to move out of bed for several days following giving birth to a baby. Psychologically depressed persons tend to reduce their physical activity to a bare minimum. The catatonic state of a psychotic individual exemplifies this case to the extreme. In a catatonic state, the individual is not able to initiate body movements, even though physical and physiological dysfunction cannot be demonstrated.

Since sorting and consolidating one's daily living experiences seems to be done by the brain during sleep, a person who is under psychological stress has increased need for rest and sleep. However, the increased cortical activity may also disrupt the person's normal sleep pattern inducing a feeling of unsatisfied sleep need. It is not uncommon for a psychologically stressed person to wake up with dreams and complain of unsatisfactory rest and sleep even after spending many hours in bed. The person's bed partner may also be a source of assessment information. For example, he or she may describe sleep behavior and possible psychologic influences, such as stress at home or on the job.

The *immediate environment* affects rest and sleep. A free nonrestrictive environment in which to move has been identified as needed for physical activity. A suitable environment for activity includes availability of space and of adequate physical and personal assistance. Unsuitable environmental factors, such as unpleasant environmental temperature and surroundings will act to restrict the person's activity. For example, encouraging daily walks for a person after a heart attack, or for health promotion and fitness for a working professional person, will be ineffective if the person is contending with severe winter weather conditions, and has no indoor alternative, or if the neighborhood seems to be an unsafe place to walk. Lack of privacy also is an immediate focal or contextual stimuli. A person may be reluctant to do exercises on a mat or in the swimming pool of a busy physical therapy department. A child placed in a playpen will have a restricted range of physical activity, which over time could affect the child's normal growth and development.

Since a human being requires an average of one-third of his or her total life time for sleep, each individual develops unique habits and patterns related to the immediate environment for sleep. Through the years, these individualized patterns take on the character of ritualistic habits. It is not uncommon for an individual to experience difficulties in falling asleep, or staying asleep, if the usual sleep habits cannot be followed, or if the bedtime schedule of activity is altered.

An unfamiliar or unsuitable environment also disrupts one's rest and sleep. Such stimuli as unpleasant noise, light, odor, and room temperature can be disturbing factors. This was likely a factor in a study which recorded the EEGs of intensive care patients for 48 hours. In these patients, only 50 to 60 percent of the 24 hours' total sleep occured at night. The remaining 40 to 50 percent occurred during the day. Patients also had less total sleep time than they would have usually had at home (Hilton 1976).

A person's use of *drugs and alcohol* acts as a focal or contextual stimuli for activity and rest. A person who is sedated with medications, or consuming large amounts of alcoholic beverages, will not be ready, either physically or psychologically, to be involved in physical activity. Alcoholic beverages, and drugs such as barbiturates, amphetamines, and opiate derivatives may be effective for initiating sleep and rest on a temporary basis. However, over time they actually induce sleep deprivation, because of their tendency to suppress REM sleep. These substances are habit forming, and as a person develops a tolerance, they become ineffective with prolonged use.

A holistic behavioral assessment and related stimuli for a person's patterns of activity and rest provide information for judgment about nursing care needs. The next step of the nursing process, then, is nursing diagnosis.

Nursing Diagnosis

Major categories of nursing diagnoses related to activity and rest needs are: (1) adequate activity and rest, (2) inadequate or impaired physical activity and disuse consequences, and (3) inadequate rest or sleep pattern disturbance. Within each of these areas, diagnoses are stated in one of the three ways suggested by the Roy Adaptation Model. Using the first method to state a nursing diagnosis that reflects adaptation, including behaviors and the relevant stimuli, an illustration is: good muscle tone and 4+ muscle strength in major muscle groups of all four extremeties due to knowledge of health benefits of fitness and commitment to regular exercise program.

Sleep pattern disturbance is an example of a summary label for a behavioral pattern in one adaptive mode. If the relevant stimuli are identified, with the label, then this is the second type of nursing diagnostic statement. For example, assessment data may show that a person has difficulty falling asleep and frequent arousals from sleep during the night, as well as reddend eyes, puffy eyelids, dark circles under the eyes, and feelings of poor sleep. This person also reports concerns about the responsibilities associated with a job promotion. The diagnosis would be stated: sleep disturbance due to a recent change in job responsibilities. Further examples of this second type of statement of nursing diagnosis are given in column 3 of Table 7–1.

Note that the Association for Sleep Disorders Centers (Sleep Disorders Classification Committee 1979) has published a diagnostic classification of sleep and arousal disorders. The original classification system had four major categories: disorders of initiating and maintaining sleep, disorders of excessive daytime somnolence, disorders of sleep-wake schedule, and parasomnias such as sleep walking and sleep terror. Each major type of disorder includes subcategories of specific conditions with their associated patterns of signs and symptoms. The 1990 edition (American Sleep Disorders Association) expands on this classification of sleep disorders.

An example of a nursing diagnosis related to activity where all adaptive modes are affected by one stimulus is the nursing diagnosis commonly referred to as *disuse consequences*. This diagnosis is considered particularly when the person's physical activity is curtailed because of medically imposed restrictions.

In the case of a fractured bone, a period of immobile therapeutic alignment preoperatively prevents further damage to the fractured bone or the surrounding soft tissues. Postoperatively, it promotes proper healing of the repaired part. In the case of a patient who is suffering acute cardiac insufficiency, absolute bed rest is one of the most important aspects of the therapeutic regime. This measure is to conserve the oxygen and energy consumption required by nonpriority physical activity, thus minimizing the cardiac load for the damaged heart muscle. The same principle applies when the nurse places a patient with a fever on bed rest. An elevation of 1° in body temperature will require a 7 percent increase in basic metabolic rate, or energy needed. The nurse uses bed rest to prevent further exhaustion of the already stressed body. At the same time, she deals with the risks of immobility by recognizing the potential for disuse consequences. Some specific consequences of physical inactivity are listed in Table 7–3. The first two columns are organized by major body functions and the underlying changes that result from a period of physical inactivity. The behavioral effect of these changes, termed disuse consequences, is summarized in column 3 (Cho 1984 and Rubin 1988). These changes from inactivity can then affect further adaptation related to activity and rest. For example, a deficit in muscle mass, tone, and strength indicates muscle atrophy which is a consequence of disuse. In turn the atrophied muscle is less effective in performing activity. The older person is especially prone to disuse consequences when immobile.

Further, looking at the effects of physical inactivity from the perspective of the Roy Adaptation Model, the nurse uses her knowledge of the other adaptive modes to recognize that the inability to move about and interact with people and the environment in one's usual pattern will greatly affect the person's self-concept, role function, and interdependence.

TABLE 7–3. CONSEQUENCES OF PHYSICAL INACTIVITY[1]

Body Function	Underlying Changes	Disuse Consequences	Preventive Interventions
Musculoskeletal	*Muscles:* autolysis of unused muscles	Muscular atrophy with decreased strength and endurance	Muscle conditioning exercises: isometric, isotonic, and resistive exercises
	Bones: increased osteoclastic process due to lack of physical stresses of weight bearing on the bones leads to increased urinary excretion of calcium	Osteoporosis and vulnerability to pathological fracture	Physical activities which would produce the stresses of weight bearing—standing and walking, pushing and pulling
	Joints: decreased pliability and increased density of the collagen mesh work leads to fibrous formation and shortening of the muscle fibers	Joint contractures with permanent loss of joint mobility	ROM (range of motion) exercises: active, assisted, or passive ROM exercises
	Nerves: denervation due to prolonged compression on nerve fibers and decreased circulation	Paralysis, foot drop, and wrist drop	Frequent change of position; use of foot board
Circulatory	Cardiac overload due to central pooling of the circulatory volume	Deconditioning leads to poor exercise tolerance	Frequent change of position, including sitting up and standing positions, if possible
	Loss of regulatory mechanism to maintain central BP (normally with position change to sitting up, the splenic and peripheral vessels constrict to maintain the central blood volume)	Postural hypotension, dizziness, and fainting in upright position	
	Sluggish venous return due to lack of pumping mechanism generated by muscular contractions of physical activity	Dependent (local) edema, especially of the lower extremities	Muscle exercises to stimulate the circulation

continued

TABLE 7–3. CONSEQUENCES OF PHYSICAL INACTIVITY (continued)

Body Function	Underlying Changes	Disuse Consequences	Preventive Interventions
	Hypercoagulability of blood (due to injury or surgery) combined with physical inactivity (see above)	Thrombus formation leads to pulmonary embolism	Well-fitting antiembolic stockings
Pulmonary	Increased intraesophageal pressure and decreased expansion of thoracic cavity in recumbent position; stasis of respiratory tract secretion	Hypoventilation	Positions of maximum chest expansion
		Hypostatic pneumonia	Frequent change of positions, and deep-breathing and cough exercises
Metabolic	Increased catabolic processes leads to increased excretion of nitrogen via gastrointestinal and urinary tract combined with poor protein intake due to poor appetite	Negative nitrogen balance leads to poor tissue healing	Ensure adequate intake of dietary protein
Eliminative	Urinary stagnation due to lack of natural position of gravity in recumbent position and loss of proprioception	Urinary retention	Frequent encouragement to void, providing adequate toilet facility and position of comfort; ideal position for male client is standing up, while sitting up is for female client
	Increased calcium content in the urine	Nephrolithiasis	Ensure adequate fluid intake with cranberry juice to acidify the urine pH level

	Decreased gastrointestinal mobility combined with dependency on others to obtain toilet facility, lack of privacy, lack of bulk in the diet, and poor abdominal and pelvic muscle tones	Constipation or fecal impaction	Avoid unnecessary use of CNS depressants; muscle toning exercise for abdominal and pelvic muscles; ensure adequate fluid and bulk intake
Integumentary	Inability to carry out daily personal hygiene measures and prolonged compression on tissues (decreased circulation)	Pressure sores and decubiti ulceration formation with secondary infection	Frequent change of position; use of protective devices (pillow, padding); frequent massaging of all bony prominences
Sensory-perceptual	Decreased environmental stimuli lead to decreased sensory stimulation; changed perceptual axis with recumbent position; inability to manipulate own environment	Anxiety, disorientation, loss of proprioception—change in body image; boredom; egocentricity	Environment structuring to provide meaningful stimuli; use of calendar, radio, TV, and wall clock can be helpful Provide opportunity to carry out meaningful conversations with others Visits from family and friends are very important

¹From chapter "Activity and Rest" by Joan Seo Cho in the second edition of *Introduction to Nursing: An Adaptation Model* by Sister Callista Roy, Englewood Cliffs, N.J. Prentice Hall, pp. 141–143, 1984.

(See Parts III, IV, and V.) The effect on the other modes takes place through the sensory perceptual processes that involve particularly anxiety, change of body image, and ego centricity. All four adaptive modes are thus affected by the stimulus of inactivity. Disuse consequences is a diagnostic term broad enough to include these effects, particularly when viewed from a specific nursing model perspective such as the one presented here and from understanding of the scientific work done related to this concept.

Given a careful assessment and the nursing diagnoses that are derived, the fourth step of the nursing follows.

Goal Setting

In using the Roy Adaptation Model, goal setting is the stating of clear outcomes for the person as a result of nursing care. As noted earlier, a complete goal statement contains the behavior of focus, the change that the nurse and patient together expect, and the time frame in which the goal can be achieved. Depending on the situation, the goal may be long term or short term.

Some general goals related to activity and rest are given in column four of Table 7–1. Consider the person with the diagnosis of good muscle tone and 4+ muscle strength in major muscle groups of all four extremities due to knowledge of health benefits of fitness and commitment to regular exercise program. If this person suddenly is hospitalized with a broken pelvis suffered in an automobile accident, an appropriate goal in the new situation of immobility is: upper extremity muscle tone will be maintained at a good level and strength will be increased from 4+ to 5+ during the four weeks of acute care. This goal is influenced by the need to prepare for use of the arms to bear weight on crutches during rehabilitation.

In the case of the person who is suffering sleep pattern disturbance related to new job responsibilities, a short-term goal is: in the next week, the person will identify in writing early in the day, the two major responsibilities that are of most concern and for the concern that is most distressing consider several alternate ways of dealing with it.

Within the activity and rest component of the physiological mode, the general overall goal is to promote adequate activity and rest for normal growth and development and for restoration, repair, and renewal of energies and effectiveness of life processes. A balance of each (not between each) is the goal, that is, activity is balanced with the need for activity, and rest is balanced with the need for rest. These goals are made specific in the many situations that nurses encounter that can interfere with meeting these needs. For example, the person's sleep needs could be adequately met in terms of length and quality, but if the individual's ongoing physical stress level is beyond the available energy level, a negative energy balance indicates the need to set a goal related to increasing the quality and quantity of rest to an adequate level. Similarly in the examples of the patient with heart disease or a fever, as noted earlier, the need for rest increases and therefore providing more rest becomes part of the goal of nursing care to achieve balance of this need. Since the nurse often sees patients during times of change that affect their activity and rest, she is in a position to set preventive goals rather than allowing consequences of imbalances in activity and rest to occur.

Based on knowledge related to activity and rest, and the specific goals for a given person, the nurse plans the related nursing interventions.

Intervention
Each step of the nursing process provides direction for the intervention stage. The goal focuses on the behavioral description of the patient situation, and the interventions address the context of the behaviors, that is, the focal, contextual, and residual stimuli. Understanding this combined effect on the patient, is the basis for assisting the person to handle the experience in the direction of positive adaptation.

Nursing measures used to promote adequate activity include: health teaching to improve motivation to exercise, removing any discomfort or restriction that is unnecessarily limiting movement, and careful planning of preventive measures for those who must be immobilized. The latter will be discussed in detail because of its importance in care of patients in hospitals, as well as the elderly or debilitated at home or in long-term care facilities.

Intervention for disuse consequences has general and specific aspects. The general aspect includes those preventive measures that promote maintenance of normal motor functions. By promoting a person's motor activity, the nurse facilitiates accomplishment of daily living tasks, and also helps provide the body with the physical stresses that are essential in maintaining the internal physiological functions.

In planning preventive nursing interventions, the nurse takes the nature and extent of medically imposed restrictions into consideration. As noted earlier, at times a period of complete bed rest or other limited movement is medically indicated, therefore the nurse cannot manage the focal stimulus, that is, the enforced physical inactivity. However, other conditions are managed so that through well-planned preventive measures disuse consequences are avoided or minimized without impeding the purpose of the needed temporary immobilization.

The general preventive nursing interventions include the following four major principles: (1) maintenance of good body alignment, (2) frequent change of positions, (3) maintenance of joint mobility, and (4) conditioning of muscles. These interventions are summarized in column four of Table 7–3.

Good body alignment is a body posture in which the body parts are arranged in an anatomically functional position and the weight distribution is well balanced in a stable manner. The normal functional standing position is shown in Fig. 7–2. Good body alignment is assumed in all body positions. For example, in supine or lying down position, one's body is in full extension, resembling the upright position. Incorrect body alignment or posture will impose undue stresses on muscles, ligaments, and joints. Frequent or prolonged use of poor body alignment can leave a permanent defect, such as flexion contracture of neck and foot drop. These outcomes are not uncommon among bedridden patients.

Disuse consequences are a direct result of static body positions for prolonged periods of time, thus *changing the patient's position* is another way to change the major stimuli for these consequences. The supine position is the most common position assumed by ill individuals. For some patients this static position becomes prolonged without spontaneous body movements, for example, persons with paralysis or who are unconscious. A frequent change of position with proper body alignment is carried out with consideration of the following: prevention of nerve damage in the pressure areas, joint contractures, pressure sores, and loss of the postural adjustment mechanism for the maintence of central blood pressure in the upright position. Within mobility restrictions, the patient's body position can include many different positions, including prone, or face-lying. Frequent changes of position not only relieve the pressure of body weight, thus promoting general circulation, but the movement of changing positions also facilitates dislodging of bodily discharges, such as mucus secretions of the respiratory tract. An active change of position to a sitting-up position is effective in maintenance of the postural adjustment mechanism and consequently prevents the symptoms of postural hypotension or lowered blood pressure upon standing.

At times it is easy for the nurse to think that sitting up in the chair is too big a task for a particular patient. However, the nurse keeps in mind that although the process of struggling to get out of the bed and moving to a chair to sit down for a minute takes a lot of effort on the part of both the patient and the nurse, the benefits of such motor activity, when within therapeutically indicated limits, are paramount. This activity provides almost all of the physical exercises that are effective in prevention of the disuse consequences.

To *maintain joint mobility* either active or passive exercises may be done. In active range of motion (ROM) exercise, the patient intitiates and completes the full range of motion. (See Fig. 7–2.) For a person who is too weak or is partially paralyzed, assisted or passive ROM exercising is done. In assisted ROM exercise, the person initiates the movement, but the nurse may complete the full range of motion. For a paralyzed or unconscious person, passive ROM exercises are done, that is, initiating and completing the full range of motion by the nurse. The involved limb is supported at all times during the motion to prevent straining the muscles and ligaments.

Passive limb movement does not require muscle contractions as in active motion. Therefore, it is not effective for muscle conditioning, but it is effective in preventing joint contractures. Joint motion exercise is never carried out beyond the point of pain or resistance.

There are several types of exercises that contribute to *muscle conditioning*. The primary purpose of muscle conditioning exercise is to prevent muscular atrophy and weakening. However, because muscle exercise provides physical stress on other structures, it aids, to some extent, in promotion of general circulation and prevention of osteoporosis.

All active body movements, such as lifting and moving objects, induce isotonic exercise. In isotonic exercise, the muscle fibers shorten during the muscle contraction. This is distinguished from isometric exercise which occurs without acutal shortening of the muscle fibers. A setting exercise is an example of an isometric exercise. Muscle setting is accomplished simply by contracting or hardening of a group of muscles for 10 seconds by purposeful intension, and then releasing to relax. This type of exercise is effective in conditioning the abdominal, gluteal, and quadriceps muscles.

The use of isometric exercise requires a certain degree of caution. During the muscle-setting period, one's intrathoracic pressure increases due to trapping air against the closed epiglottis, a phenomenon called the Valsalva maneuver. The Valsalva maneuver may precipitate cardiac arrest in a person who has a damaged heart. This untoward reaction occurs because the increased intrathoracic pressure prevents normal cardiac input and subsequently decreases cardiac output and the coronary circulation. In any case, if this type of exercise is instituted, the person is taught to exhale during the muscle-setting period.

Resistive exercise is another form of muscle conditioning exercise. This exercise is done by pulling or pushing against a stationary object. Because of its pumping effect on the venous system, this type of exercise is effective not only for muscle conditioning, but also in stimulating venous return. Simple activity such as pushing the feet against a foot board is effective in conditioning the gastronemius and quadriceps muscles. Pulling on the trapeze bar is effective in conditioning upper arms and shoulder muscles. Basic nursing skills textbooks provide detailed steps for instituting these exercises. Further, the nurse works with the health care team that may include a physiotherapist or occupational therapist who have special expertise in this area.

An illustration of specific planning of nursing interventions to meet activity needs can be given for the person who suddenly is hospitalized with a broken pelvis suffered in an automobile accident. Two nursing diagnosis for this person are: (1) good muscle tone and 4+ muscle strength in major muscle groups of all four extremities due to knowledge of health benefits of fitness and commitment to regular exercise program and (2) potential for disuse consequences related to sudden, therapeutically enforced immobility and age of 62 years. A number of long- and short-term goals are indicated, each with interventions that identify the stimuli that can be managed to reach the goal.

For the goal: upper extremity muscle tone will be maintained at a good level and strength will be increased from 4+ to 5+ during the four weeks of acute care in preparation for use of arms and shoulders to bear weight on crutches during rehabilitation, the nurse plans a series of interventions. The patient is involved in self care activities as soon as possible after admission. Such simple activity as participating in bathing, combing one's hair, shaving or putting on make-up in bed allows the pulling and weight bearing of active movement. This is effective in muscle conditioning, as well as stimulating general circulation and promoting mobility of joints. Recognizing the person's knowledge of health benefits of and commitment to regular exercise, the nurse explains that even though the exercises done in the hospital will be different from the person's usual pattern of exercise, they are even more important at this time. The nurse describes the exercises and their specific purpose. Then, the patient can be involved in setting up a schedule of muscle strengthening exercises for the upper extremities that includes lifting on a trapeze bar, increasing the number of times and the frequency gradually. Since pushing and pulling against a stationary object is important, the nurse can use ingenuity to provide such an object, such as stabilizing the over-bed table.

To maintain an effective exercise program, the nurse focuses on the person's knowledge and commitment, the scheduled use of muscles that are the primary target, providing the equipment to complete the exercises, and an environment that does not restrict the program, such as having a conflicting schedule of therapies. For this particular patient, a chart of progress of muscle strength can be made. The patient and the nurse will recognize that some unavoidable muscle weakness may occur early in the program. However, keeping the long-term goal in mind is useful. Knowing that even if this goal is not achieved, the person will be better ready to undertake the next stage of rehabilitation than if the muscle strengthening program had not been instituted and carefully carried out, can be encouraging for both patient and nurse.

Some general measures for promoting quality rest and sleep by managing the major stimuli identified in Table 7–1 include: (1) provision of the physical comfort, (2) alleviation of psychological stresses, (3) structuring daily activity schedule, (4) structuring a restful environment, and (5) controlled use of hypnotic drugs and alcohol.

Since physical pain and discomfort are among the most common causes for disruption in rest and sleep, *providing physical comfort* is a method of relief from the disruption. Appropriate choice of timing of analgesic administration are important aids to promote rest and sleep. For patients in pain, the nurse is not concerned with long-term drug dependency (see Chapter 9), however, the choice of drug is made carefully so that the person does not experience the consequences of REM sleep deprivation. Good personal hygiene aids physical comfort and thus improves the quality of one's rest and sleep. A warm bath can be relaxing. Food intake, for some persons spicy food, may interfere with sleep. This possibility as well as whether or not the person is hungry is dicussed with the person and remedied as appropriate. Soothing backrubs can be comforting and effective in inducing sleep.

As noted earlier, mere physical inactivity does not provide good quality rest. *Alleviation of psychological stress* may be necessary to allow for rest and sleep. The nurse provides the person with opportunities to ventilate feelings of fear, anxiety, and frustration. In a hospital setting, lack of knowledge or understanding of what is happening often generates feelings of powerlessness. These feelings trigger anxiety. (See Chapter 16.) Sometimes it is a misperception or incorrect understanding that causes unnecessary anxiety. The nurse is in a position to check out the patient's understanding of the situation, and the particular meaning it has for him or her. She is sensitive to a person's subtle, as well as obvious, behaviors that indicate distress that can interfere with restful sleep. From the person's perspective, then, she can help him or her deal appropriately with these factors, focal or contextual, that are interfering with rest and sleep.

For persons either at home, or in the hospital, anxiety about not sleeping may be the psychological stress that is focal in disturbing sleep. Researchers have noted that trying too hard to sleep aggravates sleep problems. When struggling with the need for sleep, and inability to fall asleep, feelings of anxiety, frustration, and anger may trigger arousal and tension. Practical interventions to deal with these situations have been suggested (Bootzin and Nicassio 1978): go to bed only when sleepy; use the bed only for sexual activity and sleeping (not reading or watching television); if unable to fall asleep in about 20 minutes, get up, go to another room until sleepy; turn the clock toward the wall; with wakefulness during the night, likewise, get up and return to bed only when sleepy; finally, awake at the same time every day and do not take daytime naps. Eventually, going to bed is associated with rapid falling asleep.

As noted earlier, physical activity induces NREM sleep, therefore adequate amounts of *physical activity,* within the indiviudal's restrictions, are worked into the daily schedule. However, any vigorous physical activity or events that trigger strong emotional responses are avoided near bedtime. Every effort is made to ensure that the sleep cycles can take their full course so that the person will not suffer from REM sleep deprivation. Treatment procedures and other activites are grouped together in such a way that the number of interruptions is kept to a minimum. Each sleep cycle takes 60 to 120 minutes. Therefore, scheduling the interruptions at longer than 2-hour intervals will allow each sleep cycle to take its full course. A large amount of food and fluid taken in the late evening will require unnecessarily frequent arousals caused by increased gastrointestinal and bladder stimulations. Any drugs that have a diuretic effect are not administered at bedtime. For healthy persons, moderate exercise used consistently can lengthen and deepen sleep.

In *structuring a restful environment,* the nurse takes into consideration the individual's personal habits and bedtime routine. The environment in general is to be free of all kinds of noxious stimuli. Room temperature, light, noise, and odor are checked out for suitability. Unavoidable, but unpleasant noise can be disguised by pleasant music. People will differ in the degree of quiet needed for restful sleep, some needing absolute quiet and others preferring some background noise. Increasingly, it is possible to arrange the environment differently for each patient as more hospital rooms are private rooms. The effects on one's sleep of a strange environment usually does not last more than 3 or 4 days and this information can help the person not have increased anxiety about changes in sleep pattern in the hospital.

Special care units present problems in establishing a restful environment by reason of their equipment and activities. Nonetheless, the nurse strives to make this environment as conducive to rest and sleep as possible. The nurse can emphasize a sense of security in the constant watchfulness of the person's condition throughout the night. The careful scheduling of activities as noted is particularly relevant in these settings. In this case, however, activity for one patient may affect another patient more readily because of the setup of many units. Sometimes it is staff conversation, a stimuli easily managed by the nurse, that is most disturbing to the patient.

Lastly, hypnotic drugs are controlled carefully and used in selected situations for sleep since they have been identified as related to quality of sleep and rest. The same is true of alcohol, particularly when it is used habitually for sleep. The nurse explains that such substances are effective on a short-term basis only and that they tend to supress restful or REM sleep. The person is encouraged to restrict their use. The nurse then assists the person to find alternate means to promote sleep.

Given the scope and variety of settings and situations that call for individually designed nursing interventions to assist persons with activity and rest needs, careful evaluation of the effectiveness of these interventions is particularly important.

Evaluation

As in each of the modes of adaptation, with activity and rest needs, the evaluation phase of the nursing process reflects the behavioral assessment. In the example given earlier, a person who is suffering sleep pattern disturbance related to new job responsibilities, returns to the clinic with the same behaviors that the nurse noted one week earlier, that is, difficulty falling asleep and frequent arousals from sleep during the night, as well as reddened eyes, puffy eyelids, dark circles under the eyes, and feelings of poor sleep. This person also reports continuing concerns about the responsibilities associated with the job promotion. As related by the patient, these concerns have been intensified by difficulty in identifying in writing the two major responsibilities that are of concern and frustration in trying to develop strategies to handle this part of the job. The person is also more anxious about the sleep disturbance and struggles with efforts to go to sleep and with concern about meeting the short term goal set for beginning to handle the difficulty. The nurse notes evidence of unclear and slightly confused thinking (see Chapter 11), possibly related to on-going sleep disturbance.

Since the behaviors of interest have not changed and the nurse is concerned about the increasing behavioral signs of the problem worsening, she provides the person with specific instructions for moderate active exercises at noontime and relaxation exercises to use at bedtime. She also decides to have the patient evaluated for prescription of a short-term hypnotic. She then asks the person to come back for a morning appointment in three days, after getting some sleep, when they can work together on the problem. The goal of identifying in writing the two major job responsibilities that are of most concern, and for the one that is most distressing considering several alternate ways of dealing with it, will again be attempted. The nurse will provide guidance in the use of a problem solving process. This example shows a revision in the intervention plan based on evaluation of an ineffective intervention and assessment of additional behaviors.

SUMMARY

In this chapter, the Roy Adaptation Model was used as a perspective from which to view activity and rest needs. A theoretical basis related to these needs was developed which includes the structures and functions involved. Each step of the nursing process was discussed and demonstrated with examples of behavior and stimuli, of nursing diagnoses, goals, and interventions, as well as associated evaluation of the effectiveness of nursing care.

Chapters in this part of the text focus on basic needs and life processes. Each is treated separately to develop as clear a background understanding of each as possible. Yet throughout the chapters the interrelatedness of each is seen. Further, it will be remembered that the understanding of the person as a whole comes only with the realization of how all human life processes act to make a living, thinking, moving, feeling person.

EXERCISES FOR APPLICATION

1. Identify the factors that influence (focal and contextual stimuli) the amount of physical activity you engaged in on a particular day in the past week.

2. Develop a tool that can be used in the assessment of rest and sleep. In your tool consider both the usual pattern and current condition.
3. Using the tool developed in item 2, assess rest and sleep needs of one person under 25 and one person over 60 years of age.

ASSESSMENT OF UNDERSTANDING

Situation

Mrs. L. is a 73-year-old widow with a social history of no known relatives or close friends who can visit her during her hospital stay. Following a major surgical procedure for a fractured left femur, she is placed on the activity restriction of complete bed rest. Without a properly planned preventive nursing intervention, Mrs. L. likely will develop some of the very serious disuse consequences.

For Mrs. L., identify the disuse consequences that can occur in three of the following bodily functions: (a) metabolic, (b) musculoskeletal, (c) circulatory, (d) pulmonary, (e) eliminative, (f) integumentory, and (g) sensory perceptual.

1. _____
2. _____
3. _____

Understanding that repair and restoration take place during rest and sleep, you are trying to improve the quality of sleep for Mrs. L. Please list at least two major nursing interventions to accomplish this.

4. _____
5. _____

6. Discuss several ways in which activity and rest are important in maintaining health.

Feedback

1, 2, and 3. Any three of the following:

a. Negative nitrogen balance
b. Muscular atrophy
   Osteoporosis
   Joint contractures
   Denervations
c. Postural hypotension
   Dependent edema
   Thrombosis
   Cardiac deconditioning
d. Hypoventilation
e. Urinary retention
   Nephrolithiasis
   Constipation

    f. Decubiti ulceration

    g. Disorientation, confusion or anxiety

4 and 5. Any two of the following:

    a. Maintain physical comfort and freedom from pain.

    b. Maintain an adequate amount of physical activity in order to induce deep sleep.

    c. Limit nightime interruptions to a minimum to allow full cycles of sleep to take place.

    d. Alleviate psychological stress which may increase need for REM sleep.

6. Activity contributes to physical fitness by promoting all the usual body processes and it prevents disuse consequences. Furthermore, it promotes adequate rest and particularly the stage of deep sleep. Although the functions of sleep continue to be studied, it is known that inadequate sleep and rest very quickly affect a person and one's ability to perform roles. Changes that occur with sleep disturbances include poor neuromuscular coordination and also signs of cognator ineffectiveness manifested as general irritability, inability to concentrate, disorientation, and confusion. Studies describing the stages of sleep, and the physical changes within the stages that lead to the assumption that the changes that occur during sleep are part of the normal daily rhythm of life. People need relaxation and restoration of energy. Activity and rest, including sleep, are part of a cycle of energy expenditure and restoration.

REFERENCES

American Sleep Disorders Association. *The International Classification of Sleep Disorders Diagnostic and Coding Manual.* American Sleep Disorders Association, Rochester, MN: 1990.

Anders, E., and E. Parmelee, Eds. *A Manual of Standardized Terminology and Criteria for Scoring States of Sleep and Wakefulness in Newborn Infants.* Los Angeles: University of California, Brain Information Service, 1971.

American Nurses' Association and American Association of Neuroscience Nurses. *Neuroscience Nursing Practice: Process and Outcome Standards for Selecting Diagnoses.* Kansas City, Mo.: American Nurses' Association, 1985.

Bootzin, R. and P. Nicassio. Behavioral treatments for insomnia, in *Progress in Behavioral Modification,* eds. Hersen R. Eisler, and P. Miller. New York: Academic Press, 1987.

Brooks, V. *The Neural Basis of Motor Control.* New York: Oxford University Press, 1986.

Cho, J. Activity and rest, in *Introduction to Nursing: An Adaptation Model,* Sr. C. Roy, p. 138–158. Englewood Cliffs, N.J.: Prentice-Hall, 1984.

Dworetzky, T. Dextor, the willowy six-footer that bends at the waist, *Discover,* (October), 18, 1987.

Hilton, J. Quantity and quality of patients sleep disturbing factors in a respiratory intensive care unit, *Journal of Advanced Nursing*, 1, 453–468, 1976.

Hobson, J. The cellular basis of sleep cycle control, *Advances in Sleep Research*, 1: 217–250, 1974.

Hodges, L., and C. Callihan. Human mobility: An overview, in *AANN's Neuroscience Nursing*, eds. Mitchell P. et al. E. Norwalk, Conn.: Appleton & Lange, 269–281, 1988.

Hollerbach, A. Assessment of human mobility, in *AANN's Neuroscience Nursing*, eds. Mitchell, P. et al. E. Norwalk, Conn.: Appleton & Lange, 283–302, 1988.

Mills, L. *Sleep Questionnaire and Assessment of Wakefulness (SQAW)*. Stanford, Calif.: Stanford Sleep Disorders and Sleep Research Program. As reprinted in Guilleminault, C. *Sleeping and Waking Disorders: Indications and Techniques*. Menlo Park, Calif.: Addison-Wesley, 383–413, 1979.

Mourad, L. Musculoskeletal system, in *Clinical Nursing*, eds. Thompson, J. et al. St. Louis: The C. V. Mosby Company, 427–541, 1986.

Opstad, P. et al. Performance, mood, and clinical symptoms in men exposed to prolonged, severe physical work and sleep deprivation, *Aviation, Space and Environmental Medicine*, 49: 1065–1073, 1979.

Oswald, I. Why do we sleep? *Nursing Mirror*, 138:71, 1976.

Pasnau, R. et al. The psychological effects of 205 hours of sleep deprivation, *Archives of General Psychiatry*, 18:496–505, 1968.

Rechtschaffen, A., and A. Kales, Eds. *A Manual for Standardized Terminology, Techniques and Scoring System for Sleep Stages of Human Subjects*. Los Angeles: University of California, Brain Information Service, 1983.

Robinson, C. Impaired sleep, in *Pathophysiological Phenomena in Nursing*, eds. Carrieri, V., A. Lindsey, and C. West. Philadelphia: W.B. Saunders Company, 390–417, 1986.

Rubin, M. The physiology of bedrest, *American Journal of Nursing*. 88:55, 1988.

Rubin, M. How bedrest changes perception, *American Journal of Nursing*, 88:55, 1988.

Sacks, O. *Awakenings*. New York: Dutton, 1983.

Sassin, J. Neurological findings following short-term sleep deprivation, *Archives of Neurology*, 39:187–190, 1970.

Schreier, A. Nursing diagnoses pattern 13, Activity and rest: Sleep pattern disturbance, in *Clinical nursing*, eds. Thompson, J. et al. St. Louis: The C.V. Mosby Company, 2099–2104, 1986.

Sleep Disorders Classification Committee, Association of Sleep Disorders Centers. Diagnostic classification of sleep and arousal disorders, *Sleep*. 2: 137, 1979.

Additional References

Bartley, D. et al. Physical fitness and psychological well being, *Health Education*, 1813: 57–60, 1987.

Ben-Shlomo L.S. et al. The effects of physical conditioning on selected dimensions of self concept in sedentary female, *Occupational Therapy-Mental Health*, 5(4): 27–46, 1986.

Canavan, T. The sychobiology of sleep, *Nursing* 84: 682, 1984.

Dement, W. The effect of dream deprivation, *Science* 131: 1705–1707, 1960.

Downs, F. Bestrest and sensory disturbances, *American Journal of Nursing*, 74: 434–438, 1974.

Dunn M. Guideline for an effective personal fitness prescription, *Nurse Practice,* 12 (9): 9–10, 1987.

Hoch, C., and C. Reynolds, III. Sleep disturbances and what to do about them, *Geriatric Nursing,* 7: 24, 1986.

Kerr, E.H. Exercise and health related fitness, *Physiotherapy.* 74 (8): 411–20, 1988.

Kryger, M., T. Roth, and W. Dement. *Principles and Practice of Sleep Medicine.* Philadelphia: W.B. Saunders Company, 1989.

Shannon, M.L. Five famous fallacies about pressure sores, *Nursing,* 84: 13–34, 1984.

Walsenben, J. Sleep disorders, *American Journal of Nursing,* 88:50, 1982.

Chapter Eight

Protection*

Marsha Keiko Sato

Protection is the last of the five physiological needs identified in the Roy Adaptation Model. The protection processes help to maintain a person's physiological integrity. The neurological, reticuloendothelial, and endocrine systems carry out complex activities that promote this integrity and defend against harmful internal and external stimuli. Protection is also a major function of the skin, although the processes involved are less complex. This chapter focuses on skin integrity and immunity as basic physiological needs that provide a protective function for the person.

OBJECTIVES

After studying this chapter, the reader will be able to do the following:

1. Describe protection as a physiological need.
2. Assess behaviors related to protection.
3. Identify major stimuli associated with the process of protection.
4. Given a situation, construct a nursing diagnosis for a patient with a disruption of the need for protection.
5. Given a situation, derive goals for a patient with protection problems.
6. Identify stimuli which may be managed as interventions in a situation of protection disruption.
7. Propose evaluative approaches to determine the effectiveness of nursing interventions.

*This chapter is a revision of the chapter "Skin Integrity" in *Introduction to Nursing: An Adaptation Model* (2nd ed.), Marsha Keiko Sato. Englewood Cliffs, N.J.: Prentice-Hall, pp. 159–167, 1984.

KEY CONCEPTS DEFINED

- *Alopecia:* continuous loss of hair in large amounts.
- *Cyanosis:* dusky blue or gray coloring for Caucasians and blue or dark brown coloring for dark-skinned people due to a lack of oxygen.
- *Immunity:* the capacity of the human body to resist almost all types of organisms or toxins that tend to damage the tissues and organs.
    Acquired immunity: the ability of the body to develop specific immunity against individual invading agents.
    Active immunity: the process by which the body is stimulated to produce its own antibodies in response to the administration of inactivated vaccines and toxoids.
    Innate immunity: immunity present at birth.
- *Jaundice:* yellow coloring of the skin caused by the breakdown of bile pigment.
- *Protection:* the process whereby the person's skin, hair, nails, and immune system function in such a manner as to help ensure body integrity and wholeness.
- *Pruritis:* severe itching.
- *Ulcer:* open crater on the skin or mucous membrane characterized by the disintegration of the tissue.

STRUCTURES AND FUNCTIONS RELATED TO PROTECTION

Protection, according to the Roy Adaptation Model, is one of five needs associated with physiological integrity. The structures involved in protection include the skin, hair, nails, and the immune system. These components serve to protect the person from internal and external stimuli that threaten body functioning and affect one's level of adaptation.

The skin, hair, and nails function as protective mechanisms for the human body by providing a physical barrier against infection and foreign matter. The skin generally serves as effective protection since the epidermis is able to repel many chemical compounds. Certain parts of the body such as the palms and soles have thicker skin to prevent the occurrence of trauma.

The entire body is covered with hair excluding the palms of the hands and the soles of the feet. Hair functions as a protective mechanism by helping to retain body heat and increasing the sensation of touch. The eyes are shielded by eyelashes and eyebrows which help to exclude foreign objects. The hair in the ears and nose have the same function.

The fingers and toes are protected by the nails, epidermal cells that have been converted to keratin. The nails function as a protective mechanism for the fingers and toes by safeguarding their sensory abilities and assisting with the manipulation of small objects.

The process of *immunity* is the capacity of the human body to resist almost all types of organisms or toxins that tend to damage the tissue and organs. Immunity, then has a major protective function for the adapting person. There are two types of immunity, innate and acquired. *Innate immunity* is present at birth and results from general processes including phagocytosis, the activity of acid secretions and digestive enzymes, and the ability of chemical compounds in the blood to attack and destroy. In addition, the human body has the ability to develop specific immunity against individual invading agents such as bacteria, viruses, toxins, and foreign tissue. This is *acquired immunity.*

There are two basic types of acquired immunity. *Humoral immunity* is the type of acquired immunity whereby the body develops circulating antibodies, that is, globulin molecules, that are capable of attacking the invading agent. The second type of acquired immunity is closely related to the first. In this process, there is the formation of large numbers of activated lymphocytes specifically designed to destroy the foreign agent. The term *cell-mediated immunity* is used for this type of active immunity. Both the antibodies and the activated lymphocytes are formed in the lymphoid tissue.

Through the process of *active immunity,* the body is stimulated to produce its own antibodies in response to the administration of inactivated vaccines and toxoids. Active immunization is one of the most effective preventative tools in maintaining adaptation against micro-organisms.

APPLICATION OF THE NURSING PROCESS

The nurse's role in relation to the need for protection is to understand the associated processes well and to plan support for these natural processes. Often this support takes the form of providing information for the person and more specific activities of health teaching. Through preventive measures, potential problems associated with protection can be avoided. When problematic situations occur, early initiation of nursing intervention and treatment can divert further complications. Two important aspects of the goal of nursing relative to this fifth physiological need are protecting the skin and promoting immunity as preventive measures.

The following section addresses each of the six steps of the nursing process as they relate to the need for protection.

Assessment of Behavior
Assessment of behavior relative to the need for protection can be divided into six major components: assessment of the skin, the scalp and hair,

perspiration, sensitivity to pain and temperature, the operative site, and the person's immunological status. Skills associated with inspection and palpation are particularly important for assessment of protection behaviors. Adequate lighting and a transparent, flexible ruler for the measurement of lesions are tools required in the assessment process.

The Skin. The nurse assesses a person's skin temperature with the back of the fingers. The normal, adaptive skin temperature is warm to the touch. Increased warmth, in general, is caused by an increase in blood flow as a result of the body's immune process. Increased coolness is frequently the result of reduced blood flow in order to supply the vital organs when in shock. Local coolness is commonly found in the extremities and is again caused by a decreased flow of blood and/or the effects of peripheral vascular disease.

The nurse observes for the presence of skin lesions which are manifest in a myriad of forms. The principal responsibility of the nurse is to describe the lesions accurately according to distribution, location, size, contour, and consistency. The adaptive behavior is a skin free of excoriations or lesions.

Skin lesions related to sexually transmitted diseases such as herpes genitalis have become of major significance to nurses and the public because of their rising incidence (Bruner and Snygg 1989). Herpes genitalis initially appears as a blister or pimple progressing to an ulcerated state and is generally located on the vagina, cervix, and female/male external genitalia.

The Scalp and Hair. The nurse observes the condition of the scalp while combing or washing the person's hair. The scalp should be smooth, moist, and clean. The presence of cysts, dandruff, or scabs would be considered unexpected or ineffective behaviors.

The distribution of the person's hair is assessed, bearing in mind that there are many normal variations. Variations that warrant further assessment are alopecia, that is, unexpected general or local hair loss, a noticeable change in the character of the hair, excessive hair growth in women, and the disappearance of body hair from an area where it normally is present. Observations also are made about the cleanliness of the hair. The expected adaptive behavior is the presence of clean hair in normal distribution and consistency on the head, extremities, trunk, pubic area, and face.

Perspiration. The nurse assesses the quantity, color, and location of perspiration on the body. Perspiration has a protective function in control of the amount of heat loss from the body. When a person has an elevated temperature, the quantity of perspiration increases in an attempt to cool the body. The adaptive behavior for perspiration is a musty, salty, or sour odor. Perspiration is termed "malodorous" if it is particularly offensive, a situation caused by the breakdown of bacterial products found on the skin.

Sensitivity to Pain and Temperature. Assessment of a person's level of sensitivity to pain and temperature is important for persons who lack this protective function since the defense mechanism of withdrawal from danger is decreased. This withdrawal behavior may be elicited for the assessment process by testing the person's perception of warm and cold objects applied to an area or by touching the person with a pin and asking if the sensation was experienced. The expected behavior is skin that is sensitive to pain and temperature.

Pain and Skin Condition Related to an Operative Incision. The nurse carefully assesses postoperative pain and skin condition as it relates to the incisional area. Persons having surgery are expected to experience pain as a protective response following an incision. The duration of the pain depends on the nature of the surgery and on the person's tolerance of pain. The presence of pain is identified through the observation of activities such as crying, tense positioning, tightening of facial muscles, and through patient statements. In describing the pain experience, the nurse must note the type, duration, and location of the pain. Further discussion of pain is found in chapter 9 on the senses.

The nurse assesses skin integrity at the operative site by observing the color of the skin, whether the sutures or adhesive strips are intact, and the presence or absence of drainage. If drainage is present, the nurse must note the color, amount, and odor. The patient's phagocytic immune response and humoral-mediated immune response operate protective functions which cause the drainage and odor.

Immunological Status. In assessment of an individual's status relative to communicable diseases, several areas of behavior are of concern. It is important to know what communicable diseases the person has had or has been immunized against. In some chronic and degenerative diseases such as leukemia and aquired immune deficiency syndrome (AIDS), the individual's immunological protection is compromised. The complications prompting the person's need for care are a result of ineffective or absent immunological responses of the body. The nurse anticipates that persons with such diagnoses will demonstrate many ineffective behaviors related to the need for protection. For example, there may be evidence of infectious processes within the body such as symptoms associated with pneumonia.

As the nurse identifies the person's behaviors relative to the need for protection, an initial evaluation is made as to whether these behaviors are adaptive or ineffective. To guide this evaluation, the nurse uses knowledge of related normal physiological functioning, established normal values, and the person's report of what is "normal" or adaptive for him or her. In consultation with the patient and/or family, the nurse establishes the tentative identification of adaptive and ineffective behaviors. With initial priorities being the ineffective behaviors, the nurses then proceeds to identify the related stimuli.

Assessment of Stimuli

Assessment of stimuli involves the identification of the factors that appear to be influencing the person's behavior. Common stimuli affecting protection include developmental stage, environmental considerations, integrity of the adaptive modes, and cognator effectiveness.

Developmental Stage. Infants are prone to skin disorders because their skin structures are functionally immature. The infant dehydrates easily because the epidermis is very permeable. Milia and cradle cap are common protective behaviors caused by the increased activity of the sebaceous glands during late fetal life and early infancy. Temperature regulation is more labile in the neonate since the skin has an immature ability to shiver in response to cold or perspire in response to heat.

During the adolescent period, the sebaceous glands become extremely active and increase in size. The condition of the skin may be disrupted by the development of acne.

The behavioral manifestations of skin integrity for an elderly person are affected by the aging process. Skin pigmentation becomes uneven due to the clustering of melanocytes. The elasticity of the skin is decreased and the skin is more delicate as a result of decreased hydration and vascularity of the dermis. Lines and wrinkles appear as a result of the loss of subcutaneous fat. The hair becomes thicker in the nose and ears while the scalp hair grays and thins. The nails become hard and brittle.

The immune process also is affected with aging. The older person encounters a greater number of infections which are more severe in nature and this may be the result of the body's inability to trigger an effective immune response. It appears that the production and function of the T- and B-cell lymphocytes are affected in some manner as the aging process proceeds.

Environmental Conditions. Many environmental stimuli influence the process of protection. For example, environmental stimuli that influence perspiration include room temperature, the amount of circulating air, and humidity. Other factors that influence perspiration include the thickness of clothing worn and personal hygiene measures, such as frequency of bathing and the use of soaps and deodorants. Increased exercise or activity and stressful or anxiety-producing situations also contribute to increased perspiration.

Cold weather as an environmental stimulus contributes to dry skin, whereas exposure to the sun may burn the skin. Poison ivy, urine, feces, soap, and some medications may irritate the skin and this may lead to the development of a rash.

Medications such as antibiotics, cytotoxic drugs, corticosteroids, and nonsteroidal anti-inflammatory drugs may suppress the immune response and are important stimuli to consider. The stimulus of radiation, as used in treatment for cancer, has the potential to cause severe disruption to the integrity of the skin. Radiation also affects the immune process by killing the lymphocytes and diminishing the number of cells available to replenish them.

Integrity of the Adaptive Modes. There are a variety of internal conditions that affect the manifestation of behaviors related to protection. The cardiopulmonary status of a person is a stimulus for the color of skin. Cyanosis reflects hypoxia caused by either heart or lung disease. Hormonal disorders may be responsible for the loss of hair. The pathological condition of diabetes is an influencing factor for decreased sensation experienced in the feet. The process of infection/inflammation alters the surface of the skin by the presence of exudate and necrosis of tissue. Infection may be the cause of thickening of the nails and infectious states or disease may cause an elevation in body temperature and influence the amount of perspiration.

Burns and other forms of trauma have the potential to alter the immune process. The skin integrity, the body's first line of defense, is disrupted. Persons with burns lose large amounts of serum which deprives the body of essential proteins and immunoglobulins. In the surgical patient, the serum cortisol level is increased from stimulation of the immunosuppressive action of the adrenal cortex.

Certain disease processes (cancer, for example) suppress the immune process. Large tumors expel antigens which attach to the circulating antibodies and render them ineffective in destroying the cancerous cells while some tumor cells are resistant to the killer T-lymphocytes (Pitot 1981).

Alteration in skin integrity relates to changes in the barrier function of the skin. The focal stimuli are probably a combination of prolonged pressure over the bony areas, anoxia, ischemia, and immobility. Poor nutrition, anemia, extreme debilitation, and edema are contributing factors. Moisture such as soiled or wet bed clothes and heat increase the likelihood of developing a pressure sore. The pulling up of patients in bed creates friction and a shearing force on the skin, a stimulus affecting the breakdown. Elderly persons are prone to the development of pressure sores because their skin is thin and fragile.

Cognator Effectiveness. The person's perception, knowledge and skill are often factors that interfere with adaptation as related to protection.

Nutritional status affects the overall condition of the skin, hair, and nails. Pale-appearing skin may be due to anemia caused by a diet low in iron. Good nutrition also is necessary for a properly functioning immune system. When the amount of protein is diminished, it causes a depressed antibody response, decreased numbers of T-cells, and ineffective phagocytic activity. Hair loss is evident in those suffering from some nutritional disturbances. Psychological disturbances are sometimes manifest through skin disruptions such as rashes, itching, and acne.

Research is beginning to demostrate relationships between emotional status and the immune system. According to Santrock (1989), research in the field of psychoneuroimmunoloy is exploring connections among psychological factors, such as emotions and attitudes, the nervous system, and the immune system. For example, depression is thought to affect adversly and suppress the immune system.

Associated with cognator effectiveness is the person's knowledge about prevention and early detection of disease processes. Prevention and health promotion increasingly are becoming a major focus of health care systems throughout the world. Immunization programs provide people with the opportunity to avoid may diseases that, in times past, claimed many lives. For example, flu immunizations are available in many areas to prevent particular strains of influenza from infecting susceptible individuals in the population.

Knowledge about communicability, diagnosis, and treatment of sexually transmitted diseases is becoming increasingly important. In many areas, programs are being mounted to assist in the education of the public relative to prevention of and protection against this widespread health problem. Of particular significance in the 1990s is acquired immune deficiency syndrome (AIDS), described by the U.S. Secretary of Health and Human Services (Marieb 1989) as the "plague of the twentieth century." According to the U.S. Department of Labor, Occupational Safety and Health Administration (1989), the incidence of AIDS has risen from less than 60 cases in the early 1980s to more than 88,000 reported cases in 1989. As Rogers (1989) indicated, by 1992 it is projected that there will be 365,000 reported cases of AIDS and as many as 263,000 deaths attributed to the syndrome.

AIDS is characterized by its overwhelming effect on the body's immune system. As Marieb (1989) described, "the whole immune system is turned topsy-turvy": a profound deficit of normal antibodies develops, suppressor T-cell activity often is enhanced and abnormal antibodies are produced. "The course of AIDS is inexorable, finally ending in complete debilitation and death from cancer or overwhelming infection (Marieb 1989)."

Education of the public is important in the prevention of AIDS and early detection of other disease processes. For example, breast and testicular self-examination have been demonstrated effective in the early detection and treatment of cancerous tumors. It is important for the nurse to assess the person's understanding and practice of these preventive and health promotion activities.

Once the stimuli associated with the ineffective and adaptive behaviors have been identified, the nurse, in consultation with the patient, establishes their focal, contextual, or residual influence on the person. This classification assists the nurse in setting priorities in the subsequent steps of the nursing process. The information obtained in the assessment steps is then used to formulate nursing diagnoses.

Nursing Diagnosis

As noted earlier, Roy has described three ways of stating a nursing diagnosis: (1) as a statement of the behaviors within one mode with the most relevant influencing stimuli, (2) as a summary label for behaviors in one mode with relevant stimuli, or (3) as a label that summarizes a behavioral pattern when more than one mode is being affected by the same stimuli. The nursing diagnosis thus relates behavior and stimuli in an attempt to describe the major areas of concern for adaptation of the person.

Indicators of effective adaptation relative to the need for protection would be evident in nursing diagnoses statements such as "intact skin free of excoriations and lesions due to nutritious diet and conscientious hygiene," or "profuse perspiration due to outside temperature of 102°F." In the latter situation, perspiration is the body's method of adapting to warm temperatures in the external environment.

Common adaptation problems, or broad areas of concern, within the component of protection include pressure sores (decubitus ulcers) and itching (pruritis). Pressure sores occur frequently in the elderly and those who are immobilized; they result from disrupted circulation to the affected tissue. (Issues related to immobility are discussed further in Chap. 7.) A relevant nursing diagnosis for this adaptation problem could be "pressure sore on left lateral ankle due to prolonged pressure and immobility." Indicators of positive adaptation related to the problem of pressure sores would be the maintenance of skin integrity with the absence of skin infection.

Alteration in comfort related to skin lesions is often termed "itching." The focal stimulus for itching may be a skin disorder resulting from a systemic disease or pregnancy. An allergic reaction (immune response), local lesion, dry skin, and emotional upset are other influencing factors. The time of day is a contextual stimulus since itching is often worse at night when there are fewer things on which to focus. A warm environment also increases the desire to itch. A nursing diagnosis reflecting this adaptation problem is "itching related to contact with poison ivy." Once the nursing diagnoses have been established, the nurse proceeds to the next step of the nursing process—goal setting. The priority nursing diagnoses, those relating to the ineffective behaviors and the focal stimuli, would be given initial consideration although the importance of maintaining adaptive behavior is acknowledged.

Goal Setting

Goal setting within the Roy Adaptation Model involves the establishing of clear statements of behavioral outcomes of nursing care for the person. Goals may be either short term or long term but must identify specific behaviors to be demonstrated by the person as well as the time frame and the manner in which the behavior will change. As with each previous step of the nursing process, the person must be involved in whatever way possible in the fomulation of these goals.

In the example of the nursing diagnosis "pressure sore on left lateral ankle due to prolonged pressure and immobility," a relevant goal would focus on the pressure sore. A short-term goal could be, "Within one week the pressure sore on the left ankle will decrease in diameter from 1 inch to 1/2 inch." In this goal, the behavior relates to the size of the pressure sore and the healing that is expected to occur, the time frame is "within one week" and the change is the decrease in the diameter of the sore.

Another example of goal setting illustrates the importance of focusing on the maintenance of effective adaptation. The situation pertains to the postoperative status of the incision (a disruption in skin integrity that could lead to ineffective adaptation should an infection develop). The nursing diagnosis indicates that the patient has an incision with a dressing resulting from surgery to the abdomen. A goal statement focuses on the status of the incision: "Within two days, incisional edges will be approximated with evidence of normal healing and the absence of infection." Here, the behavior focuses on the healing of the incision, the time frame is within two days, and the change expected is the evidence of normal healing, the approximation of the wound edges, and the absence of infection.

Although the goals illustrated pertain to situations in which skin integrity has been disrupted, it is important for the nurse to derive goals aimed at preservation of the protective functions of the body. Within this context are many preventive and health promoting goals relating to protection. A nurse in a community agency may establish a goal for an infant that pertains to immunization status at a particular age. For example, "At four years of age, the child will demonstrate active immunity against the common communicable childhood diseases." The behavior associated with this goal is "immunity."

Once the behavioral goals have been established, the nurse proceeds to identify the nursing interventions most likely to assist in the achievement of the desired outcomes.

Intervention

Nursing intervention in the Roy Adaptation Model involves the management of stimuli through the selection and implementation of approaches.

In order to promote adaptation, it may be necessary to change the focal stimulus or to broaden the adaptation level by managing other stimuli present in the situation. Management of stimuli may involve altering, increasing, decreasing, removing, or maintaining stimuli. In selecting approaches, the nurse considers possible alternatives and then selects the approach with the highest possibility of obtaining the desired results.

Frequent positioning of the immobilized patient assists in promoting circulation by ensuring that bony prominences are cushioned against pressure. The body's internal protective response is facilitated through programs of immunization in the community agencies. Many health promotion programs have been designed to assist individuals in protecting and promoting their own health by early detection of disease processes. Each of these examples can be viewed as attempts to manage stimuli that compromise the person's protective processes.

Many of the nursing interventions associated with aseptic technique are directed at the control of micro-organisms and the minimization of inflammatory and infectious responses of the body. For example, preoperative skin cleansing and shaving are attempts to manage the opportunity for foreign substances (hair and micro-organisms) to enter the incisional site. Both are aimed at the prevention of infection.

Specific interventions are directed at control of adaptation problems related to protection. Interventions to control itching include soothing baths, trimming the nails, and the use of firm pressure instead of scratching. For localized itching, the application of cool, wet compresses may be used. Temperature control and the use of diversionary activities such as watching television are other suggested interventions.

There are many interventions applicable to the care of pressure sores. Frequent changing of the person's body position, at least every two hours, is an important nursing measure. In addition to the right and left lateral and dorsal positions, the person should be placed in the prone position also unless it is contraindicated. The prone position allows pressure to be relieved from the bony prominences such as the sacrum and promotes air circulation to the area. If the person is fairly immobilized, the nurse can give back rubs and massage the bony prominences at every shift. Adjusting the person's body weight by using a small folded towel or sheepskin under a hip or shoulder has been effective in promoting blood return to the area. Foot cradles, heel protectors, and egg crate mattresses are also useful aids to reduce pressure on the skin. Many hospitals are supplied with air-fluidized beds or low-air-loss beds which greatly relieve the pressure experienced by the body in the lying position.

The nurse observes the skin color of the person and notes localized areas of red, blue, or mottled skin, which indicate decreased circulation. Rubbing around these areas helps restore circulation. If the skin integrity becomes disrupted as in the case of a pressure sore, then other interventions are necessary. Consider the goal cited: "Within 1 week the pressure

sore on the left ankle will decrease in diameter from 1 inch to 1/2 inch."
Interventions aimed at achievement of this goal are directed at the stimuli causing the problem, that is, immobility, lack of circulation to the area, and the further complicating possibility of infection from microorganisms.

Pressure sores need to be cleansed as an intervention to fight the infectious process and help in the regeneration of epithelium. Necrotic tissue may be removed through the application of proteolytic enzymes (substances composed of streptokinase, fibrinolysin, and collagenase). After debridement, the pressure sore is flushed with the prescribed solution and a topical medication can be applied. A wet-to-dry dressing or a moist dressing is placed over the pressure sore to protect the new tissue growth from infection and to maintain hydration.

Nursing interventions may be directed at the prevention of pressure sores. To decrease the stimulus of moisture on the skin, the patient and bed need to be clean and dry. Lifting persons instead of pulling and keeping the bed wrinkle free decrease the problem of friction. A diet high in protein and vitamins is essential to the repair of tissue. The application of lotion helps to keep the skin soft and intact.

Protection is a component of the physiological mode where nursing interventions often focus on the maintenance of adaptive behaviors in an effort to prevent adaptation problems. Thus, many interventions are protective and preventive in nature. Specifically, nurses are very conscientious in their efforts to minimize the opportunity for infectious processes to enter the body. For example, herpes genitalis is a sexually transmitted disease and much can be done in the form of prevention. Nurses are functioning in positions where they can help to prevent the spread of such infections through a program of counseling and education. It is important that nurses maintain current knowledge regarding sexually transmitted diseases and their treatment.

Protective and preventive interventions are particularly important as they pertain to the increasing incidence of AIDS mentioned earlier in this chapter. Nursing measures associated with the prevention of the spread of AIDS and the care of the increasing numbers of hospitalized person's in the final stages of the disease are vitally important and have widespread implications for nurses functioning in all aspects of practice. As Rogers (1989) pointed out, "prevention is the only approach to dealing with this epidemic [AIDS]." This intervention includes providing information to persons regarding protection from and prevention of the disease including preventing its spread to self, other patients, and staff through the use of universal blood and body fluid precautions such as those set forth in Flynn and Hackel (1990).

The success of the interventions such as those described in assisting the person to achieve the preset behavioral goals is determined through evaluation. This is the sixth step of Roy's nursing process.

Evaluation

Evaluation involves determining the effectiveness of the nursing inter-vention in relation to the person's behavior. Was the goal that was set in the fourth step of the nursing process attained? To make this decision, the nurse assesses the behavior of the person after the interventions have been implemented. As in the initial assessment steps, observation, mea-surement, interview, and interpersonal skills are used. The nursing inter-vention would be considered effective if the person's behavior aligns with the preset goals.

Looking back to the goal related to the pressure sore, it was identified that the diameter of the lesion should reduce from 1 inch to 1/2 inch within 1 week. If the nursing interventions described were assisting with the healing process, it would be noted by the nurse that the size of the pressure sore had decreased. If no change were noted, the nurse would proceed through the nursing process again, perhaps establishing that the goal was unrealistic or that there were other interventions that may be appropriate to try.

Expected outcomes for the protection component would be the mainte-nance of skin integrity and effective processes of immunity. The person's skin should be intact and free of discomforts such as itching. It may be helpful for the person to acquire knowledge regarding skin care and its importance in the area of protection. Indicators of positive adaptation related to the problem of itching would include patient statements indicat-ing relief of discomfort, a skin free from scratch marks and abrasions, and an intact skin surface. Indicators of positive adaptation related to the problem of pressure sores would be the maintenance of skin integrity with the absence of skin infection.

Once the effectiveness of the nursing intervention has been deter-mined, the nurse returns to the first step of the nursing process to look more closely at behaviors that continue to be ineffective. It is important to recognize that the nursing process is ongoing and simultaneous. Also, it is necessary to discuss each aspect as a separate entity but one must bear in mind that each aspect is related to and affected by the other.

SUMMARY

In this chapter, the skin, hair, and nails were described as physical barri-ers functioning as protective mechanisms to maintain adaptation. The immune process was viewed as contributing to the person's adaptation level by protecting the body from foreign substances or micro-organisms.

The assessment of protection behaviors and stimuli were addressed as were nursing diagnoses and adaptation problems, goals, interventions, and evaluation in terms of the nursing process according to the Roy Adap-tation Model. In providing for the person's need for protection by maintaining skin integrity and an adaptive immune process, the nurse contributes to the overall integrity of the person.

EXERCISES FOR APPLICATION

1. Identify activities that you engage in, as a healthy adult, that are directed at your adaptation relative to the need for protection.
2. If you were immobilized in skeletal traction, what nursing interventions would you require to assist you in the maintenance of adaptation relative to protection?

ASSESSMENT OF UNDERSTANDING

1. List four physiological structures that provide protective functions for the body.
   a. _____
   b. _____
   c. _____
   d. _____
2. In behavioral assessment of an operative site, which of the following factors would be important to note/measure?
   a. approximation of wound edges
   b. temperature of skin at wound edge
   c. color of skin at wound edge
   d. presence of discharge
   e. pain in the incisional area
3. Developmental stage is an important stimulus affecting protection behaviors. Label the following behaviors according to the developmental stage to which they pertain.

   I—infant
   A—adolescent
   O—older adult

   a. _____ uneven skin pigmentation
   b. _____ epidermis very permeable
   c. _____ nails become hard and brittle
   d. _____ subaceous glands active and increase in size
   e. _____ temperature regulation labile

Situation

A 3-year-old child has been brought to the doctor's office with an elevated temperature and a reddened, itchy rash on the upper chest and back. The mother has stated that several children in the day-care center have been sick with the measles.

4. Construct a nursing diagnosis focusing on the need for protection

using the first method, that is, a statement of behavior with its most relevant influencing stimulus.

5. Derive a goal related to the nursing diagnosis developed in the previous item.

6. Identify three nursing interventions that are approaches in dealing with an itchy rash and the associated stimuli that are being managed with such interventions.

	Intervention	**Associated stimulus(i)**
a.	_____	_____
b.	_____	_____
c.	_____	_____

7. Which of the following behaviors would indicate that the nursing intervention had been effective in goal achievement?
   a. cessation of scratching
   b. evidence of scratch marks on skin
   c. "It's still itchy."
   d. sleeping
   e. contentedly watching television

Feedback

1. a. skin
   b. hair
   c. nails
   d. immune system
2. a, c, d, and e
3. a. O
   b. I
   c. O
   d. A
   e. I
4. Example: "Itchy rash on upper trunk and back related to exposure to and possible infection by measles virus."
5. Within 1 hour, the child will not be scratching and will state that the rash no longer itches.

6. | **Intervention** | **Associated stimulus(i)** |
   |---|---|
   | a. soothing baths | soothes irritated nerve endings |
   | b. application of moist cloths to rash | assists in temperature control |
   | c. diversionary activity | preoccupation with rash |

7. a, d, and e.

REFERENCES

Bruner, L.S., and D. Snygg. *Textbook of Medical-Surgical Nursing*. Philadelphia: J.B. Lippincott, 1989.

Flynn, J.M., and R. Hackel. *Technological Foundations in Nursing*. E. Norwalk, Conn.: Appleton & Lange, 1990.

Marieb, E.N. *Human Anatomy and Physiology*. Redwood City, Calif.: The Benjamin/Cummings Publishing Company, 1989.

Pitot, H.C. *Fundamentals of Oncology*. Second Edition Revised and Expanded. New York: Marcel Dekker, Inc., 1981.

Rogers, B. AIDS and ethics in the workplace, *Nursing Outlook*, 37 (6): 254–255, 1989.

Santrock, J.W. *Life-Span Development* (3rd ed.). Dubuque, Iowa: W.C. Brown, 1989.

U.S. Department of Labor, Occupational Safety and Health Administraton. Occupational Exposure to Bloodborne Pathogens. Proposed rule and notice of hearing. (29 CF Part II 1910) *Fed. Reg.* 54:23053, May 30, 1989.

Additional References

Adams, A. External barriers to infection, *Nursing Clinics of North America*. 20 (1): 145–149, 1985.

Bates, B. *A Guide to Physical Examination*, Philadelphia: J.B. Lippincott, 1987.

Bullock, B.L., and P. Philbrook. *Pathophysiology: Adaptations and Alterations in Function*. Boston: Little, Brown and Co., 1984.

Cohen, J.J. Stress and the human immune response: A critical review, *Journal of Burn Care Rehabilitation*. 6 (2): 167–173, 1985.

Gurevich, I. The competent internal immune system, *Nursing Clinics of North America*. 20 (1): 151–162, 1985.

Gee, G. and T.A. Moran. *AIDS: Concepts in Nursing Practice*. Baltimore: Williams and Wilkins, 1988.

Mertz, G., and L. Corey. Genital herpes simplex infections in adults, *Urology Clinics of North America* 11 (1): 103–119, 1984.

Seiler, W.O., and H.B. Stahelin. Recent findings on decubitus ulcer pathology: Implications for care. *Geriatrics*. 41 (1): 47–57, 1986.

Chapter Nine

Senses*

Sister Callista Roy

The senses play an important role in the adaptive process. They are a person's channels for the input necessary to interact with the changing environment. The model of integrated cognitive processing presented in Chapter 11 indicates that immediate sensory experience is the focal stimuli to be processed. Sensations, and the resulting perceptions, are influenced greatly by who the person is and one's environmental, cultural, and other background experiences. In the Roy Adaptation Model, these influences are contextual and residual stimuli, including adaptation in the other modes. In turn, one's life functioning depends on intact sensory function and adapting to the effect of temporary or permanent disabilities related to sensation.

A theoretical background related to the primary senses of seeing, hearing, and feeling will be discussed. The nursing process will be described as it relates to the senses and particularly to the sensory experience of pain, which nurses encounter frequently in clinical practice.

OBJECTIVES

After studying this chapter, the reader will be able to do the following:

1. List the three primary senses and describe briefly the function of each.
2. Identify at least two common theoretical principles for all the sensory systems.

*This chapter is a revision of the chapter, "Regulation of the Senses," Jeanine R. Dunn, in the first edition of *Introduction to Nursing: An Adaptation Model,* Sister Callista Roy, Englewood Cliffs, N.J.: Prentice-Hall, 1976, pp. 133–150 and the chapter, "The Senses," Sheila Driscoll, in the second edition (1984) pp. 168–188.

3. Distinguish between sensation and perception and list common stimuli that affect each.
4. State two nursing diagnoses related to the senses.
5. Derive two goals for a person with a recent, permanent loss in one of the senses.
6. Specify nursing interventions to be used to assist persons experiencing pain.
7. State behaviors of persons experiencing pain that will be observed for change in evaluating whether or not nursing interventions have achieved the goal of pain relief.

KEY CONCEPTS DEFINED

- *Acute pain:* discomfort which is intense but relatively short lived and reversible.
- *Chronic pain:* discomfort which is of long duration and which may not be reversible.
- *Pain level:* intensity or degree of discomfort which can be experienced from different stimuli.
- *Pain threshold:* level of stimulus intensity at which discomfort is reported.
- *Pain tolerance:* level of pain intensity that one can endure.
- *Perception:* the interpretation of a stimulus and the conscious appreciation of it; result of activity of cells in the cortex.
- *Primary senses:* the channels of seeing, hearing, and feeling by which one receives information and thereby interacts with the environment.
- *Sensation:* process by which energy in the environment is detected by a sense receptor and transduced into information.
- *Sensory deprivation:* absolute reduction in sensory stimulation.
- *Sensory distortion:* stimuli that have no order or predictability.
- *Sensory monotony:* stimuli that are never changing, being repeated and continous.
- *Sensory overload:* increased stimulation to the point of too much to process appropriately.

STRUCTURES AND FUNCTIONS RELATED TO THE SENSES

The primary senses of seeing, hearing, and feeling are channels by which one receives and exchanges information needed for life's activities, including relating to others. As noted in Chapter 11, Guyton (1987) considered the sensory division as one of the four complex networks whereby neurological function is fulfilled. This network initiates most neural activity with stimuli acting on the visual, auditory, tactile (on the surface of the body), or other kinds of receptors. Sensation is the process whereby energy, for example, light, heat, mechanical vibration, and pressure, is transduced into neural activity in the form of either graded potentials or action potentials. A particular characteristic of sensation is that it can cause an immediate reaction, or its memory can be stored in the brain for minutes, weeks, or years and then can help to determine the bodily reactions at some future date.

Visual System. The retina is the visual receptor. Light enters the eye and is bent slightly by the cornea. It is then bent further by the lens so that images are focused on the receptors at the back of the eye. The human retina has two types of photoreceptor cells, the rods that are sensitive to dim light and used for night vision and the cones that transduce bright light for daytime and color vision. The axons of ganglion cells (the third type of cells) leave the retina to form the optic nerve and after crossing over, most go to the opposite hemispheres of the brain. A number of separate visual pathways are formed. This is how different parts of the visual field are represented in different parts of the brain. Thus a person may have varying visual disturbances after brain damage, for example, from a stroke, depending on areas of the brain affected. If the stroke affects the left side of the brain, the person may not be able to see in the right visual field.

To understand how the brain cells representing vision act, researchers have used microelectrodes to record the activity of these cells in anesthetized cats and monkeys while visual stimuli are presented on a screen placed in the animals' visual fields. These cells seem to differ in two ways (Kolb and Whishaw 1985). The receptive fields (areas of responding cells) seem to be larger at each succeeding level of cortex. Thus complexity increases at higher brain levels. Secondly, cells in different levels of the visual system respond to different properties of visual stimulation. For example, there are cells that respond to the corners of objects and others that respond to objects moving.

The Auditory System. The anatomy of the ear provides the basis for understanding how the ear transduces sound waves into action potentials. The eardrum vibrates when sound waves strike it. Transmission of the vibrations is by way of three small bones in the middle ear to the fluid of the inner ear. One of the bones, the stirrup, drives the fluid back and forth in the rhythm of the sound waves. The movements of the fluid cause a thin membrane, the basilar membrane, to resonate. It is this movement of the basilar membrane that causes movements of the auditory receptors. These receptors are the hair cells in the organ of Corti, whose cell membrane potentials are altered, resulting in neural activity. Different frequencies of sound are coded by way of the structure of the spiral-shaped cochlea which holds the basilar membrane and organ of Corti.

Axons of the hair cells leave the cochlea to form the major part of the auditory nerve, the eighth cranial nerve. After projecting to the level of the medulla in the lower brainstem, synapses are formed and two distinct pathways emerge. One pathway projects to the primary auditory cortex and the other to the secondary regions. Representation of each cochlea in both sides of the brain is one way these pathways differ from the visual pathways. Less is known about the auditory cortex than about either the visual or the somatosensory. In general, it appears that in each subfield that has been mapped, low tones are represented farther back, with high tones more forward. Single neurons in the auditory system code the frequency or pitch of sounds with different neurons having their greatest sensitivity to different sound frequencies. Below the level of the cortex, generally, cells are responsive to a broader band of frequencies than are cells higher in the central nervous system.

The Somatosensory System. The somatosensory system includes the nervous system mechanisms that receive information from the body. It is a multiple sensory system composed of several submodalities: (1) touch and pressure, which is elicited by mechanical movement of body tissue; (2) position sense or kinesthesia, resulting from mechanical changes in the muscles and joints, both the sense of static limb position and the sensation of limb movement; (3) heat and cold showing discharges related to skin temperature changes; and (4) pain that is activated mainly by factors that damage tissue.

In describing the somatosensory pathways, one can simplify the complexities involved by considering that there are two subsystems (Kolb and Whishaw 1985). The first is for fine touch, pressure, and kinesthesis, and the other is for pain and temperature. The first system has fibers that leave the receptors and ascend the dorsal columns of the spinal cord to synapse in the lower brainstem. These fibers cross over and terminate in the thalamus and from there projections go to several areas of the cortex. The second subsystem follows a different pattern. The fibers related to pain and temperature leave the receptors to synapse in the dorsal horn of the spinal cord. These cells then cross over to the other side of the cord and form a new tract. This tract terminates primarily in two areas of the thalamus. Finally, projections go to various areas of the cortex, as is the case with the other sensory systems.

The results of work of numerous researchers have suggested that at least five basic sensations are coded in the somatosensory system: light touch to the skin, deep pressure to the fascia below the skin, joint movement, pain, and temperature. Specific cells in the thalamus respond to only one mode of stimulation. At the level of the cortex there is response also to a specific stimulus, but a given cell is responsive to a smaller region, thus making it possible to locate the stimulus on the skin. Other cells, even at the skin surface have more complex properties, such as those of the hand, which respond to movement and precise orientation of stimuli. These properties make it possible to explore shape and three-dimension tactily.

THEORETICAL BASIS OF SENSATION

Based on understanding the structure and function of the senses as a division of the nervous system, some common theoretical principles for all the sensory systems are identified. These can be summarized briefly as follows: (1) specialized receptors, whereby sensory energy is transduced into neural activity in the form of graded potentials or action potentials; (2) receptive fields, which allow stimuli to be located in space or on the body surface; (3) localization and detection, determined by receptor density and overlap; (4) neural relays of three or four neurons, connected in sequence from receptor cells to cortex; (5) information transmission, involving the coding of action potentials from all sensory systems and carrying that information along nerves, then tracts of the brain and spinal cord; (6) sensory subsystems that include multiple pathways such as diffent pathways to the cerebral cortex for color perception and for tracking moving objects; and (7) multiple representation, whereby there are both primary and secondary re-representation of each sensory field on the cortex (Kolb and Whishaw 1985).

Meiss and Tanner (1982) note that reducing an enormous array of environmental factors and influences to the single common language of the nervous system is a first and very important step in enabling us to cope with a highly complex world. There are a large variety of sensory receptors in the human body and a continuous stream of stimulation to these receptors. Sensory receptors act as both detectors and transducers. They detect the presence or absence of some component of the environment. Then as transducers, they sample a portion of the energy associated with the particular component and convert the sampled energy into an electrical signal containing information such as the intensity of sound.

Sensation gives rise to another complex process that involves the central nervous system and is a process of the cognator subsystem postulated by the Roy Model (see Chapter 1). Perception is the interpretation of a stimulus and the conscious appreciation of it. It has been noted here that sensation is a result of activity of receptors and their associated pathways and corresponding cortical sensory areas. Perception rather is the result of activity of cells in the cortex beyond the first synapse in the sensory cortex. From the perspective of the Roy Model and a nursing view of information processing (Roy 1988), one considers that the immediate sensory experience is transformed into a perception by links with such factors as education and experience; that is, the focal stimulus is processed in the light of contextual and residual stimuli. Perception includes providing meaning to what is sensed. For example, knowing that the latch on a gate outside one's house is loose, a person will attach a nonthreatening meaning to the sound of the gate swinging open at night. As noted earlier, previous sense experiences may be stored as part of the interpretation of a present sense experience.

APPLICATION OF THE NURSING PROCESS

Understanding the processes by which the senses play an important role in perceiving and interacting with the world, the nurse can more competently assess and plan care related to the person's use of the senses. Any loss of function can affect the person greatly. However, as the Roy Adaptation Model clearly emphasizes, people have great capacities to adapt to changed circumstances. The nurse assists persons with temporary or permanent sensory losses to achieve and maintain the highest level of adaptation of which they are capable.

In addition to the effect a sensory loss may have on the person, loss of a functioning sense can change the way others, including health professionals, view a person. For example, legally blind persons often report that store clerks, waiters and waitresses, and others rarely address them directly when they are accompanied by a sighted person. In a hospital situation a hard-of-hearing person may be labeled as confused or disoriented when they do not give what are considered appropriate responses to the queries of hospital staff. The confusion suddenly clears when the nursing staff recognize the person's sense limitation and make efforts to compensate for the loss. The application of the nursing process is the formalized way that the nurse makes these assessments and plans appropriate care to promote adaptation and mastery related to the senses.

Assessment of Behavior

Behavioral assessment of this physiological mode component involves physical assessment skills using both observation and measurement. In addition, the nurse uses sensitive interviewing and his or her own perceptiveness. At times the nurse may conduct baseline assessments of a given sense, for example, performing eye screening tests for school children. At other times, these assessments may be more precise and complete as when a tuning fork is used by a nurse practitioner to measure two dimensions of hearing acuity in the annual physical examination of an older person. Besides the skills of assessment related to each of the primary senses, other approaches, including questions are used to assess general behaviors in this mode component.

Primary Senses. The external, or functional, examination of the *eye* includes its ability to move in its orbit and the reaction of the pupil to light and accommodation. The function of the eye may be tested by use of the *Snellen Chart,* where the person is asked to identify illuminated letters or objects of varying sizes. The acuity of each eye is measured separately while the other eye is covered with an opaque card. The expected response is that the person can identify letters of the 20 line at 20 feet when asked to read the chart.

A *perimeter* is the instrument used to test peripheral vision. This indicates how far to the side the person can see without moving the eye. The test is conducted with the person's vision fixed with test objects moved in from the far periphery. Sometimes this can be done electronically with lights on a 180 degree field on the wall. Other times, the moving object is a piece of chalk on a string so that a mark is made on the spot where the person first reports seeing the object in the line of vision. A response ineffective for visual adaptation is reporting limited vision at the sides. To test *color vision,* the person is asked to identify colored figures or colored light patterns that can be discriminated only if the person has the ability to identify colors.

Internal examination of the structural part of the eye is done in several ways. A *tonometer* is used to measure the intraocular pressure, which normally is 11 to 22 mm Hg. The interior of the eye may be seen with an ophtalmoscope, which directs a small beam of light through the pupil. Refraction tests ascertain the ability of the lens and cornea to focus on the retina.

Testing to ascertain the degree and type of *auditory function* or hearing loss may be carried out by an audiologist, a physician, a nurse, or other appropriately trained health care personnel. Selecting an auditory screening test depends on the age of the person. Hearing tests for the infant (1 to 3 months) require the infant to respond to some sound, for example, shaking a rattle out of sight. Behaviors indicating that the sound has been heard may be subtle, such as moving or stopping a movement or widening the eyes. From 3 months to 1 year the child is expected to respond to localized sound; from 1½ to 2 years to respond to a voice test; and from 1 to 2 years to respond to specific requests. The parents' reports of how the child responds to ordinary sounds are particularly important. Audiometric screening tests may be performed for children as young as 3 years of age and are generally used for 5-year-olds and older. Play audiometry also can be used between ages 1½ and 5 years (Hill 1987). The child first learns a specific task such as putting rings on a peg, then is instructed to do this whenever a sound is heard through the earphones.

The most common hearing test to determine the specific type of hearing defect is the audiogram. The basic instrument for the measurement of hearing is called the *audiometer.* Two types of stimuli (pure tones and actual words) are presented to measure the sensitivity (acuteness of hearing) and discrimination (how clearly the ear distinguishes different sounds) of the person's hearing. An adaptive hearing response is hearing selected spoken words correctly over 50 percent of the time. Indications of difficulty are such comments as "You are speaking too softly; I don't understand you," or "He (or she) just mumbles; the words are loud enough but I can't make out what he (or she) is saying." The criterion adaptive response for the audiometer is hearing selected tones correctly over 50 percent of the time.

There are two additional tests related to hearing function. The *Rhinne test* is used to compare bone conduction with air conduction of sound. The tone produced by the tuning fork is generally heard approximately twice as long by air as by bone conduction. The *Weber test* is used to compare hearing in the two ears. In this test the tone produced by the tuning fork is heard with equal loudness by both ears. In addition to the behaviors noted on testing, the nurse is also alert to other behaviors that may indicate difficulty hearing such as: faulty speech, inattentiveness, unresponsiveness, strained or intense facial expression, and a tendency toward withdrawal in social situations.

Assessment of *somatosensory* integrity has many facets. Light touch is tested by touching the skin with a wisp of cotton. The person's eyes are closed and they state when and where they are being touched. Joint movement is tested by having the person identify the position of fingers as up or down as the examiner moves them. The sense of pain is estimated by pin prick occasionally substituting the blunt end of the saftey pin. The person reports whether the stimulus is sharp or dull. Two test tubes filled with hot and cold water may be used to test temperature. As the person reports temperature changes, the examiner charts the areas of loss with oblique lines, one way for heat and the other direction for cold.

The ability to perceive the stimulus is the basic behavior assessed with each of the sense modalities. Bates (1983) makes some general suggestions about assessment of the sensory system. Compare the symmety of sensation on the two sides of the body. With pain, temperature, and touch compare distal and proximal areas of the extremities. If vibration and position are normal in the fingers and toes, then one may safely assume that the more proximal areas will also be normal. The examiner scatters the stimuli and varies the pace of testing so that most major peripheral nerves are covered and so that the patient does not merely respond to a repetitive pattern of testing. If an area of sensory loss or hypersensitivity is detected, the examiner maps out the boundaries in detail. Textbooks on physical assessment and general clinical nursing practice are available to provide additional details on assessment of the senses.

Assessment of Stimuli

The theoretical basis for understanding the function of the senses has highlighted the fact that sense experience becomes perception in the con-

TABLE 9–1. QUESTIONS FOR NURSING ASSESSMENT OF SENSORY IMPAIRMENT

1. Is sense impairment temporary or permanent?
2. Is impairment recent or of long standing?
3. Is more than one impairment present?
4. How does the person view the loss of function?
5. How is the person affected in the current environment?
6. What is the person's level of knowledge, the knowledge needed, and readiness for teaching?

text of one's total life experience. As with each mode of the Roy Adaptation Model, in addition to assessing the behaviors, the nurse looks carefully at the total life experience relative to adaptation of the senses. Neurological pathology is generally the focal stimulus for altered sensation. Understanding such pathology is one way the nurse uses knowledge from medical science in her clinical practice. A major focus of the nursing assessment related to behaviors of altered sensation, however, will be on the stimuli that affect the person's experience of altered sensation. Guidelines for assessing focal, contextual, and residual stimuli will be summarized in six basic questions (see Table 9–1) by which the nurse can assess the person's life experience.

An important factor influencing the person's adaptation is whether the impairment is temporary or permanent, or is this an unanswerable question at the current time. An example may involve the nurse's encounter with three persons newly admitted to a hospital neurological unit. They all have paralysis and loss of sensation in their right arms and hands. In reviewing the medical reports and in interviewing these people, the nurse determines by first- and second-level assessment (see Chapter 2) that one of them has a probably correctable situation. He has been admitted for workup before brain tumor surgery, which is thought to have good possibilities for correcting the loss of arm sensation. The second person sustained the loss of sensation in a sky-diving accident 5 years ago, and the loss appears permanent. The third person had a cerebral vascular accident 3 days ago, and it is uncertain at this time whether or not sensation will return to the right limb. It is clear that without incorporating this kind of information in assessment data, it would be difficult to complete the remaining steps of the nursing process with these persons.

The second question closely follows the first, as it is fundamental to assessment: "Is the impairment recent or of long standing?" When an 80-year-old man casually comments that he has not been able to hear anything with his left ear since he was young, the nurse may register this information with a sense of significance different from her response to another person's complaint of sudden loss of hearing after a period of unconsciousness caused by a malfunction of scuba-diving equipment.

The third question raises the concern: "Is more than one impairment present?" Perhaps a person with diabetes is learning to adjust to pares-thesia (or loss of feeling) affecting both feet, but is also experiencing retinal degeneration causing pronounced loss of vision.

Throughout the assessment, the nurse is incorporating information regarding the fourth question: "How does the person view the loss of function?" There is a wide range of reactions regarding both old and new problems involving the major senses, and these reactions are based on all the contextual and residual factors that make the person unique. For example, the slightest danger of a potential loss of hearing could be very threatening to a musician, whereas a person who works around jet air-craft might take it in stride as an expected component of the job. Nurses assess how persons feel about newly developed losses, and also try to understand how persons are coping with long-standing incapacities. Does the blind person confront the loss of vision with continued anger, forced resignation, or matter-of-factness? Some people, for example, may still require a great deal of help in reaching a level of adaptation even many years after becoming blind, while others may be at a stage of knowing they have met such a challenge with the best possible adaptation.

The nurse deals with the fifth question and considers it of immediate relevance in all nursing encounters: "How is the person affected in the current environment of home, work, school, clinic, or hospital?" The per-son's comfort in these settings is very important, but even more funda-mental are safety factors. The nurse is very careful to assess the sense with a view to potential safety problems. To what degree does the person not see, hear, or feel, and what hazards does this present? Can the school child with retinitis pigmentosa safely play sports in the bright sunlight, or would school gym sports such as tumbling and swimming be better choices? Does the hard-of-hearing hospitalized person tend to smile and nod even when addressed by a name other than his own? Does the patient with cataracts see well enough to ambulate safely around obstacles in the long-term care facility? The nurse learns quickly that nursing according to the Roy Adaptation Model fosters and encourages physical indepen-dence. However, responsibility in assessing the senses is rooted in a sharp awareness of potential situations that could result in harm to the person. In particular, the combination of a new environment, as when a person is admitted to the hosptial, and the stress of illness may change the context so as to reduce the safety level for a usually adapted person.

The sixth assessment question follows naturally from the other five, and helps the nurse finalize the assessment: "What is the person's level of knowledge, the knowledge needed, and readiness for teaching?" Do we need to teach for long-range purposes, as, for example, the proper method for inserting contact lenses, or how the newly diagnosed glau-coma patient will instill daily eyedrops? Is the concern short-term spe-cific bits of information, such as safety precautions while one eye is bandaged? Is it appropriate for one nurse to conduct all the teaching, or do notes need to be made on charts, care plans, or home care flowcharts so that more than one nurse can contribute to teaching information and reinforcing the learning that has been accomplished? Are persons significant to the patient also to be involved in health teaching? How much can the person be expected to absorb, and on which senses can one rely? The nearly blind person will learn little from a teaching film, and the person who is in the process of adapting to a hearing aid will profit little from a small-group discussion.

From the data that is generated by these questions, the nurse can identify which factors are most immediately influencing the person, that is, what is focal; and which are contextual or contributing to adaptation of the senses and any alterations in their functioning. Finally, the nurse may note stimuli that need further assessment because they may be affecting the person's ability to respond positively to the situation, but they have not yet been verified by the nurse or the patient. Basically, many of the problems of altered sensation are medical problems with associated medical interventions to treat the many possible disruptions to the structures and functioning of the senses. The nurse's total assessment of the person's behavior and stimuli, provides the understanding of the person's life experience from which the nursing diagnoses are derived.

Nursing Diagnosis

Diagnoses in this physiological mode component proceed in the same way as discussed throughout this text. One method for stating a nursing diagnosis according to the Roy Model is for the nurse to identify the specific behavior and the most relevant stimuli. An example for a 9-year-old boy with a sports related eye injury is: No vision in left eye, left eye sutured and closed with patch, and states he unexpectedly bumps into objects due to recent, sudden, and permanent loss of sight by being struck with a baseball that caused retinal damage.

The second approach to diagnosis is to provide a summary label for behaviors in one mode with relevant stimuli. Some summary labels that are commonly used for problems related to sensation are: potential for injury, potential for impairment of skin integrity, body image disturbance, partial self-care deficit, potential for disorted communication, stigma, sensory deprivation, sensory overload, and pain. In a given clinical situation, each of these can be described better by adding a statement of the relevant stimuli. For example, in the situation described, the nurse later makes the diagnosis: decreasing potential for injury due to assistance from brother and training from Junior Blind Club.

The third alternative for making a nursing diagnosis within the Roy Adaptation Model is to use a commonly accepted term that summarizes a behavioral pattern when more than one mode is affected by the same stimuli. Two examples are: (1) sensory disturbance: input deficit or input excess, and (2) pain.

Sensory Disturbance. Sensory input, that is, all the stimuli received by the senses, varies in both amount and predictability. Continuous input of meaningful sense cues is necessary for adaptive human behavior. Problems occur when a person is receiving cues at either end of the continuum of absolute reduction in sensory stimulation (sensory deprivation) or increased stimulation to the point of too much (sensory overload). Qualitatively input ranges from stimuli that have no order or predictability (distortion) to stimuli that are never changing, being repeated and continuous (monotony). The amount of deprivation, overload, distortion, and/or monotony that affects a given person depends on the person and the other factors of the situation. In Roy Model terms, this means the effect of sensory input changes depending on the person's integrity of adaptive modes and adaptation level, made up of focal, contextual, and residual stimuli.

Specific examples of variation of sensory input (focal stimuli changes) that nurses may encounter are: (1) deprivation—blindness, eye patches, deafness, isolation, and traction; (2) distortion—one eye patched, scarred cornea, partial deafness, tinnitus, and strange hospital noises; (3) overload—admission day and special care units; and (4) monotony—same position and respirator.

Behavioral responses to sensory deprivation extend from mild to extreme. Mild reactions to reduced or increased sensory input include: boredom, restlessness, irritability, fatigue, drowsiness, mental confusion, and occasional anxiety. In more extreme cases—for example, when researchers have placed subjects in a black, soundproof box—drastic cognitive responses include delusions, primary process thinking, and inability to think. Emotionally, subjects became labile, or unstable. Perceptual hallucinations were frequent.

One important contextual factor influencing the behavioral response to variation in sensory input is the amount of concurrent social contact. In the black box experiments, the subjects had less drastic effects if they were in contact with the experimenter. If input through one modality is reduced, for example, if the eyes are patched, then input in other modalities are contextual stimuli. One researcher found that eye-patched clients with hearing impairments had greater reactions to the deprivation than eye-patched clients with normal hearing. Others have noted that immobility at the time of deprivation increases its effect. Some studies have shown that certain drugs have been precipitating factors in responses to deprivation. Some investigators have validated the expectation that length of time of deprivation is significant. For clients whose eyes were patched for less than 24 hours, only 35 percent had one or more mental symptoms. However, when the time was increased, as in the case of surgery following a detached retina, 100 percent had one or more symptoms of deprivation. One study found that knowledge of the length of time deprivation will last also lessens the symptoms.

Residual factors which may possibly affect behavioral responses to variations in sensory input are: age—older persons seem more suscepti- ble; sex—women seem to tolerate disturbance longer than men; and premorbid personality factors, as for example, the compulsive person has a greater need to structure the environment.

Pain. Pain involves input to certain sense receptors and deserves special consideration because the phenomenon of persons experiencing pain is one of the most significant areas of nursing practice. Varying degrees of discomfort usually accompany the conditions for which people seek health care. The nurse constantly encounters persons in pain, and all the ad- vances of science have not, to date, eliminated the experience of pain. This fact is distressing, but the novice quickly realizes that the ability of the nurse to provide comfort and alleviate suffering is a fundamental component of nursing responsibility. The experienced nurse never forgets this responsibility and strives throughout his or her career to improve abilities to provide comfort-giving measures.

Numerous publications provide evidence of research that opens new perspectives on understanding the experience of pain. The reader is re- ferred to McCaffery's seminal work that appeared in 1979 and to other sources for indepth discussion of topics related to pain which can be dealt with only in a limited way in this text.

A practical and comprehensive statement by McCaffery (1979) about pain has been widely used as a definition of pain. It states that pain is "whatever the experiencing person says it is, existing whenever he says it does." There are also more technical definitions based on theories of how pain is neurologically transmitted, perceived in one's present conscious- ness, and recorded in memory. Neuroscience research has been widely influenced by the gate control theory of pain proposed by Melzack and Wall (1965, 1970, and 1989). In this theory, both the peripheral and cen- tral nervous systems are involved. The primary processing area, or gate, is located in the dorsal horn of the spinal cord. Ascending and descending pain pathways have been identified that provide for understanding both excitatory and inhibitory neurochemical activity. This theory has been used to explain persistent pain in the absence of peripheral stimulation.

Pain can be a frightening and at times overwhelming experience, not only for the suffering person, but also for the persons witnessing it. Ef- forts to gain some insight into their own feelings regarding pain can help nurses have a level of personal comfort when coping with the pain experi- ences of patients. As difficult as it may be to witness suffering, people in pain cannot be helped when care-givers avoid them. Feeling confident regarding what is effective nursing care for people experiencing pain helps alleviate the nurses's own apprehensions.

While various categories of pain are recognized, the focus here is on pain felt on a physiological level that also affects the other three adaptive modes, self-concept, role function, and interdependence. Pain may be acute or chronic, and the assessment and interventions for each can be quite different, as the literature increasingly reveals. *Acute pain* is relatively short-lived, intense, and reversible. It may have a useful component, as when it alerts a person to an illness or injury, and the symptom of pain may aid the health care personnel to determine the nature of the problem. Short-term pain can also accompany many therapies and diagnostic procedures. Perhaps the most common example of this is postoperative surgical incision pain. *Chronic pain,* which does not offer hope of predictable time limit, serves no useful purpose, and so creates situations frustrating to patients and nurses alike.

Understanding some common terms used in relation to the pain experience—pain levels, threshold, and tolerance—can be useful in nursing practice. However, understanding the subjective definition given by McCaffrey (1979), and the holistic and individualized perspective of nursing, assures that the terms are used correctly and not to pass negative judgment on any person's individual experience and his or her interpretation of it.

Pain levels simply means that various stimuli provoke varying amounts or degrees of pain. For example, a small area of burned tissue does not hurt as much as more extensive burn trauma, and although a surgical incision can always be uncomfortable, a high abdominal incision that is aggravated by deep breathing and coughing may produce a more intense level of pain. There are also *thresholds of pain,* which means that the beginning of the experience of pain, in relation to the stimulus, varies from person to person. Finally, there is *tolerance for pain,* which has to do with how much pain a person can endure at a given time. Two persons may experience pain at the same threshold, but the higher-pain-tolerant person may more readily incorporate the pain into overall sensations at the time without it becoming a major focus of attention.

Given the individual nature of the pain, the nurse who compares the pain experience of various people or clouds pain assessments with a personal standard of what pain levels it is acceptable to respond to and for how long, does patients an injustice. Rather the nurse will want to accept the challenge of learning more about the complexity of pain and the individual person.

Some basic guidelines for assessment of pain can be followed even though the phenomenon is complex and presents itself in multiple forms. Whether the school nurse encounters a 5-year-old child complaining of a stomach ache, the hospital nurse answers the call light of a post-operative patient, or the home care nurse visits a person afflicted with chronic rheumatoid arthritis or terminal cancer, certain information is useful to plan for promoting adaptation. As in assessment of the senses in general, the nurse obtains a behavioral description of the person's pain experience

TABLE 9–2. QUESTIONS FOR NURSING ASSESSMENT OF PAIN EXPERIENCE

1. Location of pain: obvious or concealed cause?
2. Is more than one source of pain involved?
3. Onset and duration?
4. Constant or intermittent?
5. Intensity and type, including acute versus chronic aspects?
6. What does person think is causing pain?
7. What does person believe will give relief?

and the factors influencing it. Basically one wants to know: the location of pain, if more than one source is involved, the onset and duration, if it is constant or intermittent, the intensity and type of pain, what the person thinks is causing the pain, and what the person thinks will give relief. (See Table 9–2.)

A logical place to begin to assess the person's pain is *location*. Sometimes part or all of someone's pain is derived from an obvious problem such as a fracture or deep cut. However, the fact is that nurses sometimes erroneously assume that they know the source of a person's pain complaint. For example, a 65-year-old man recovering from laminectomy surgery complained of being uncomfortable. The nurse assumed that he was experiencing surgical-incision-site pain and administered the potent intramuscular analgesic that was prescribed. After the injection, the patient commented: "At home I just take a couple of aspirin when I have a headache like this." It is also common for a person to have pain in more than one location at the same time, so it behooves the nurse to confirm the source of the person's pain each time she is assessing the situation.

Whenever possible, ask to have indicated exactly where each pain is. The person who complains of stomach pain may point to the left lower quadrant, or the headache may be cervical neck pain when the site is demonstrated. In addition, pain in an expected location may be derived from a newly developing problem, as when a person with an uncomfortable cast in place comments regarding increased pain in the cast area. The alert nurse may discover, by her careful questioning regarding the exact location of pain, that a newly developing infection under the cast has become a concern.

It is also important to assess the *duration and onset* of pain. This is especially important during initial assessments to determine the acuteness or chronicity of the pain, but can also elicit helpful information whenever a complaint of discomfort is voiced. The simple question, "When did you start noticing the pain?" may prompt the person to relate a certain position in bed or the ingestion of a particular food or medication to the discomfort they are feeling.

An aspect that is related to onset and duration is the constancy of the pain, and the individual is certainly the best judge of this. One person being treated for severe gastroenteritis complained of pain around the site of an intravenous infection. There was no problem apparent to the nurse, but when the question of whether it hurt all the time was asked, the puzzle was solved. It was related that the discomfort started when the most recent intravenous-feeding bottle was hung, but was not present when the arm was held in a slightly bent position. The nurse realized that the higher dose of potassium in the most recent bottle was causing the pain, and it was relieved when the person bent his arm and so slowed down the rate of infusion. Rather than subjecting the person to the stress of an unnecessary intravenous restart, communication showed that a slower infusion rate, which the physician approved, kept the person comfortable.

Intensity and type of pain are further areas to explore. Let people tell you, in their own descriptive words, how strong the pain experience is and also give information about the type of pain. They may choose terms such as burning, stabbing, sharp, dull, aching, feels like a boil, or feels like a lot of pressure. Try to avoid labeling the pain yourself, as the person may latch onto your terminology. If they don't come forth with a term, always give a choice of terms: "Would you describe it as a sharp pain or a dull pain?" Be alert to references or comparisons to past episodes of illness or pain: "It's a lot like the last time I came to the emergency room," or "Once I had distress like this after a big Italian meal," or "Of course, I've had stomach problems all my life, but this time it's pretty bad." These kinds of comments can be followed through to obtain a thorough assessment and can help establish whether the individual's pain experience is acute or chronic in nature.

Usually, people with acute pain show some visible signs of distress even when they may be trying to mask it. Anxiety is almost always present, and they will wince with certain movements, tense muscles, moan, register increased blood pressure and pulse rates, or show other individualized behavioral manifestations of their discomfort. People who have long endured chronic pain, even when it is severe, may have accommodated themselves to the feeling of pain and demonstrate little outward response. Also, depression often accompanies chronic pain, and this may serve to drain energy and cause the person to avoid both displays of pain and speaking of it due to feelings of helplessness or an "Oh, what's the use" attitude. Sometimes there may not even be any visible body part that looks affected. For example, the pain connected with some disorders of the pancreas is of such a chronic nature that a person may be observed watching television or talking casually on the phone even while experiencing severe pain.

Another point in assessing the type of pain is that persons with acute or chronic pain may not volunteer information about pain, as they assume the nursing staff knows their situations and needs. It may, in fact, be puzzling to patients that some nurses will quiz them about pain and others never mention it. One person, admitted for a kidney stone, thought that he was expected to have pain only in the late afternoon and evening hours, as the evening-shift nurses were the only ones who frequently checked his level of comfort. Other people will not rely on the solicitude of the nursing staff, and will readily share their response when they are hurting. The nurse must incorporate into her assessment this understanding not only of the individualized experience of pain, but also the very individualized methods of expressing it. She is also aware that her own behavior affects that expression.

The nurse should try to accumulate information without intially referring directly to pain. "How are you doing today?" and "Tell me how you're feeling this morning" types of comments accompanied by an interested and direct look at the person (as opposed to the tubes, bedside flowers, or the nurses' notebook) are successful in eliciting information regarding discomfort.

The final part of the assessment is a double check with the person to see if both of you have the same idea as to what is causing the pain. This has been discussed earlier in this text as validating the focal stimulus. An example of this process might be as follows. The nurse says to the patient: "It seems to me that you're a little more uncomfortable today. Is it because you didn't rest well last night?" "Well, that is partly it, but I was out of the back traction most of yesterday having x-rays and I can sure tell the difference today." This is also the time to check what the person thinks will give relief. Recalling that pain is a subjective experience, the nurse recognizes that the person is the only authority about the pain that he or she experiences, just as he or she is the only one to tell whether or not techniques intended to bring comfort have been effective.

When people are hurting, many aspects of normal physiology and human activity and interaction including eating, walking, sleeping, moving, communicating, and sexual function may become less effective. Thus pain is a nursing diagnosis affecting the other physiological mode components and other adaptive modes. Behavior observed will thus include behavior in any of the modes, but the goal to be set and treatment approach of choice for dealing with all modes affected will be to relieve the pain.

In considering the common diagnostic categories for pain within the cognitive-perceptual pattern, Gordon (1987) lists alteration in comfort: pain; alteration in comfort: chronic pain; and pain self-management deficit (acute, chronic).

Goal Setting

In setting goals using the Roy Adaptation Model, the nurse makes a clear statement of outcomes expected for the person as a result of nursing care. This statement often stems from the nurse's summary with the patient of the assessment data and possible nursing diagnosis. A clear statement is one that contains the behavior of focus, the change or stability expected, and the time frame for achieving the goal. In dealing with altered sensation, the nurse considers both short- and long-term goals. Often a long-term goal is made up of several successive short-term goals.

Given the example of the child with blindness in one eye, the clinic nurse may establish with the child and his mother the goal that he will travel to and from school safely by himself one day this week. The long-term goal is that he will be independent in participating in classroom and school activities safely and effectively. Each goal will have appropriate stategies planned to meet the goal.

The outcome criteria established by the American Association of Neuroscience Nurses (AANN, in Mitchell, et al. 1988) for persons with uncompensated sensory deficits, particulary of vision, hearing, and tactile sensation, are: the individual communicates a sense of comfort and security within the environment; the individual uses assistive devices and compensatory techniques correctly; and the individual sustains no burns, falls, wounds, or pressure injuries.

Intervention

The goal of the nursing care plan focuses on the behaviors noted in the nursing process assessment. The interventions, rather, are designed based on the related stimuli that have been assessed. Although management of the focal stimulus is a preferred method of promoting adaptation, the loss may be focal and many sensory losses cannot be altered. Nursing interventions thus deal with the person's adaptation level that is made up of focal, contextual, and residual stimuli. These are the stimuli that affect the person's experience of altered sensation. In understanding the person's total experience, the nurse can better design appropriate interventions.

Nursing measures used for the 10-year-old with recent loss of vision in one eye, to facilitate safety and need for independence in traveling to and from school, would include providing the child and his parents with a booklet on safety for the partially sighted, determining the distance and terrain to be covered on the way to school, 10 minutes a day practice walking in an area with obstacles, and having his brother accompany him on the first few walks.

For persons with one or more sensory impairments, the AANN lists the following general nursing measures: orient the individual to the environment, utilizing the intact senses; modify the environment and daily routines in such ways as, permanent placement of furniture and articles and adaptation of the telephone, door bells, and warning devices; provide detailed information and instruction related to the disability and compensatory devices as appropriate in care activities; and institute appropriate safety precautions such as providing assistance and supervision and eliminating or reducing environmental hazards.

In considering interventions for adaptation problems evolving from sensory deprivation and overload, an especially tangible and immediate change in or managment of stimuli is used. When a person is deprived of adequate sensory input, as could happen when blind or deaf or both, in an isolation room, confined in traction or on a respirator, the nurse may make direct use of personal contact on a scheduled basis; television, radio, and tapes, and judicious choice of roomates and room location are some interventions designed to increase stimulation. If the adaptation problem evolves from an overdose of stimulation, as can occur with hospital admission days, prolonged outpatient testing procedures, a noisy location on the unit, or intensive care unit situations, the nurse will again intervene. This time the plan may provide for uninterrupted rest periods, a move to a quieter location, rescheduling tests so that they occur over a period of days, and similar measures designed to reduce the amount of new experiences with which the person is confronted in a given time period. This may be especially important for an older person or a person who is confused (see Chapter 11).

There are a number of options available when relief from pain and discomfort is the goal. Based on the cause of the pain the nurse selects one or more interventions. Common pain-relieving activities are listed in Table 9–3. These are particular ways of managing the focal and contextual factors contributing to the pain experience. It should be emphasized that the importance of more than one intervention is often overlooked. The person with cholecystectomy incision site pain may require an intramuscular analgesic, but a short ambulation to relieve gas accumulation also may be warranted. A refreshing bath, a lotion backrub, and some local heat or cold application may be the best combination for a person experiencing a flareup of spinal osteoarthritis.

The context in which the pain management strategies are presented is important to their effectiveness. People want relief and the nurse always

TABLE 9–3. COMMON PAIN-RELIEVING ACTIVITIES

1. Repositioning person, bed, wheelchair
2. Realignment of pillows, covers
3. Warm or cool baths or showers
4. Ambulation
5. Analgesic administration
6. Other drug therapies
7. Backrubs
8. Reassurance
9. Distraction, including the use of humor
10. Dressing changes
11. Local heat or ice application
12. Staying with person in close physical proximity—touching arms, hands, shoulders

suggests interventions to the patient in a positive manner, conveying the idea that pain relief is the specific goal. Even when persons have to be denied what they see as a relief measure, a positive approach can help, as in the following example. A person was admitted at 2:00 AM to a surgical unit with the medical diagnosis of rule-out appendicitis. The emergency room physician wrote orders for close observation, intravenous fluids, and "no pain medication until seen in AM by surgeon." The patient asked the nurse for a shot for pain. Instead of responding flatly that she could not give the medication, the nurse carefully explains that potent medications would mask symptoms and make the process of medical diagnosis more difficult. Other measures that the nurse could use include staying with the patient for several minutes and incorporating such comments as the following in their conversation: "You'll be able to rest better now that you have been admitted to your room. I'll check on you frequently throughout the night, but I feel that you'll be able to sleep now. You were dehydrated and the intravenous fluid will take care of that problem."

Drug therapy is often used in control of pain. Nurses have the responsibility for making judgments about drug administration, for giving the medication, and for teaching patients about their drugs, as well as about the use of other pain relieving measures. Analgesics are common drugs of choice when pain relief is the goal, even though they treat only the symptom of pain and not the cause. These are categorized as narcotic or nonnarcotic, addictive or nonaddictive, prescription or over-the-counter, strong or weak, and peripheral or central acting (Curtis 1986). An ideal analgesic would have the strength matched to the extent of the pain, be nonaddicting, and would have few side effects.

Peripheral action drugs interfere with the transmission of painful stimuli from body sites, whereas central acting drugs alter perception, and consequently responses, to pain on a cortical level. Narcotics, such as morphine, are the more potent of the oral and intramuscular agents. They interact with the opiate receptors in the body. The nonnarcotic agents, such as aspirin, acetaminophen (Tylenol, Datril, Tempra), and aspirin-like nonsteroidal anti-inflammatory drugs such as ibuprofen (Motrin, Advil, Nuprin), are considered less strong and do not have opiate receptor affinity. However, specific properties of these drugs such as anti-inflammatory action, make them very effective for certain painful conditions, for example, arthritis. More detailed information about the properties of analgesics and about other drug therapies for pain can be found in pharmacology sources.

Although morphine is an addictive narcotic for some persons, fears about addition, by the patient in pain or health care workers planning pain relief interventions, are generally misplaced. This issue has intensified with high-social concern for drug abuse and its consequences for the individual, family, and community. Melzack (1990) notes that concern over addiction has led many nations in Europe and elsewhere to outlaw virtually any uses of morphine and related substances. Many care givers in countries where morphine is legal for medical therapy, including North America and Great Britain, are afraid of turning patients into addicts and therefore deliver amounts that are too small or spaced too widely to control pain. Malzack notes that undertreatment leads to the tragedy of needless pain and agony. Based on numerous studies that validate the distinction, he urges health care workers to distinguish between the addict who craves morphine for its mood-altering properties and the psychologically healthy patient who takes the drug only to relieve pain.

Nursing judgment of a high order is used when medications are part of planned interventions for pain relief. This is especially true when several options are prescribed. There may be oral and intramuscular preparations ordered; several different drugs and various doses for the same drug. An example is the case of a 34-year-old man admitted to an orthopedic unit after sustaining several fractures and various lacerations during a motorcyle accident. After surgery to insert a pin and cast application, his pain relief medications were as follows: Demerol 75 to 100 mg IM every three to four hours for severe pain; Demerol 50 to 75 mg IM every three to four hours for moderate pain; Visteril 50 mg IM may be added to Demerol doses prn; Tylenol grains 10 p.o. every four hours prn; Mylanta 30 cc p.o. every four hours prn.

Decisions involve differentiating between moderate and severe pain, deciding if Vistaril will be of help to this person, administering Tylenol and Mylanta when the need is assessed, and determining the appropriate interval between each injection of Demerol for this person in the context of the pain experience at that time. In addition to assessing the kinds of discomfort the person is experiencing at a given time, the exact hour and amount of the last pain medication and how it affected him, how he perceives the pain, and his size and weight are relevant to nursing judgments.

The typical prn drug order essentially means that the drug is given only after the pain returns. Enough evidence has now been collected to demonstrate that this approach, based on the fear of addiction, is not valid (Melzack 1990). Rather there is another more humane way to treat pain that is slowly gaining acceptance. In this approach the pain is controlled continuously by doses that are given regularly, according to a schedule that has been determined to prevent recurrence of the individual's pain. With this preventive administration of medication before pain becomes extreme, patients seem to require fewer doses and are better able to resume regular activities earlier (Curtis 1986). This method was pioneered in the treatment of cancer patients.

Other interventions for pain include: acupuncture, transcutaneous electrical nerve stimulation; distraction, relaxation and biofeedback; imagery and hypnosis and enrollment in a pain control center. The latter have provided innovative help to people troubled by chronic, incapacitating pain. These centers emphasize the proper use of nutrition, medication, exercise, relaxation techniques, and insight therapy. A multidisciplinary team helps the person make changes in attitude and lifestyle. The goal is to change the main focus of one's life away from the pain. The end result may be a life style and self-concept that is more satisfying to the person, and yet realistic about the physical pain which cannot be totally eliminated.

Evaluation

The effectiveness of nursing interventions are evaluated by determining whether or not the goals of the plan for care have been accomplished. The goal has stated the behavior of focus, the change or stability desired, and the time frame.

Considering the goal described earlier for the child with a recent loss of sight in one eye: travel to and from school safely by oneself one day this week, the behavior of interest is the child's trips to and from school. If he has in fact made at least one trip by himself this week, without injury, the goal has been accomplished. If this goal was not accomplished, the nurse will assess the situation further to see if all relevant factors in designing the intervention have been considered, for example, inspite of his stated eagerness to try this task, the child may be more afraid than he will admit, particularly if he thinks older boys will take advantage of his vision limitation. Another possibility is that the interventions have not been used long enough; the child may need more practice navigating on his own street, with someone nearby to give feedback and warn him if he is about to make a mistake.

In evaluating interventions for pain, the main criterion is pain relief. The patient's report of relief is the most important behavioral indicator. The person is observed for decrease in nonverbal cues of discomfort as well, for example, clenched teeth, tightly shut lips, furrowed brow, biting the lower lip, grimacing, and rhythmic or protective body movements. Relief may be in different degrees. If an intervention has been partly effective, it may need to be modified in some way. For example, the person may require a larger dose of analgesic, increased ambulation, more frequent position changes, reinforcement of relaxation techniques, or a combination of interventions to obtain more complete relief. In addition the nurse will evaluate whether or not the person is experiencing any negative effects from the intervention, such as decreased respirations from an analgesic or pressure on a body part from special positioning.

SUMMARY

This chapter has focused on the senses as a component of the physiological mode and channels for receiving information and thus interacting with the environment by way of complex neurological networks. Theoreti-

cal principles for all sensory experience and basic knowledge related to
the senses of vision, hearing, and feeling were presented briefly. Then the
nursing process based on the Roy Adaptation Model was applied to assessing and responding to nursing diagnoses related to the senses.

EXERCISES FOR APPLICATION

1. For two hours, restrict the use of one of your senses by patching
   one eye. Go about your usual activities and after the two hours,
   write down any difficulties you had. Include any particular feelings related to these difficulties or the experience in general.
2. Spend a few minutes reflecting on the greatest intensity or degree of
   physical pain you have ever felt. Describe this experience to a friend.
3. Devise a way to assess pain in a school-aged child.

ASSESSMENT OF UNDERSTANDING

1. Identify three major structures associated with the primary senses.
   a. _____
   b. _____
   c. _____
2. Which of the following general principles are common for all sensory systems?
   a. specialized receptors
   b. neural relays from receptor cells to cortex
   c. perimeter testing
   d. interpretation of a stimulus
   e. information transmission along nerves, and tracts of the brain
      and spinal cord.
3. Name three stimuli that affect both sensation and perception.
   a. _____
   b. _____
   c. _____

Situation:

A patient has just had surgery to remove a tumor between the inner ear
and the brain stem (acoustic neuroma). He has lost hearing on the affected side. He complains of distorted sound, being unable to tell direction
of sound, being fearful of adequately monitoring his environment, and
difficulty in relating to his grandchildren because he cannot understand
what they are saying.

4. State a nursing diagnosis for this patient.
5. Derive a goal statement that contains the behavior of focus, the
   change expected, and the time frame involved.

6. Give at least five basic considerations for nursing judgment when administering medication for pain relief.

   a. _____

   b. _____

   c. _____

   d. _____

   e. _____

7. Which is the most important criterion for evaluating whether or not nursing interventions have achieved the goal of pain relief?

   a. the person's statement of comfort

   b. the time and amount of medication given

Feedback

1. Any three of the following: visual system—retina, cornea, lens, rods, cones, axons, optic nerve; auditory system—eardrum, bones of the middle ear including stirrup, basilar membrane, organ of Corti, axons, auditory nerve; somatosensory system—muscles, joints, skin and other tissue, fibers for fine touch, pressure, and kinesthesis and fibers for pain and temperature.

2. a, b, and e.

3. a. person's total life experience

   b. sensory impairment that is permanent or temporary, recent or long standing

   c. person's view of any loss of function

   d. the current environment

   e. level of knowledge and readiness for teaching

4. Examples: Uncompensated auditory deficit; or: stated difficulty dealing with environment and important relationships due to sudden, recent, and permanent loss of hearing in one ear.

5. Example: Within the next week the patient will report enjoying a visit with his grandchildren when he gave them the opportunity to be at the level of his hearing ear and to see his new device for transmitting sound from the deaf side to the hearing ear.

6. Any of the following: the location of the pain; the source; onset and duration; constancy; intensity and type as reported by the person; person's experience of this pain and previous experiences; whether a combination of approaches can bring relief; size of the person; exact time and amount of last pain medication administration, as well as evaluation of relief obtained; and the type of medication available.

7. a

REFERENCES

Bates, B. *A Guide to Physical Examination* 3rd ed. Philadelphia: J.B. Lippincott Company, 1983.

Kolb, B., and Whishaw, I. *Fundamentals of Human Neuropsychology* (2nd ed.). New York: W.H. Freeman and Company, 1985.

Gordon, M. *Nursing Diagnosis: Process and Application.* New York: McGraw-Hill, 1987.

Guyton, A. *Human Physiology and Mechanisms of Disease.* Philadelphia: W.B. Saunders Company, 1987.

Hill, C. Sensory functions and alterations, in *Nursing Management of Children,* eds. Servonsky, J., and S. Opas, 26: 1221–1261. Boston: Jones and Bartlett Publishers, 1987.

McCaffery, M. *Nursing Management of the Patient with Pain* (2nd ed.). Philadelphia: J.B. Lippincott Company, 1979.

Meiss, R., and Tanner, G. Sensory receptors, in *Basic Physiolology for the Health Sciences,* ed. Selkurt, E. Boston: Little Brown pp. 115–159, 1982.

Melzack, R. The tragedy of needless pain, *Scientic American,* 262 (2): 27–33, 1990.

Melzack, R., and P. Wall. Pain mechanisms: A new theory, *Science,* 150: 971, 1965.

Melzack, R., and P. Wall. Psychophysiology of pain, *International Anaesthesia Clinics,* 81 (1): 3, 1970.

Melzack, R., and P. Wall. *The challenge of pain.* Revised edition. New York: Penguin, USA, 1989.

Mitchell, P., et al. eds. *AANN Neuroscience Nursing: Phenomena and Practice,* E. Norwalk, Conn: Appleton & Lange, pp. 501–515, 1988.

Roy, C. Altered cognition: An information processing approach, in *AANN Neuroscience Nursing: Phenomena and Practice,* eds. Mitchell, P. et al. E. Norwalk, Conn.: Appleton & Lange, 1988.

Additional References

Abu-Saad, H., and M. Tresler. Pain, in *Pathophysiological Phenomena in Nursing,* eds. Carrieri, V., A. Lindsey, and C. West. Philadelphia: Saunders, pp. 235–269, 1986.

Bruera, E. et al. Influence of the pain and symptom control team (PSCT) on the patterns of treatment of pain and other symptoms in a cancer center, *Journal of Pain and Symptom Management,* 4 (3): 112–116, 1989.

Melzak, R., and R. Wall. *Textbook of Pain* (2nd ed.) Churchill Livingstone, 1989.

Perry, S. & Heidrich, G. (1981). Placebo response: myth and matter. *American Journal of Nursing, 4,* 720–725.

West, B.A. Understanding endorphins: our natural pain relief system, *Nursing '81,* 81: 50–53, 1981.

Wilson, F., and B. Elmassian. Endorphins. *American Journal of Nursing,* 81, 722–725, 1981.

Zborowski, M. *People in Pain.* San Francisco: Jossey-Bass, 1969.

Chapter Ten

Fluids and Electrolytes*

Karen Jensen

Fluid and electrolyte balance is identified in the Roy Adaptation Model as one of four complex processes associated with the physiological mode. Maintenance of body fluids and electrolytes in correct proportion is vital for the integrity of the individual. This chapter provides an overview and brief description of this complex physiological process and identifies the associated structures and functions. The nursing process as it applies to fluids and electrolytes is explored.

OBJECTIVES

After studying this chapter, the reader will be able to do the following:

1. Describe fluid and electrolyte balance as a complex physiological process.
2. State behaviors that indicate fluid and electrolyte imbalance.
3. List common stimuli that lead to fluid and electrolyte imbalance.
4. Given a situation, construct a nursing diagnosis for a patient with fluid and electrolyte imbalance.
5. Derive goals for a patient with fluid and electrolyte imbalance in a given situation.
6. Identify stimuli which may be managed as interventions to bring about fluid and electrolyte balance.
7. Propose evaluative approaches to determine the effectiveness of nursing interventions.

*This chapter is a revision of the chapter "Fluids and Electrolytes," Nancy Zewen Perley in the first edition of *Introduction to Nursing: An Adaptation Model,* Sister Callista Roy, Englewood Cliffs, N.J., Prentice-Hall, 1976, pp. 87–108 and the chapter "Fluid and Electrolytes," Nancy Zewen Perley, edited for the second (1984) edition by Sally Valentine, pp. 189–237.

KEY CONCEPTS DEFINED

- *Acidosis:* a decrease in pH (excess of hydrogen ion concentration) related to accumulation of acid or loss of base.
- *Alkalosis:* an increase in pH (deficit of hydrogen ion concentration) related to accumulation of base or deficiency of acid.
- *Calcemia:* a suffix pertaining to calcium in the blood.
- *Electrolytes:* ionic (charged) substances such as salts, acids, and bases.
- *Fluids:* internal body fluids located within and outside body cells.
- *Homeostasis:* a state of body equilibrium, or the maintenance of a stable internal environment of the body (Marieb, 1989).
- *Hyper:* a prefix meaning excess or above normal value.
- *Hypo:* a prefix meaning deficit or below normal value.
- *Kalemia:* a suffix pertaining to potassium in the blood.
- *Natremia:* a suffix pertaining to the sodium in the blood.
- *Volemia:* a suffix pertaining to volume of plasma in the body.
- *pH:* a measure of hydrogen ion concentration and thus of acidity or alkalinity.

STRUCTURES AND FUNCTIONS RELATED TO FLUIDS AND ELECTROLYTES

Adaptation relative to fluids and electrolytes is referred to as the process of homeostasis. Marieb (1989) defined homeostasis as the maintenance of a stable internal environment of the body. Relative consistency of body fluids can be maintained by responses that promote adaptation. A wide variety of body systems including the respiratory, circulatory, gastrointestinal, renal, nervous, and endocrine systems play a regulatory role in the maintenance of fluid and electrolyte balance. Without this balance, disruptions occur in the cellular and, therefore, systemic bodily functions. These disruptions result in changes in many components of the physiological mode.

Marieb (1989) described fluid and electrolyte balance in terms of three major categories: water, electrolytes, and acid/base. These fluids and electrolytes exist in intra- and extracellular compartments. Intracellular fluid is the fluid existing within the cell walls while extracellular fluid refers mainly to plasma, the fluid portion of blood within the vessels, and the interstitial fluid which is the fluid in the spaces between tissue cells.

Water Balance
Water within the body serves as the universal solvent in which electrolytes and non-electrolytes are dissolved. The concentration of these solutes in water influences water balance between intracellular and extracellular compartments.

The balance of water within the body is related to intake and output. Water is taken into the body in the form of beverages and moist food, and is a product of metabolism. Water is lost from the body through excretion of urine and feces, perspiration, and respiration. The thirst mechanism regulates intake: plasma osmolality triggers the thirst mechanism and the release of antidiuretic hormone from the hypothalamus. Output of water is regulated by the kidneys.

Disturbances of water balance in the body can be described in terms of (1) excessive water loss (dehydration), (2) excessive intercellular water retention, and (3) accumulation of fluid in the interstitial compartments (edema). Water volume is closely tied to sodium levels since sodium functions as a magnet for water, controlling extracellular fluid volume and water distribution in the body.

Electrolyte Balance

Electrolyte balance relates to salt balance within the body. The major elements forming salts within the body fluids are sodium, potassium, and calcium. These major elements are addressed briefly to provide the reader with an overview of their roles within the body, the associated control mechanisms, and the major effects of excesses and deficits.

Sodium. Sodium plays a central role in fluid and electrolyte balance by controlling extracellular fluid volume and water distribution in the body. Changes in plasma sodium levels affect plasma volume and blood pressure as well as volumes of the intra- and extracellular fluid compartments.

Sodium regulation involves a variety of neural and hormonal mechanisms. Aldosterone from the adrenal cortex constitutes a major hormone in the process of sodium balance by enhancing sodium reabsorption by the kidneys; water follows the movement of sodium by osmosis. Antidiuretic hormone [ADH] produced in the posterior pituitary and stimulated by the hypothalamus increases the permeability of the collecting tubules of the kidney and thus enhances water reabsorption. In addition, pressoreceptors in the heart respond to changes in blood volume and stimulate the hypothalamus and posterior pituitary in the production of ADH.

Stimuli that produce significant changes in blood pressure and volume include, for example, prolonged vomiting or diarrhea, excess perspiration, blood loss, severe burns, and pathological vasodilation associated with bacterial shock. These stimuli serve to increase blood osmolality. Through increased concentration of urine and increased water reabsorption, the body attempts to adapt by increasing blood volume and blood osmolality. A decrease in sodium ion concentration (hyponatremia) inhibits the release of antidiuretic hormone and allows more water to be excreted in the urine. An increase in sodium levels (hypernatremia) for example, caused by decreased blood volume, stimulates the release of antidiuretic hormone and results in less water in the urine.

Potassium. Potassium is required for normal neuromuscular functioning and metabolic activity. The role of potassium in the synthesis of protein is particularly important. Even a slight alteration in potassium levels affects neurons and muscle fibers. In turn, there can be profound effects on other body functions such as cardiac muscle function and cognitive function.

Regulation of potassium is accomplished primarily by renal mechanisms. When concentrations of potassium fall below normal levels, the kidneys conserve potassium by reducing its secretion. There is, however, limited ability of the kidneys to retain potassium. Thus, ingestion of appropriate levels of potassium is important. Three major factors determine the rate and extent of potassium secretion: tubule cell potassium content, aldosterone levels, and the pH of the extracellular fluid.

Potassium excess in the extracellular fluid (hyperkalemia) increases neuron and muscle fiber excitability and causes depolarization. Deficits (hypokalemia) causes hyperpolarization and nonresponsiveness. Both situations may lead to abnormal cardiac rhythm and cardiac arrest. Confusion is the manifestation in the brain of these situations of potassium imbalance.

Calcium. Most body calcium is found in the bones but a small percentage is required in the extracellular fluid for normal clotting of blood, cell membrane permeability and secretory functions. Muscular excitability also is affected by calcium.

Calcium is regulated by parathyroid hormone and its antagonist, calcitonin (produced by the thyroid gland). Parathyroid hormone affects calcium release from bone, absorption of calcium by the small intestine, and kidney reabsorption of calcium. Low levels of calcium (hypocalcemia) result in increased excitability and muscle tetany. High levels (hypercalcemia) inhibit neuron and muscle cell activity.

Other minor elements such as magnesium and chloride have important functions within the body. Their actions are complex and often poorly understood. Further information is found about these elements and those previously described in physiology resources.

Acid/Base Balance

The acid/base status of body fluids is related to the concentration of hydrogen ions and described in term of pH, normal values of which range from 7.35 to 7.45. Concentration of hydrogen ions is regulated by chemical buffers in the blood, the respiratory center in the brain stem, and renal mechanisms. Buffer systems are important in resisting a change in pH in one or more fluid compartments while respiratory and renal mechanisms rid the body of excess acid or retain hydrogen ions. Abnormalities in acid/base balance can be respiratory (associated with the respiratory system control of pH) or metabolic (control that is nonrespiratory in nature) and result in acidosis or alkalosis. Marieb (1989:887) described acidosis as "a state of abnormally high hydrogen ion concentration in the extracellular fluid" and alkalosis as "a state of abnormally low hydrogen ion concentration in the extracellular fluid." Respiratory acidosis occurs when gas exhange in the lungs is hampered by disease or inadequate inspiration. The result is the accumulation of carbon dioxide in the blood. Alkalosis occurs when carbon dioxide is released in excessive amounts, for example, through hyperventilation. Acidosis results in central nervous system depression and may result in coma and death while alkalosis results in over excitement of the nervous system and may lead to muscle tetany, extreme nervousness, convulsions, and respiratory arrest leading to death.

Full discussion of the complex structures and functions related to fluid and electrolyte balance is not within the parameters of this text. A basic physiology source, for example, Marieb (1989) reviews the intricacies of these mechanisms.

APPLICATION OF THE NURSING PROCESS

As Perley (1984:190) described,

> The nurse caring for a person must have an understanding of behavioral norms indicating fluid and electrolyte balance and be a skilled observer. The nurse is in an excellent position, due to frequent contact with the person, to assess both subtle and overt behaviors and changes in these behaviors that indicate ineffective body responses. It is easier to prevent imbalances if the nurse has knowledge of stimuli that influence balance. The nurse then uses this knowledge to predict and monitor the person for potential imbalances.

After reviewing the patient's history, the nurse proceeds with a systematic assessment of fluids and electrolytes focusing on the needs and processes associated with the physiologic mode of the Roy Adaptation Model as a guideline for the assessment.

Assessment of Behavior

In assessing fluid and electrolyte balance, the nurse obtains both subjective and objective data relative to all modes of the model with particular emphasis on the physiological mode. Related to the need for oxygenation are behaviors indicative of respiration and circulation within the body. The particular behavioral manifestation will depend on the stimuli. For example, cardiac arrhythmias may be a manifestation of potassium excess in the blood. Problems with blood volume are manifest in the characteristics of the pulse and blood pressure. Therefore, assessment of fluids and electrolytes as related to the need for oxygenation would involve assessment of the pulse, blood pressure, respirations, and change in skin color.

Associated with the nutritional need and related to fluid and electrolyte balance are appetite, thirst, symptoms of nausea and vomiting, and the condition of the tongue. Increased thirst may be indicative of excessive amounts of sodium or potassium in the body. A dry, furrowed tongue signals a deficit in fluid volume in the body.

The amount and characteristics of urinary and intestinal output and bowel activity are important behaviors related to fluid and electrolyte balance. Urinary output is an important indicator of fluid volume while diarrhea may influence both fluid volume and electrolyte balance. Levels of intake and output in situations of fluid and electrolyte imbalance constitute an important behavioral indicator. A decrease in bowel sounds evident on abdominal auscultation may indicate problems with potassium levels in the body.

Imbalances in fluids and electrolytes will also affect the person's need for activity and rest and their report of "how they are feeling." Complaints of fatigue, malaise, drowsiness, restlessness, agitation, and irritability may be behavioral indicators of ineffective adaptation related to fluids and electrolytes, particularly where calcium levels are concerned. Disruptions in bone integrity also may indicate calcium problems.

Related to the processes of physiological protection is the condition of the skin and the skin in turn reflects fluid and electrolyte balance. The nurse would expect to find abnormalities in skin temperature, turgor and color in situations of fluid volume alterations. Peripheral and peri-oral sensation may be affected by calcium deficits with patients reporting "tingling" of fingers or lips. With decreases in fluid volume, one would expect to find diminished reflexes and decreased tearing and salivation.

Fluid and electrolyte imbalance may result in neurological manifestations including belligerence, apathy, confusion, disorientation with reports of headache, and progressive alteration in the functioning of the central nervous system.

An important behavioral validation in the assessment of fluid and electrolyte balance is the results of laboratory tests, in particular, those related to concentrations of elements and ions in the blood and urine. Hemoglobin and hematocrit levels are important indicators of blood volume and specific gravity of urine is an important indicator of body sodium levels.

Once the nurse has completed the behavioral assessment of fluid and electrolyte balance, a tentative judgment as to whether the behaviors are adaptive or ineffective is made. As was identified in Chapter 2, normal values are available to guide this judgment, as are general expectations relative to the identified behaviors. In other situations, pronounced regulator activity with cognator ineffectiveness may provide the key to the identification of ineffective adaptation. By obtaining the indication of whether the person is maintaining an appropriate balance of fluids and electrolytes, priorities can be established with respect to the next level of the nursing process—assessment of stimuli.

Assessment of Stimuli

Of the common stimuli affecting adaptation, lack of integrity of the physiological mode is the most common source of fluid and electrolyte disruptions. In particular, disease pathology associated with acute or chronic illness or injury is frequently the focal stimulus causing ineffective processes of fluid and electrolyte balance. Consider the following examples. Disruption of skin integrity from a burn with the subsequent loss of extracellular fluid and release of cellular potassium has pervasive effects on body homeostasis. Excessive calcium in the body may result from the breakdown of bone calcium in pathological conditions such as metastatic cancer of the bone, multiple myeloma, or leukemia. With renal disease, the kidney has limited or no ability to excrete hydrogen ions, potassium, or water. Diabetes is another chronic condition that can adversely affect hydrogen ion concentration within the body. Deficient aldosterone production by the adrenal glands is an acute condition that results in loss of sodium and conservation of potassium. Each of these situations has a profound effect on fluid and electrolyte balance and adaptation.

Associated with integrity of the physiological mode and affecting fluid and electrolyte balance is loss of specific body fluids through vomiting, diarrhea, wound drainage, or medical interventions such as gastrointestinal suctioning. Fluid and electrolyte imbalance may be instigated by the administration of medications or other medical regimens. For example, excessive administration of intravenous solutions may overload the body with fluids. Use of potent or inappropriate diuretic medications without fluid replacement results in loss of fluid, potassium, and sodium. To assist with this problem, some diuretics have been developed with the feature of enabling potassium conservation within the body. Overuse of antacids and laxatives also serves to disrupt electrolyte balance, the former inhibiting the absorption of vital elements, the latter contributing to excessive loss.

Cognator effectiveness, as associate with the person's knowledge level, may constitute a stimulus contributing to the fluid and electrolyte imbalance in situations where there is inappropriate use of the medical interventions. For example, a person may be precipitating excessive intestinal absorption of calcium with the overuse of Vitamin D. Or the person's dietary intake may be deficient in one or more of the vital elements, either because of lack of knowledge about a balanced diet or disorders such as anorexia.

Other common stimuli that may affect adaptation relative to fluids and electrolytes are developmental stage and environmental factors. In the very young and elderly, fluid and electrolyte balance are particularly influenced by nutritional status. Environmental factors such as intense heat or inaccessibility of water also affect the body's ability to maintain fluids and electrolytes in appropriate balance.

Once the stimuli influencing fluid and electrolyte balance have been identified, the nurse proceeds to suggest whether they are focal, contextual, or residual in their effect on the person's physiological integrity. The focal stimulus is the one most immediately confronting the person. The stimuli identified represent possible focal stimuli for the complex process of fluid and electrolyte balance. Contextual stimuli are all other internal or external stimuli evident in the situation and contributing to the behavior caused by the focal stimulus. Residual stimuli represent those stimuli whose effect on the person has not or cannot be validated.

Within the process of fluid and electrolyte balance, it is evident that, in some situations, certain behaviors can be stimuli for other behaviors. For example, vomiting may be classified as a behavior since it constitutes an action under specified circumstances. However, vomiting may also be considered a stimulus where fluid and electrolyte balance is concerned since persistent vomiting may lead to excessive fluid loss and imbalance in vital elements needed by the body. At times it may not be clear as to whether a particular activity is a behavior or a stimulus and in many cases, it may indeed be both. Since the remainder of the nursing process is contingent on factors identified in both parts of the assessment, it may be of value to document the term as both a behavior and a stimulus to ensure that the concept is not lost as the nursing process proceeds. Experience will clarify the most appropriate method of documenting when such dilemmas are encountered in the assessment of the patient.

Nursing Diagnosis

Once the nurse has identified the person's adaptive and ineffective behaviors and has assessed and classified the relevant stimuli in the situation, the information is interpreted in the form of a nursing diagnosis. As was explained in Chapter 2, Roy has suggested three alternatives for stating nursing diagnoses: (1) a statement of the behaviors within one mode with their most relevant influencing stimulus, (2) a summary label for behaviors in one mode with relevant stimuli, or (3) a label that summarizes a behavioral pattern when more than one mode is being affected by the same stimulus(i).

It is important to remember that it is possible to state nursing diagnoses that reflect adaptive behavior in the particular component of focus. In fluid and electrolyte balance, a nursing diagnosis illustrating adaptation could be "stable processes of water balance and of salts in body fluids due to adequate hydration, good nutritional status, and integrity of other physiological components." In situations of fluid and electrolyte disruption, it is important that the essence of the disruption be conveyed in the nursing diagnosis in such a manner as to provide direction for subsequent steps of the nursing process. This is facilitated by identification of the specific behaviors that are of concern and the relevant stimuli that are influencing them. An example of a nursing diagnosis using the first method suggested by Roy could be "urinary output of 5 cc in eight hours due to no oral fluid intake, traumatic injury to leg with excessive loss of body plasma, and lack of fluid replacement."

A disruption in fluid and electrolyte balance would likely yield many nursing diagnoses relating to each of the ineffective behaviors. A detailed approach, as dictated through the first alternative for structuring the statement, may facilitate thorough interpretation of the data.

Using summary labels to assist with conveying the essence of the problem may be the appropriate method, however. For example, the term "dehydration" conveys, for the experienced nurse, a variety of symptoms including such behaviors as poor tissue turgor, dry mucous membranes, weight loss, decreased urine production, accelerated heart rate, and disorientation. With meaningful terminology such as this, nurses convey to each other and to other health professionals a great deal of information in a word or brief phrase. To complete a nursing diagnosis in this fashion, the nurse might state as a nursing diagnosis, "dehydration due to excessive use of diuretics."

A label that summarizes a behavioral pattern when more than one mode is being affected by the same stimuli normally involves a very complex concept and assumes the background knowledge associated with an experienced practitioner. The concept of "shock" provides an example of this method of stating a nursing diagnosis. The diagnosis statement could be "shock due to hemorrhage from gastric ulcer." Much information is contained in the terms "shock" and "hemorrhage" that would provide meaningful direction for the experienced nurse but may be less meaningful and provide less direction for the person with less clinical and theoretical background.

It is tempting for the nurse, in situations of fluid and electrolyte imbalance, to focus on the pathophysiology involved rather than the behaviors and stimuli that are related to what is happening physiologically in the person's body. Knowledge of pathophysiology is important to assist the nurse in the identification of behaviors and stimuli related to fluid and electrolyte balance but, with the framework that the Roy Adaptation Model provides, behaviors and stimuli pertain to the person's behavioral manifestation of the problem and the factors that appear to be causing them. In turn, the nursing diagnosis also focuses on behaviors and stimuli rather than on the pathophysiological condition(s). Once the nursing diagnosis is formulated, the nurse proceeds to the fourth step of the nursing process—goal setting.

Goal Setting

Goal setting as described in the Roy Adaptation Model is defined as the establishment of clear statements of behavioral outcomes of the nursing care for the person. The goal should address the behavior, the change expected and the time frame in which the goal should be achieved. Goals may be long term or short term and these time frames are relative to the situation involved.

In the example provided, a patient was observed to have only 5 cc of urinary output in an 8-hour period. This is considered to be ineffective behavior when compared to normal and expected urinary output of a healthy person. A goal for this patient could be, "The patient's urinary output will increase within the next hour." This would constitute a short-term goal, the behavior of which is "urinary output," the change expected is "increase," and the time frame is "the next hour."

Consider a situation where a person has been diagnosed with "diarrhea due to excessive use of laxatives." A long-term goal in this situation may be, "The patient will have regular bowel functioning without the use of laxatives within a two-week period." Here the behavior is "bowel functioning," the expected change is designated by "regular" and "without the use of laxatives" and the time frame is "within a two-week period."

Generally, the goal of the nurse relative to fluids and electrolytes is to re-establish an adaptive state of balance. This goal is operationalized by the identification of the specific goals that address each of the ineffective and potentially ineffective behaviors identified in the person.

Another goal during the acute phase of fluid or electrolyte imbalance is to protect the individual from any potential injury or untoward occurrence. In this respect, the importance of anticipating potential problems associated with the person's condition is evident. The necessity of involving the person, where possible, in the establishment of the goals is a principle that must be remembered if the goals are to be realistic and if the patient is to be committed to their attainment. The nurse then proceeds to identify and implement nursing interventions to assist the patient in achieving the behavioral goals.

Intervention

Once the goals have been established relative to behaviors that will promote adaptation, the nurse determines how to assist the person in attaining these goals. Just as the focus of goal setting is the person's behavior, the focus of intervention is the stimulus(i) influencing the behavior. According to the Roy Adaptation Model, *intervention* is, thus, the management of stimuli and involves either altering, increasing, decreasing, removing, or maintaining them.

In the previous situation involving the patient with limited urinary output in eight hours, interventions could focus on the oral fluid intake, the injury to the leg, and the lack of fluid replacement—all stimuli identified in the nursing diagnosis. By identifying and analyzing possible approaches, the nurse selects the approach(es) with the highest probability of achieving the goal. Giving the person oral fluids may resolve the problem but if surgery is imminent, oral intake may jeopardize the scheduling of an operation.

It so happens that the injury to the leg is scheduled for surgical repair. To assist with the management of this stimulus, the nurse would be involved in preparing the patient for the operating room. Intravenous replacement may be something that could be initiated immediately. The nurse may be involved in initiating the infusion and in monitoring its administration and subsequent effect on the patient.

In the situation where the patient was diagnosed by the nurse as having "diarrhea due to excessive use of laxatives," the nursing intervention could focus on the excessive use of this type of medication. It may be that knowledge and understanding the potential effects of such action would be the stimulus requiring management and attention by the nurse. Once nursing interventions have been implemented, their effects on the patient's behavior are evaluated. This is accomplished in the sixth and last step of the nursing process—evaluation.

Evaluation

In evaluation of the effectiveness of the nursing interventions on the patient's adaptation relative to fluid and electrolyte balance, the nurse assesses the extent to which the goals established in the fourth step of the nursing process have been achieved. The focus of the evaluation thus becomes the person's behavior.

In considering the previously identified goal: "The patient's urinary output will increase within the next hour," the nurse, in evaluating the effectiveness of the interventions would, within the hour, measure the urinary output. Had there been no urinary output, the absence of urine would be an indication that the patient was not progressing towards the goal and that the behavior continued to be ineffective. This would necessitate immediate action on the part of the nurse with prompt and continued reassessment and further intervention.

SUMMARY

This chapter has focused on the application of the Roy Adaptation Model nursing process on the complex physiological process of fluid and electrolyte balance. A brief overview of the structures and functions associated with the process was provided as was insight into the manner in which the model would be applied in relation to the six steps of the nursing process according to the model.

The interrelationship of fluid and electrolyte balance with other components of the physiological mode are evident. For example, disruptions in fluid and electrolyte balance may cause oxygenation problems. In turn, problems with oxygenation, for example, gas exchange may influence adversely fluid and electrolyte balance. That is, a behavior in one mode or component may constitute a stimulus for another.

EXERCISES FOR APPLICATION

1. Develop a tool to assist you with the assessment of fluid and electrolyte balance. Address in the tool important behavioral indicators and stimuli that commonly affect fluids and electrolytes.
2. Using the tool developed in item 1, assess your own status relative to fluids and electrolytes. Re-read the relevant sections of this chapter to identify the adequacy of your tool.

ASSESSMENT OF UNDERSTANDING

1. Which of the following systems are primarily involved in maintenance of fluid and electrolyte balance?
   a. respiratory
   b. endocrine
   c. circulatory
   d. skeletal
   e. neurological
   f. gastrointestinal
   g. reproductive
2. In assessment of behaviors related to the complex physiological process of fluid and electrolyte balance, which mode(s) is/are of particular concern?
3. List five common stimuli that lead to fluid and electrolyte imbalance.
   a. _____
   b. _____
   c. _____
   d. _____
   e. _____

Situation

Joe is a 20-year-old diabetic patient admitted to hospital after having a "24-hour flu" with nausea, vomiting, and headache. On assessment, the nurse identifies that he has not eaten nor had anything to drink in two days. He reports scant urinary output twice in the last 24 hours.

4. Construct a nursing diagnosis using the first method, that is, a statement of behavior within one mode with its most relevant influencing stimulus.

5. Derive a goal related to the nursing diagnosis you developed in the previous item.
6. Management of which stimulus(i) might assist in achievement of the goal set in the previous item?
   a. management of the nausea and vomiting by securing an order for antiemetic medication.
   b. management of the diabetic condition by investigating blood sugar level.
   c. management of intake with intravenous infusion.
7. If the goal developed in item five was, "The patient will have a urinary output of 50 cc within four hours," what would be the key to evaluating the effectiveness of the intervention?

Feedback

1. a, b, c, e, f
2. the physiological mode
3. a. disease pathology
   b. cognator effectiveness
   c. developmental stage
   d. environmental factors
   e. medical interventions
4. Examples: "Decreased urinary output due to inadequate intake of fluids," or "Inadequate intake due to nausea and vomiting."
5. Example: "The patient will have increased urinary output within 8 hours."
6. Any or all responses may apply.
7. The measurement of urinary output in four hours

REFERENCES

Marieb, E.N. *Human Anatomy and Physiology*. Redwood City, Calif.: The Benjamin/Cummings Publishing Company, 1989.

Perley, N.Z. Fluid and electrolytes, in *Introduction to Nursing: An Adaptation Model*. Englewood Cliffs, N.J.: Prentice-Hall, Inc. 1984.

Additional References

Barta, M.A. Correcting electrolyte imbalances, *RN*, February 1987: 30–34.

Chambers, J.K. ed. Common fluid and electrolyte disorders, *Nursing Clinics of North America*, 22, no. 4, (December 1987): 749–861.

Delaney, C.W., and M.L. Lauer. *Intravenous Therapy: A Guide to Quality Care.* Philadelphia: J.B. Lippincott Company. 1988.

Mahon, S.M. Symptoms as clues of calcium levels," *American Journal of Nursing*. no. 3 (March 1987): 354–356.

McAdams, R.C., and K. McClure. Hypovolemia: When to suspect it, *RN*, (December 1986): 34–41.

Metheny, N.M. *Quick Reverence to Fluid Balance*. Philadelphia: J. B. Lippincott Company. 1984.

Silinsky, J.J. Serum electrolyte studies. *RN*, (August 1984): 79–81.

Toto, K.H. When the patient has hypokalemia, *RN*, 50, no. 3 (March 1987): 38–42.

Toto, K.H. When the patient has hyperkalemia, *RN*, 50, no. 4 (April 1987): 38–42.

Chapter Eleven

Neurological Function*

Sister Callista Roy

Neurological function plays a key role in a person's adaptation. Both the regulator and the cognator subsystems are related to neurological functioning. Intact neural channels affect regulator processing. Similarly, perceptual/information processing, learning, judgment, and emotion are cognator processes with a neurological basis. Understanding of the complexities of neurological functioning is rapidly growing in the multidisciplinary neurosciences today. This chapter focuses specifically on how this knowledge can help one understand the thinking, feeling, moving, and interacting person who is adapting within the changing world. Applications are made to the use of knowledge of neurological function in the nursing process.

OBJECTIVES

After studying this chapter, the reader will be able to do the following:

1. Describe the major structures of the central and peripheral nervous systems.
2. Discuss the principles of integrated cortical functioning and neural plasticity.
3. Identify the three behaviors assessed with the Glasgow Coma Scale.
4. Discuss how the adaptive modes act as stimuli to affect neurological function.
5. Recognize the most significant signs of decreased level of consciousness related to increased intracranial pressure.

*This chapter is a revision of the chapter, "Neurological Function," Marsha Milton Roberson in the second edition of *Introduction to Nursing: An Adaptation Model*, Sister Callista Roy, Englewood Cliffs, N.J.: Prentice-Hall, pp. 211–237, 1984.

6. State specific goals for a patient with memory deficit and derive nursing interventions for this person.

KEY CONCEPTS DEFINED

- *Action potential:* rapid changes in the cell membrane potential of the neurons associated with potassium within the cell and sodium outside the cell.
- *Coma:* the state of unconsciousness from which a person cannot be aroused to make purposeful responses.
- *Consciousness:* level of arousal and awareness, including orientation to the environment and self awareness.
- *Integrated neural functioning:* integrated brain activity due to centers for many functions being widely distributed and interconnected throughout the brain.
- *Neural plasticity:* the adaptive capacities of the central nervous system; the ability to modify it's own structural organization and functioning.
- *Neuron:* structural and functional unit of the nervous system which carries information in the form of impulses.
- *Synapse:* the junction point of one neuron to the next.

STRUCTURES AND FUNCTIONS RELATED TO NEUROLOGICAL FUNCTION

The neuron is the structural and functional unit of the nervous system. Messages are carried throughout the body in the form of impulses through a succession of neurons. Anatomically, the links between neurons are highly organized in the complex structures of a nervous system. Figure 11–1 illustrates the major components and Table 11–1 lists the structures of the nervous system: (1) The central nervous system with the major divisions of the brain and the spinal cord, and (2) the peripheral nervous system that is made up of 12 pairs of cranial nerves and 31 pairs of spinal nerves (see Table 11–2). The functioning of the peripheral nervous system has afferent and efferent components. The efferent component includes what is called the autonomic nervous system (this term may be misleading since it is a subdivision of the peripheral nervous system and not another system).

Activation of the autonomic nervous system (ANS) occurs mainly by centers located in the spinal cord, brain stem, and hypothalmus. The relationship of two divisions of the autonomic nervous system to the cranial and spinal nerve structures is seen in Figure 11–2. The ANS is commonly considered the essential neurogenic regulatory system for maintaining the internal environment of the body at an optimal level

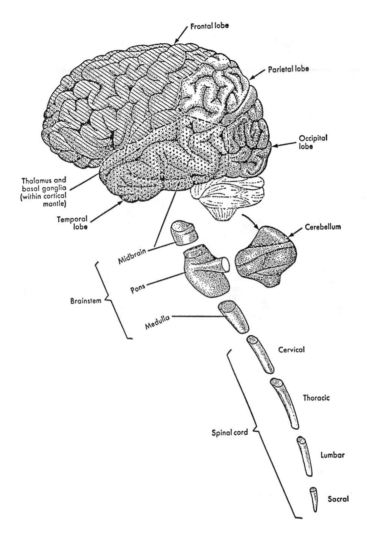

Figure 11–1. Major components of the central nervous system *[From Cohen, D.H., and S.M. Sherman. (1988) The nervous system, in Berne, R.M. and M.N. Levy, (eds.) Physiology. St. Louis: C.V. Mosby, p. 74. Redrawn from Kandel, E.R., and J.H. Schwartz, (1981).* Principles of neuroscience. *New York: Elsevier Science Publishing Co. Used with permission.]*

called homeostasis (Selkurt 1982). The significance of the autonomic activity can be seen in Table 11–3 which describes the effects of sympathetic and parasympathetic action on the body organs.

Nerve signals are transmitted throughout these structures by action potentials, that is, rapid changes in the cell membrane potential of the neurons. These events, action potentials, can be understood by the physics related to potassium within the cell and sodium outside the cell (explained

TABLE 11—1. STRUCTURES OF THE NERVOUS SYSTEM

I. Central Nervous System	II. Peripheral Nervous System

A. Brain
  1. cerebral
  2. cerebellum
  3. medulla
B. Spinal cord
  1. cervical
  2. thoracic
  3. lumbar
  4. sacral
	A. Basic structures
	  1. cranial nerves
	  2. spinal nerves
	
	B. Functional networks
	  1. afferent
	    a. receptor neurons[a]
	    b. pathways of flexion[a]
	    c. swallowing reflexes[a]
	  2. efferent
	    a. somatic
	    b. autonomic

[a]Examples of afferent functioning

TABLE 11—2. SUMMARY OF CRANIAL AND SPINAL NERVES AND THEIR FUNCTIONS

Cranial Nerves	Function	Spinal Nerves	Function
I. Olfactory	Sense of smell		Sensation, movements and sweat secretions by muscles in regions:
II. Optic	Visual acuity		
III. Oculomotor	Pupils/	C1-5	Neck
	Extraocular	Phrenic plexis	Diaphragm
IV. Trochlear	eye movement	C5-7	Shoulder
VI. Abducens	(EOM)	C5-7	Arm
V. Trigeminal	Facial	C5-8	Forearm
	sensation and	C7-8	Hand
	jaw movement	L1-5 & S1	Pelvis
	Corneal reflex	L2-5 & S1, 2	Thigh
	(used more	L4-5 & S1, 2	Leg
	frequently in	S1, 2	Foot
	assessing the	S3, 4, 5	Perineum
	comatose	S2, 3	Bladder
	patient.)		
VII. Facial	Facial movement and taste sensation (anterior two-thirds of tongue)		
VIII. Acoustic	Gross hearing		
IX. Glosso- pharyngeal	Gag reflex and ability to swallow		
X. Vagus			
XI. Spinal accessory	Head movements		
XII. Hypoglossal	Tongue		

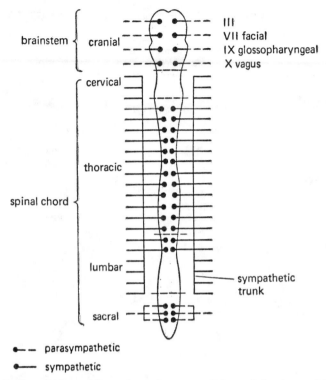

brainstem { cranial

III
VII facial
IX glossopharyngeal
X vagus

cervical

thoracic

spinal chord {

lumbar

sympathetic
trunk

sacral

●– – parasympathetic

●——— sympathetic

Figure 11–2. Two divisions of the autonomic nervous system relative to cranial and spinal cord nerves *(From Vander, A.J., J.H. Sherman, and D.S. Luciano. Human Physiology. New York: McGraw-Hill. Used with permission.)*

further in basic physiology texts). The nerve signals spread in the nervous system by way of the synapses. The synapse is the junction point from one neuron to the next. Some of the most recent and significant discoveries in the neurosciences relate to studies of the chemical synapses of the central nervous system. This work involves the identification of neurotransmitters (more than 30 to date) that are secreted by the first neuron at a synapse. In turn this chemical acts on receptor proteins in the membrane of the next neuron to excite it, to inhibit it, or to modify its sensitivity in some other way. The synapses, then, can perform selective functions (Guyton 1987) in carrying the nerve signals through the system.

Neurological function is carried out by way of a complex network of neuronal circuits for the transmitting of the nerve signals. One way to examine the general design of this complex network is to look at the major functions it fulfills. These include: (1) the sensory division (see Chapter 9), (2) the motor division (see Chapter 7), (3) the division for processing of information, and (4) the division for storage of information (Guyton 1987).

TABLE 11–3. FUNCTIONS OF THE AUTONOMIC NERVOUS SYSTEM DESCRIBED BY EFFECTS ON BODY ORGANS

Organ	Effect of Sympathetic Stimulation	Effect of Parasympathetic Stimulation
Eye: Pupil	Dilated	Constricted
Ciliary muscle	Slight relaxation	Constricted
Glands: Nasal	Vasoconstriction and	Stimulation of copious
Lacrimal	slight secretion	(except pancreas)
Parotid		secretion (containing
Submandibular		many enzymes for
Gastric		enzyme-secreting
Pancreatic		glands)
Sweat glands	Copious sweating (cholinergic)	None
Aprocrine glands	Thick, odoriferous secretion	None
Heart: Muscle	Increased rate	Slowed rate
	Increased force of contraction	Decreased force of contraction (especially of atrium)
Coronaries	Dilated (β_2); constricted (α)	Dilated
Lungs: Bronchi	Dilated	Constricted
Blood vessels	Mildly constricted	Dilated
Gut: Lumen	Decreased peristalsis and tone	Increased peristalsis and tone
Sphincter	Increased tone (most times)	Relaxed (most times)
Liver	Glucose released	Slight glycogen synthesis
Gallbladder and bile ducts	Relaxed	Contracted
Kidney	Decreased output and renin secretion	None
Bladder: Detrusor	Relaxed (slight)	Excited
Trigone	Excited	Relaxed
Penis	Ejaculation	Erection
Systemic arterioles:		
Abdominal	Constricted	None
Muscle	Constricted (adrenergic α)	None
	Dilated (adrenergic β_2)	
	Dilated (cholinergic)	
Skin	Constricted	None
Blood: Coagulation	Increased	None
Glucose	Increased	None
Basal metabolism	Increased up to 100%	None
Adrenal medullary secretion	Increased	None
Mental activity	Increased	None
Piloerector muscles	Excited	None
Skeletal muscle	Increased glycogenolysis	None
	Increased strength	

(From Guyton, A. (1987). Human Physiology and Mechanisms of Disease. Philadephia: W.B. Saunders Company, p. 443. Used with permission.)

In today's society the processing of information is a major resource for both the individual and for any group within the society. The world is rapidly changing and requires purposeful and changing interactions and responses. The human nervous system acts as a control mechanism for such interactions and responses. It literally receives millions of bits of information from different senses, integrating and interpreting these, and initiating a response. The incredible speed of the processing is seen at every level of function, from the pupilary reflex of the eye and quick evasive action when spotting a hazard on the road to the sensing of the tone of a group on entering a room. The complexity of the processing is seen, for example, when a nurse cares for a dying patient. She is able to take in more than bits of information and experiences with the person the gamet of emotions that lie in the meaning to both of them of life and its ultimate purpose.

THEORETICAL BASIS OF NEUROLOGIC FUNCTION

Knowledge developed in anatomy, chemistry, physics and physiology, including neurobiology, contributes to understanding all of the functions of the nervous system. Key theoretical concepts of neurologic function related to the senses and activity and rest have been described in earlier chapters. The remaining theoretical concepts in this component of the physiological mode deal with processing and storage of information. The complex transmitting of signals as described is just the beginning of human activities that provide meaning to life experiences. The integrated higher functions that emerge make it possible for one to connect past experiences with the present and relate both past and present to the future. This function is particularly important since it acts as a regulator of life events. Futhermore, in the Roy Adaptation Model, understanding cognitive and emotional processing by the cognator subsystem is essential in understanding and relating to the adapting person.

Models of information processing have developed from early applications such as telephone switchboards in the 1940s to recent artificial intelligence models with computer simulations. Basically, these models describe input, central processing, and output stages. A given model may emphasize one stage more than another depending on the purpose of the model. Das and his colleagues (Das et al 1975 and 1979, and Das, 1984) developed an information integration model based on studies by Luria (1973, 1980) of head injury patients. In this model, the structure is the brain, the processes are neuropsychologic, and the knowledge base is provided by the experience and education of the person.

Roy (1988) has proposed a related nursing model for cognitive processing (see Figure 11–3). This model draws from knowledge in the neurosciences and from the needs of clinical practice. The model shows that the

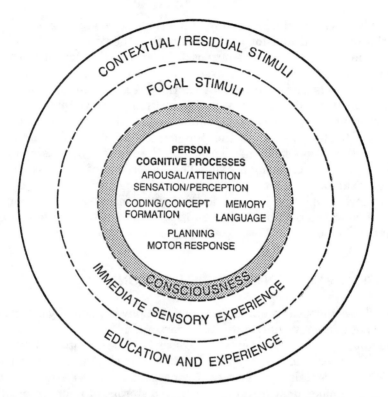

Figure 11–3. Nursing model for cognitive processing *(From Roy, C. "Alterations in Cognitive Processing," AANN's Neuroscience Nursing Phenomena and Practice. E. Norwalk: Appleton & Lange, p. 188. Used with permission.)*

basic cognitive processes occur within a field of consciousness. Consciousness is characterized by both arousal and awareness, particularly awareness of self. As noted earlier in this text, some authors consider expanding consciousness equivalent to health. The environment for cognitive processing is based on an understanding of environment as defined in the Roy Adaptation Model. More specifically the environment for cognitive processing includes: (1) focal stimuli as immediate sensory experience, and (2) contextual and residual stimuli, considered primarily in terms of education and experience. Principles basic to Roy's (1988) cognitive processing model are integrated neural functioning and neural plasticity.

Integrated neural functioning is manifested in several ways. Knowledge of exactly how thinking and feeling processes occur at the neurologic level is still limited. Scientists continue to pursue the question and one major conclusion is that it appears that many brain areas participate and interact in these processes. Cortical and subcortical areas are involved and processes of consciousness, attention, and perception are intimately interrelated. The principle of integrated neural functioning is operating when the person selects important stimuli from among all possible stimuli present and then channels these stimuli to the relevant brain centers for an appropriate response.

Increasing data is being presented to show that relevant brain centers for many functions are distributed throughout the brain. Mountcastle (1979) reviewed a century of work that had used various approaches to obtain functional maps of the brain. He recognized that each area of the cortex has distinctive layers and columns of cells, however, it also has its own unique set of extrinsic connections. Through these widely and reciprocally interconnected systems, integrated activity is the very essence of brain function. Mountcastle's conclusion supports Luria's (1980) insights gained from 40 years of working with patients from World War II.

The principle of integrated neural functioning calls into question the notion of localization (functions located in specific structures), lateralization (separate functions for each cerebral hemisphere), and stimulus-response learning (responses from reflexes chained together). Similarly, in relation to the storage of information, Willis and Grossman (1981) identify that from what is known about higher processing functions, the storage of information is a function of the brain as a whole. This is likely to remain a key part of understanding memory, even when neuroscientists know more about the electrophysiological changes called memory traces. Such a holistic formulation of cerebral function is useful in nursing assessments and interventions related to cognator activity.

The second principle that provides a theoretical basis for understanding the taking in and processing of information is the principle of *neural plasticity*. Plasticity refers to modification of structures with functional changes. Neural plasticity refers to the adaptive capacities of the central nervous system—its ability to modify its own structural organization and functioning. One may think of plasticity as the second fundamental property of the nervous system. According to the first property, a nerve excitation makes a rapid change that leaves no trace. Plasticity, on the other hand, permits enduring and functional changes to take place.

The enduring changes of the developing nervous system have three specific characteristics. These plasticities occur at critical periods, can last over a lifetime, and seem to lack what is usually defined as motivation and reinforcement for their establishment. A well-studied example of molding the structure and function of the nervous system by environmental changes is the development of vision and hearing in animals. Limiting sensory input at a given time can result in lack of later ability to have full use of a given sense.

Plasticity is greater in early years, with multiple new patterns of structure and function possible. The reservoir of plasticity decreases across the life span. Still recent studies are focusing on plasticity of the adult brain, the aging brain, and particularly the person with brain injury. There is evidence of greater potential for retaining and restoring nervous system functional effectiveness than was previously thought (Bignami et al 1985, Diamond et al 1975, and Finger and Stein 1982). Many mechanisms of neural plasticity have been identified, including sprouting of remaining nerve fibers after injury. Though this work is incomplete and currently limited in clinical application, the knowledge that neural plasticity exists provides incentive for nursing research and practice in this area of promoting adaptation with neurologically injured patients at all phases of recovery.

APPLICATION OF THE NURSING PROCESS

Neurological function is at the core of human behavior and interaction. In promoting adaptation the nurse will use extensive knowledge of this component of the physiological mode in conjuction with knowledge of the other modes of adaptation. Assessments of neurological function are at times subtle and often critical for all the goals of adaptation from survival through mastery. The detail and outcome of the initial neurological assessment varies according to the person's condition. For example, a nurse in the emergency room may assess decreased level of consciousness with other significant neurologic signs in an accident victim and summon a neurosurgeon. The nurse in a well-baby clinic may be observing the developing integrated neural activity of a child over time making detailed assessments of sensory, motor, and cognitive functioning and use this data in planning care with the family.

Assessment of Behavior

Two key domains for assessing neurological function indicated by Roy's nursing model of cognition in Figure 11–3 are consciousness and cognitive information processing. Sensory and motor evaluation are other neurologic related components that are to be evaluated and these are discussed in Chapters 7 and 9.

Level of Consciousness. Unequivocally the major assessment factor to determine neurological status is level of consciousness. It has been said, "The brain does not fail unannounced." Rather a predictable set of behaviors occur and can be identified. Slight changes in level of consciousness are significant. Increasing forgetfulness or slight lethargy may be the first behavioral indicators of increasing intracranial pressure.

Level of consciousness may be classified in a number of ways. Mitchell (1988) notes that the amount and kind of stimulus required to arouse a person and the nature of the response are basic dimensions used in all classifications. Therefore these are the key factors to assess. One approach that quantifies arousal is the Glasgow Coma Scale (GCS), (Jennett and Teasdale 1977). It has become the most frequently used approach in the acute care setting. The behaviors noted at regular intervals are eye opening, verbal response, and motor response. The examiner's voice is the stimulus, but if there is no response, then pressure may be applied to the person's finger tip. The best response in a given time period determines the score because this has been found to be the most reliable score. The maximum cumulative score of 15 indicates a fully conscious, alert person, whereas the minimum score of 3 indicates coma. Coma is also described as the state of unconsciousness from which a person cannot be aroused to make purposeful responses. Figure 11–4 shows how a person's GCS may be noted on a flow sheet and the level of progress determined and evaluated over time. At the same time the nurse may note a decrease in score that indicates worsening of neurologic status and requires rapid attention.

The quality of motor response is an important behavioral indicator of neurological status. Neuro control of basic motor functioning is tested first by asking the person to squeeze the examiner's two hands simultaneously. Then the person is asked to push both feet against the nurse's hands (if in bed), and he or she assesses for equality of strength. The general equality of all movements is also noted, as decreased muscle strength is a frequent behavioral indicator of neurological disruptions.

If consciousness is impaired the quality of motor response to pain is particularly important. This can be evaluated during a routine procedure that includes the use of noxious stimuli, such as endotrachcheal suctioning. The following possible responses to pain are listed in order of increasingly disrupted neurological functioning.

1. *Purposeful movement.* Movement is made away from the pain stimulus.
2. *Nonpurposeful movement.* A random movement is made in response to pain.
3. *Decorticate rigidity.* The legs extend and rotate internally with the feet plantar flexed. The arms adduct and are pulled into the chest with the wrists and fingers flexed. Indicates interruption of cortical motor fibers but intact pathways through the brain stem.
4. *Decerebrate rigidity.* As in decorticate posturing, the legs extend, the arms extend, the wrists and fingers are flexed. Indicates disruption of motor fibers in the midbrain and brain stem.

Decorticate and decerebrate posturing may at first be unilateral and then become bilateral, the former being less serious. The posturing may occur first only with noxious stimulation. As the dysfunction increases, the posturing is continual. With severe neurological dysfunction, there is no response to pain. This is usually a grave sign.

Consciousness has been referred to as involving both level of arousal and awareness. Awareness includes level of orientation and level of self-awareness. The *oriented* person knows time, place, person, and purpose, that is, where he or she is, his or her name, and why he or she is here. The

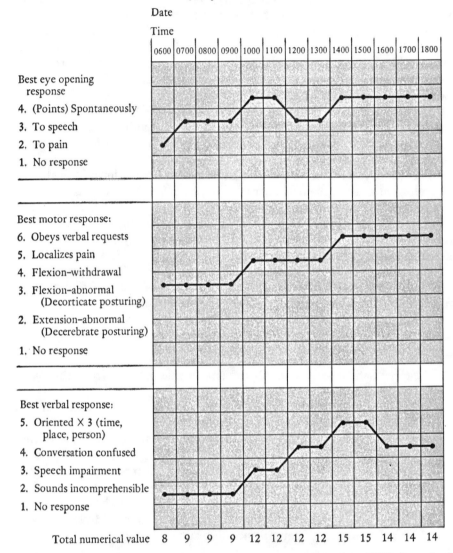

Figure 11—4. Glasgow Coma Scale. *(From Jennett, B., and G. Teasdale. (1977). "Aspects of Coma after Severe Head Injury," in* Lancet, *pp. 878–881. Used with permission.)*

confused person appears dazed and in varying degrees, either continuously or intermittently, is not oriented to time, place, person, or purpose. Consciousness as self-awareness is reflected in the person as an individual as well as in relationships with others. The nurse observes the person's mood, expressions, grooming, mannerisms, and speech. Behaviors of the self-concept, role function, and interdependence modes are relevant for this assessment.

Information processing. Ways to assess processing and storing information are even more diverse than those for assessing consciousness. Each is based on its own organization of cognitive functions and understanding of how these processes take place. In conjuction with the nursing model for cognitive processing proposed by Roy, major functions are outlined in Table 11–4. The nurse collects meaningful data during interview and observation, particularly including a careful history of change in functioning over time. Behaviors for each processing function are noted in a global way. Family and patient observations of functioning provide important clinical data needed for both medical diagnosis and nursing care planning. Nursing assessments related to integrated neurological functioning lead to identifying dysfunctions that have an impact on daily living

TABLE 11–4. MAJOR FUNCTIONS OF COGNITIVE PROCESSING WITHIN A NURSING MODEL

I. Input Processes
  A. Arousal and attention
    1. Selective attention
    2. Speed of processing
    3. Alertness
  B. Sensation-Perception
    1. Primary sense processing
    2. Pattern recognition
    3. Naming and associating
II. Central Processes
  A. Coding
    1. Registration
    2. Consolidation
    3. Synthesis
  B. Concept formation
    1. Integrated recognition
    2. Abstraction and flexibility
    3. Calculation
  C. Memory
    1. Simultaneous
    2. Successive
  D. Language
III. Output Processes
  A. Planning
  B. Motor response
    1. Motor planning
    2. Initiating action
    3. Regulating action

(Cammermeyer 1988). Specific deficits and behavioral manifestations of each of the functions listed in Table 11–4 are described in detail elsewhere (Roy, 1988). An assessment can be made of each one of these functions by observing the person involved in one ordinary task. For example, the nurse assesses the normal cognitive processing of a toddler when the child reaches out and calls for his mother. The mother has been selected out from other stimuli in the room; the child perceives she is there, recognizes a pattern, and makes an association. Coding, early concept formation, memory and language have all been involved and the motor response follows.

For more specific screening of level of functioning, a number of tests exist that are appropriate for clinical use. For example, the Mini-Mental State (MMS) (Folstein et al 1975, Anthony et al 1982) tests orientation, registration, attention, calculations, recall, and language. It takes five minutes to administer and has proven reliable in identifying dementia and psychiatric disorders. By noting subtle difficulties that a person is having in information processing, the nurse can identify needs for formal neuropsychologic evaluation. The person's frustration in ordinary situations or making excuses for simple mistakes may be initial cues of processing difficulties.

Assessment of Stimuli

The identification of factors that contribute to changes in neurological status is part of the nursing assessment of this physiologcial mode component. As with behavioral assessment, the nurse may contribute significant information about the circumstances of changes in functioning. On initial presentation, she talks with the patient, family, and/or witnesses to the onset of behaviors. In the case of an automobile accident, did the person lose consciousness first and then collide with another car? Was the homeless person complaining of dizziness and without meals that included adequate protein before collapsing on the street? Did a painter simply fall from the ladder or did he clutch at his chest first? The focal and contexutal stimuli may be related to the medical condition of the person or they may stem from the person in any of the four modes of adaptation. These factors are briefly outlined in Table 11–5.

Medical-Related Stimuli

Often a given neurological medical diagnosis is the focal stimulus for the behavior the nurse observes. For example, a tumor located near the cerebellum will affect the person's ability to stand on one foot. Trauma, infection, neuromuscular disease, vascular disturbances, and developmental disorders result in varying degrees of changes in neurological functioning. A vascular spasm may cause a brief and temporary headache that has little effect on the person's adaptive potential. On the other hand, conditions such as cerebrovascular accidents (strokes) and multiple sclero-

TABLE 11–5. FACTORS AFFECTING NEUROLOGICAL FUNCTION

I. Medical-related stimuli
- A. Neurological disruptions
  1. Trauma
  2. Infection
  3. Neuromuscular disease
  4. Vascular disturbances
  5. Developmental disturbances
- B. Treatment modalities
  1. Medication
  2. Surgery
- C. Laboratory values

II. Integrity of the adaptive modes
- A. Physiological
  1. Nutrition
  2. Fluid and electrolyte balance
  3. Activity
  4. Position
  5. Stress
- B. Self-concept
  1. Body image
  2. Self-expectancy
- C. Role function
  1. Age
  2. Environment
- D. Interdependence
  1. Family
  2. Significant others

sis can result in extensive changes that require great and prolonged efforts to maximize adaptive potential.

Similarly, the nurse recognizes that various treatment modalities, including medication and surgery, affect neurological functioning. For example, drugs categorized as anticonvulsants, cerebral vasodilators, and narcotic analgesics all affect level of arousal. Dramatic changes in neurological function follow certain forms of treatment, for example, a return to consciousness following removal of a subdural hematoma or the cessation of formerly intractable seizures following surgical treatment.

Two of the laboratory values that have the greatest immediate effect on neurological functioning are arterial blood gases and hemoglobin levels. The partial pressure of CO_2 in the arterial blood and PaO_2 effect cerebral blood flow which thus affects level of consciousness. Similarly, if hemoglobin is low, the oxygen-combining capacity of the blood is reduced and cerebral hypoxia is exacerbated. If the hemoglobin is above normal, there is a greater tendency for clot formation, resulting in vascular obstruction and therefore ischemia.

Integrity of the Adaptive Modes

Stimuli that affect neurological function can also be categorized in each of the four adaptive modes of the Roy Model, that is, physiological needs, self-concept, role function, and interdependence. In the examples discussed here we see the kaleidoscopic aspect of the model by which behaviors can become stimuli and one stimulus affects another.

Nutritional behaviors can affect neurological functioning. For example, the nurse considers that obesity increases one's risk of hypertension and having a cerebrovascular accident. Similarly, certain nutritional deficits affect one's neurological status. For example, thiamine deficiency results in disturbances in the metabolism of nerve tissue. The tissue is then unable to utilize appropriately carbohydrates, resulting in the neurological effects of weakness, muscle pain, and tenderness. *Fluid intake* may affect neurological status in such ways as decreased fluid intake reducing intracranial pressure, and increased intake hastening recovery in certain neurological infections.

In neuromuscular disruptions, *activity* may either exacerbate or relieve particular behavioral manifestations of the condition. For example, tremors in Parkinson's disease decrease with activity and increase with rest. The distressing behavior of increased muscular fatigability in myasthenia gravis increases with activity and decreases with rest. Although coughing is an important activity after many surgeries, it is inadvisable in many cranial surgeries, because it increases intracranial pressure. Deep breathing and turning instead can promote adaptive ventilation.

The nurse can use knowledgeable *positioning* to enhance neurological and adaptive functioning. For example, after a thrombotic or embolic cerebrovascular accident, keeping the patient in a side-lying position decreases the risk of aspiration, and keeping the head of the bed low for the first few days may promote cerebral circulation. Keeping the head of the bed slightly elevated and the head in alignment with the body are important for the patient with increased intracranial pressure. If the head is out of alignment with the body (that is, the body is flat and the head turned to the side), venous return from the brain is impaired and pressure increased further.

The *neuroendocrine* and behavioral response to stress is discussed in Chapter 12. Some specific applications of this concept as it affects neurologic adaptation are noted here.

Stress may take the form of painful procedures, emotional trauma, or a lowered body resistance from fatigue and malnutrition. Such stress factors serve as a stimulus for aggravating neurological behavior. For example, the noxious stimulation of suctioning or a venipuncture can cause intracranial pressure to increase. As this pressure increases, we see neurological behavioral manifestations worsening, such as lethargy progressing to a stupor. In a neuromuscular disruption, such as multiple sclerosis and myasthenia gravis, the stress factors of fatigue, malnutrition, cold, damp weather, and even pregnancy exacerbate the behavioral manifestations of those diseases, that is, neuromuscular weakness.

One's expectations of a neurological disruption may be inappropriately negative. If so, anxiety, fear, depression, and hopelessness may be the result. Expectancies are related to knowledge level. For example, brain tumor erroneously signifies death to many, although death occurs only in some cases. Paralysis may signify sterility, which is not usually the case in the female. It is therefore essential that the nurse have knowledge about the particular disruption and that she understands the specifics of the individual case and medical prognosis. The exchange of information between doctor and nurse can be a key factor in the patient developing realistic self-expectations.

For all disruptions, the nurse must assess the patient's and family's understanding. Assessing this stimulus is important for the intervention phase of planning care. Information is given according to the level of comprehension. Teaching is initiated when the acute period has subsided and learning readiness is evident: for example, lack of denial of medical facts, lack of excessive anxiety, pain in control, and so forth.

Teaching measures include a discussion of what one should expect in terms of physiological changes as well as modifications in one's self-concept, interdependence, and role function. To prevent complications or possible recurrence, the nurse informs the family and the individual of behaviors to report to the physician. Adjustments to changes in neurological functioning can be made more successfully, with less stress, when one can distinguish between expected changes and indications of complications in what one experiences in one's body. The nurse helps clarify these expectations.

An adaptive *self-concept* is of utmost importance in dealing with chronic neurological impairments. Once the individual has been able to grieve the loss of function, integration of a new body image is essential. This reintegration is necessary to move forward with the tasks of rehabilitation. An adapted body image can make the difference between one's relearning to walk, speak, and generally live up to one's potential or being prone to progressive debilitation.

Within the *role function mode*, we consider developmental level as the determinant of primary role. In the context of this chapter, specific neurological disruptions are more common at certain ages than others. For example, multiple sclerosis occurs most frequently in the young adult, whereas Parkinson's disease and cerebrovascular accident occur more frequently in the elderly adult. Disorientation is more prevalent in the elderly due in part to sensory impairments and vascular degeneration.

Role changes often involve changes in environment. The environment may positively or negatively affect one's adaptation. In the case of a disoriented person, the hospital environment itself can greatly accentuate ineffective behavior. Artificial lighting, the noise of foreign machinery, and altered time schedules all contribute to a person's confusion. Once such persons are medically stable, returning them to the familiar surroundings of their homes can promote adaptation. Noise is an important stimulus, as it can further increase intracranial pressure. Even the lack of clutter in the environment serves as a stimulus. In the case of a person who has had a cardiovascular accident, uncluttered surroundings in the home or hospital promote the behavior of orientation.

The *interdependence adaptive mode* highlights the importance of significant others and support systems in the life of an individual. For the person with difficulties in neurological functioning, family members hold unusual prominence in the person's ability to cope with these changes. Many of the behaviors associated with changes in neurologic function are chronic. To be contended with situations of altered communication ability, muscular weakness, and disorientation requires a great deal of patience. If the family and/or significant others offer support and understanding, this can act as a stimulus to help the person's ability to cope. In some instances the family may not be able to change a particular behavioral manifestation of neurological dysfunction (such as progressive muscular weakness in Duchenne's dystrophy), but their support can help prevent complications in all four adaptive modes. With the encouragement of the family, the patient may be better motivated to strengthen new muscle groups as other muscles are affected. This action not only affects the physiological mode in helping prevent the complications of inactivity, but the person's self-concept is better maintained. Similarly, feelings of independence are encouraged as one is better able to carry out some of the responsibilities of previous roles by the simple fact of being more physically mobile.

Whenever possible, the nurse assists the neurologically impaired person to maintain his or her role in the family. In the paralyzed individual, cognitive processes such as contributing to family decision making are promoted. The nurse assists the family in identifying the remaining adaptive behaviors and promoting these. If neurological impairments are irreversible, the nurse assists the family in preventing complications.

The nurse who is assessing stimuli affecting a person's neurological functioning, then, considers carefully the family and significant-other relationships that are primary factors influencing how the person will be able to deal with changes in neurological function.

Nursing Diagnosis

During the nursing assessment of neurological function, the nurse notes the positive functioning of this intricate system of thinking, feeling, moving, and interacting. At the same time, changing functioning and any deficits are noted. This behavioral assessment together with data about stimuli provides a basis for nursing diagnoses in this mode component. Because of the subtleties of behavior changes that are important, Roy's first method of diagnosis often is the most appropriate, that is, statement of the behavior with the relevant stimuli. For example, the nurse might note that the 13-year-old in her sixth day of coma following a car accident has flickered her eyelids when the overhead lights were turned on. Summary labels for behaviors, the second method of nursing diagnosis, in this mode component might include, for example, deficits related to the ability to take in the environment called decreased consciousness and coma. A deficit in ability to process one's experience by storing and retrieving information is generally termed memory deficit.

Neurological function is the basis for cognator activity and thus affects nursing diagnoses in all of the adaptive modes and across modes, therefore, there are numerous possibilities for the third type of diagnosis, summary of a behavioral pattern with more than one mode affected by the same stimuli. An example of such a diagnosis might be, "adapting to neurological changes and loss of physical self due to slow progress of myasthenia gravis and the ongoing support of family."

Two diagnoses of particular concern in nursing care, decreased consciousness and memory deficit, will be discussed next. A patient may have the diagnosis of *decreased level of consciousness* due to increased intracranial pressure. The anatomical bases for consciousness are divided into two regions: the cerebral hemispheres above the tentorium and the reticular formation of the brain stem extending from the midpons through the diencephalon. Understanding this problem requires an understanding of the condition of increased intracranial pressure (IICP). This condition can be seen in many neurological disruptions, such as central nervous system tumors, brain abscess, hydrocephalus, aneurysms, and traumatic brain injury with contusions or hematoma. Changing pressures within the cranium affect level of consciousness, because the skull is a nonflexible bony structure. The brain takes up 80 percent of the space inside the skull. Cerebrospinal fluid and the blood in the cerebral arteries and veins occupy the remainder of the space. A change in the volume of any one of these components brings about compensatory changes to maintain ICP at a normal level. However, if pressure within the skull increases, there is little room to accommodate the change. IICP refers to an increase in pressure in the subarachnoid space, where cerebrospinal fluid (CSF) circulates around the brain and spinal cord and in the ventricles.

One bodily mechanism to attempt adaptation by immediately relieving IICP, is brain herniation, that is, the brain protruding into another compartment or area, taking advantage of any spaces where brain structures meet. The brain itself is not rigid and can make shifts with fairly predictable patterns, each associated with characteristic clinical signs. This compensation is usually short lived, however, and quickly becomes life threatening.

The several compartments of the cranium are separated by sheets of dura. Pressure shifts brain tissue from one area where pressure is high to another where pressure is lower. There are three major patterns of brain shift (Plum and Posner 1982). Shifts across the intracranial cavity force the brain tissue under the dura that divides the two hemispheres (midline shift). In downward displacement, the hemispheres and the basal nuclei go through the tentorium where the midbrain passes (central herniation). Displacement and compression of blood vessels further contribute to disturbance of ICP and to cerebral hypoxia. Severe brainstem changes result. Finally there is herniation through the foramen magnum where all the structures are being pulled downward (uncal herniation). The latter is signaled by warnings from structures that lie outside the brain parenchyma. Of particular clinical importance is the fact that the third cranial nerve, which controls pupil response and extraocular eye movements (EOM), may be caught between swollen structures and ligaments. Thus the lethal effects of compression of the medulla can be prevented by the nurse's observation of a change in the size of the pupil of the eye.

In diagnosing decreased level of consciousness, the nurse notes the related neurological signs that indicate changes in intracranial pressure. Figure 11–5 shows the sequence and progression of behavioral responses to IICP. Accurate observations of behaviors and relevant stimuli are crucial for patients with decreased intracranial adaptive capacity (Mitchell, 1988). Nursing judgments in these acute situations can be life saving.

Memory deficits stem from the complex working systems for reception, coding, and storage of information, as well as retrieval of information. Brain structures such as the hippocampus may be involved in particular stages, for example, sorting, assembling, and supplying information that is emotionally significant. Short-term changes in synaptic function have been identified in work on habituation and conditioning, but how such changes might be converted into long-term memory lasting for years is not known. Metabolic activity or protein synthesis might be important in these processes. It has been noted that an overriding principle of cognitive processing is the integrated functioning of the brain as a whole. This characteristic makes the memory storage and retrieval processes most sensitive to changes that occur throughout the brain.

Focal stimuli for memory deficits include metabolic changes, infection, tumors, seizures, stroke, and toxic reactions. The retrieval process seems most affected by these pathologies. The memory disturbance that generally follows closed head injury has particular characteristics. These patients may have a period of coma followed by a period of confusion. During the length of these two intervals, current events have not been stored. This time frame is commonly called the period of posttraumatic amnesia and its duration is often used as an index of closed head injury severity.

Degenerative brain pathology, as sometimes occurs in alcholism and other drug use, has long been known to produce defects of memory. Korsakoff's syndrome describes a cluster of six characteristics of this type of pathology (Talland 1965): (1) Anterograde amnesia in which patients

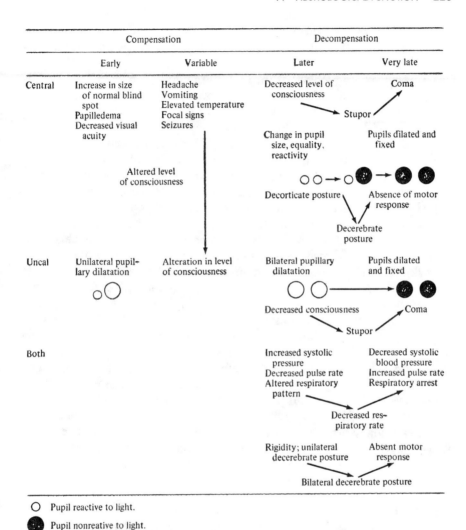

	Compensation		Decompensation	
	Early	Variable	Later	Very late
Central	Increase in size of normal blind spot Papilledema Decreased visual acuity	Headache Vomiting Elevated temperature Focal signs Seizures	Decreased level of consciousness	Coma
			Stupor	
		Altered level of consciousness	Change in pupil size, equality, reactivity	Pupils dilated and fixed
			Decorticate posture	Absence of motor response
			Decerebrate posture	
Uncal	Unilateral pupillary dilatation	Alteration in level of consciousness	Bilateral pupillary dilatation	Pupils dilated and fixed
			Decreased consciousness	Coma
			Stupor	
Both			Increased systolic pressure Decreased pulse rate Altered respiratory pattern	Decreased systolic blood pressure Increased pulse rate Respiratory arrest
			Decreased respiratory rate	
			Rigidity; unilateral decerebrate posture	Absent motor response
			Bilateral decerebrate posture	

○ Pupil reactive to light.

● Pupil nonreative to light.

Figure 11–5. Behavioral responses of supratentorial IICP; classified by stage of appearance and herniation syndrome. *(From Moidel Harriet. (1976). Nursing Care of the Patient with Medical Surgical Disorders. New York: McGraw-Hill, p. 868. Used with permission.)*

are unable to form new memories, (2) retrograde amnesia, that is, the patients have global impairment of remote memory for most of their adult life, (3) confabulation where information is made up to cover up memory loss, (4) meager content in conversation indicated by little spontaneous conversation, (5) lack of insight that is particularly difficult because patients are virtually unaware of their memory deficit, and (6) apathy manifested by indifference and incapacity to persevere in ongoing activites.

Alzheimer's disease is another degenerative brain disorder that has generated interest recently for both clinical and scientific reasons. It accounts for about 50 percent of patients diagnosed as demented and it provides a good model for the study of senility in general. Changes in the brain structures are being looked at in relation to neurochemical changes, particularly relative to acetylcholine. This condition leads to marked deficits in memory, language, and perception as well as symptoms of depression.

Persons with memory deficits may be deprived of the richness of their own past. They can feel lost in the unfamiliar world of the here and now. They are suspicious of what may happen to them because of the inability to understand and predict events as yet unfolding. Adaptation problems related to memory may occur transiently, as in concussion, or for a prolonged period as with Alzheimer's disease. The deficit may be continual or intermittent. It may have qualitative aspects such as defective spontaneous recall, lack of ability to integrate information into a whole as a basis for a modulated response, or conceptual inflexibility. In general the nurse is working with a diagnosis of memory deficit, but always recognizing that observations of behaviors and stimuli, together with updated knowledge in the field, provide the basis for planning care.

The American Association of Neuroscience Nurses (AANN) has published process and outcome standards for selected diagnoses of high relevance to their practice (Mitchell et al 1988). In developing both broad diagnostic categories and specific nursing diagnoses, this group began with the list of the North American Nursing Diagnosis Association. They combine consciousness and cognition in one large diagnostic category. Subcategories within this which relate to the discussion include: high risk of secondary brain injury; altered level of responsiveness: decreased; altered level of responsiveness: heightened; altered level of responsiveness: inappropriate behaviors and moods; and, uncompensated cognitive deficit (specify type of deficit).

Goal Setting

In using the Roy Adaptation Model, goal setting involves working with the patient and family to establish clear outcomes for nursing care. The goals address the behavior, the change or level of stability expected, and the time to accomplish the goal. Any patient may have either long-term or short-term goals that relate to neurologic functioning. However, when working with patients with disorders of the nervous system, characteristically the goals tend to take the extremes of being very immediate, as in critical care, or very long term, as in rehabilitation and care of the elderly. The focus of goals for the two diagnoses, decreased level of consciousness and memory deficits, will be addressed, then examples given of specific goal statements.

For the patient with decreased level of consiousness due to increased intracranial pressure, the general goal of care is to minimize intracranial pressure and prevent secondary brain injury and complications of coma, with eventual progression to a higher level of responsiveness. Prevention of secondary brain injury includes the following process criteria identified by the AANN Standards (Mitchell et al 1988): (1) to identify the individual's baseline level of brain function, including responsiveness, size and reaction of pupils, brainstem reflexes, respiratory rate, and behavior, and (2) to institute measures to promote cerebral perfusion, including avoiding hypoxia, hypercapnia, hypo, or hyper tension.

An example of a specific goal for a person in a trauma intensive care unit who has decreased level of consciousness due to increased intracranial pressure can be stated: the intracranial pressure reading on the monitor will remain below 15 for the next 30 minutes before the patient is suctioned for tracheal secretions. The focus of the goal is the behavior of IICP; the criteria for meeting the goal is the specific reading on the monitor, and the time frame is 30 minutes.

For patients with memory deficits, the general goals of nursing care: to provide for safety and other basic needs, to establish a sense of trust and confidence, to help the person and family understand the person's abilities and limitations, to improve memory function, and to develop and use methods to compensate for deficits. A specific goal for the family of a person with Alzheimer's disease might be: before the nurse's home visit next week, the husband will devise two ways to remind his wife not to go outdoors alone and at that time will report on the effectiveness of their use. The focus of the goal is on the husband's development and use of effective memory devices for his wife's safety. The criteria will be whether two methods were devised that worked. The time frame is one week.

Intervention

Interventions are carried out to meet the stated goals. According to the premises of the Roy model, altering the stimuli that make up the adaptation level is a way to promote adaptation. Managing focal stimuli is often the intervention of choice when dealing with neurological functioning and these cover a wide range of the person's internal and external environment. Nutritional and fluid intake can be altered according to its effect on neurological functioning, for example, limiting fluids after cranial surgery. Another example of managing focal stimuli is providing tactile and auditory stimulation for the patient in coma.

Contextual and residual stimuli can also be the focus of interventions to broaden the range of coping ability. Measures to reduce stress and fatigue are used to minimize the neuromuscular weakness of exacerbations of such conditions as multiple sclerosis and myasthenia gravis, as well as to control episodes of seizure activity in persons with epilepsy. While teaching a mother specific exercises for her child with cerebral palsy, the nurse may also refer her to a support group for parents of children with disabilities to help her manage other contextual and residual factors affecting the situation.

Some of the key interventions related to the nursing diagnoses discussed will be outlined. Basic medical-surgical textbooks and books on the neurosciences for nurses and other clinicians can be consulted for other specific interventions related to neurological functioning and all its complexities in the many situations of normal development and disruptive changes that the nurse may see.

When the person has *decreased level of consciousness* due to increased intracranial pressure, the nurse recognizes the significance of the intracranial pressure and carries out the following interventions:

1. Fist priority—maintain an open airway, adequate ventilation, and circulation.
2. Observe and report slight neurological changes, especially changes in pupils, motor response, verbalizations, and vital signs.
3. Maintain a quiet environment.
4. Elevate the head of the bed 30° with the head in alignment with the body (turning the head alone can result in constriction of vessels in the neck and decrease venous blood return from the brain).
5. Prevent sudden increases in pressure (from vigorous coughing, isometric exercises—contraction and relaxation of a muscle without mechanical work—straining during defecation, which can bring on the Valsalva maneuver).
6. Minimize emotional and physical trauma (spaced family visits with instructions given to avoid emotional upsets).

Varying degrees of coma require attention to all physical nursing measures. It is the nurse's responsibility to prevent complications of the comatose state, such as decubiti, stomatitis, and atelectasis. The patient is turned and repositioned every two hours and given back massage. Turning alternates the pressure to different areas of the skin as well as enhancing respiratory ventilation. Various devices such as gel pads, egg crates, sheepskin, alternating pressure pads, and waterbeds, help prevent decubiti. An alternating pressure mattress is particularly effective because pressure in various areas is frequently altered. A rubber doughnut placed around the decubitus actually serves one function, to create further decubiti. This is caused by the increased pressure on the skin beneath the doughnut. The nurse uses foot supports or a foot board to prevent foot drop, that is, falling of the foot due to flexor paralysis of the ankle.

If the eyes are open and blinking is absent, artificial tears may be used but patching protects the eyes better. A usual approach is to wet eye patches in a sterile water or saline solution and gently cover the eyes with the lids closed. The nurse removes the patches to do pupil checks and allow for possible sensory input for short periods. In cases of coma, a neurological assessment is done every two to four hours. For cranial nerves, checks are done on III (pupils), V (corneal reflex), and IX and X (swallow and gag). Any voluntary movements and responses to pain are noted. A check is made for the plantar reflex. As in all other conditions, an open airway is a top-priority concern. The patient's trachea is suctioned if breath sounds are congested and/or the airway obstructed. The nurse assesses for incontinence and abdominal or bladder distention. Mouth care is provided every two hours to prevent infection, such as stomatitis, respiratory tract infection, and aspiration. The nurse explains to the patient what she is going to do, and never discusses a negative prognosis at the patient's bedside. The sense of hearing is often present although no other neurological faculties appear intact.

The interventions for *memory deficits* will be tailored to the particular person, the deficit noted, as well as to the person's remaining abilities. The nurse works with the family to plan care for the person. Both family and nurse will avoid confusing the person with details beyond the immediate. They can provide frequent reassurance when the person shows fear of the unfamiliar. Developing a sense of trust and confidence can be enhanced by simple measures such as putting the name of the primary care nurse readily in view at the patient's bedside or attached to the person if he or she is ambulatory. Useful, orienting information is given often, such as the time of day, how long until the next meal or bedtime. Simple routines for care in daily living are developed and used. The steps for dressing can be written out. A daily schedule is posted or put on audio tape for those with vision problems or attached to the armrest of a wheelchair for those up in the chair.

The nurse and other care-givers use a calm, matter-of-fact approach when the patient needs the same information given repeatedly or when he or she shows signs of confabulation or lack of insight. The person also can be guided toward productive and satisfying activity after simple self-care needs are met. For example, the list of daily activities may include watering a plant. The particular plant listed is changed according to which plant needs to be watered and the patient is not burdened with having to remember which plant was done the day before.

For some persons it may be necessary to provide protection and supportive supervision. Structures such as doors and stairwells will be checked and altered to prevent unsupervised wandering and falling. The psychological comfort of the environment can be enhanced by activities such as reminiscent groups. In the long term care of persons with memory deficits, especially those that are progressive, the nurse may recommend resources to provide relief for caregivers. The nurse can be helpful as a knowledgable and caring person when a family needs assistance with the issues related to long-term institutional care.

Earlier in this chapter the principles of integrated neural functioning and neural plasticity were described. Based on evidence that multiple networks in the brain can carry on the same function, and that there are possibilities for modifying central nervous system structural organization and function, in many conditions there is hope for recovering or improving memory function (Bach-Y-Rita 1978). Persons who suffer brain injury from stroke or head injury present difficult problems of memory deficit and levels of recovery are often uncertain. There may be continued inability to remember conversations or instructions, telephone numbers, written material, television shows, or even faces for several months after the stroke or accident. The person may lose track of what he or she is saying in midsentence. This is especially true if there is any distraction or interruption such as a phone ringing or someone speaking and interrupting the train of thought.

In designing interventions for improving memory, two principles that have already been mentioned are used, that is, they are individualized to the person and to the deficit. The nurse is in a good position to do this especially for the settings where these persons will be (Sisson 1988). Based on frequent contact with patients and their families the nurse observes the specific deficits and reactions to them. In this way, meaningful and individualized intervention techniques and strategies can be developed. In some settings, the nurse also has available formal evaluation of memory deficits by the health care team including neuropsychology. In other cases she bases her care primarily on the nursing assessment of the memory deficit.

Interventions are further individualized by the total nursing assessment which includes the influences of the other adaptive modes. Specific factors might be: tolerance to fatigue, for example, immediately after head injury a ten-minute session of memory exercises at the bedside may be the patient's limit; and when working with young adult male patients (representing nearly 80 percent of the head injury population), one can devise memory exercises using playing cards so that the activity is more acceptable to patient's primary role.

A final major principle in designing interventions for improving memory is that the efforts of the nurse, family, and other health care personnel are based on a specific theoretical approach to understanding cognitive function. The notion of integrated brain functioning and the model of an information processing system can be helpful here. The Das/Luria model has been used by Roy (1989) to define further her proposed cognitive information processing model. In the work of these authors (Das, Kirby & Jarman 1975 and 1979 and Luria 1973 and 1980), the basic information processing functions of sensory input, perception, memory, concept formation, and output have simultaneous and successive properties. Simultaneous means that the input is received all at once such as seeing the picture of a house and synthesizing the separate parts of it into a whole. Successive processing refers to processing elements in serial order. For example, in hearing human speech, one hears one word after another and makes a sentence from the order of words.

The same simultaneous and successive dimensions are present in planning functions as well. One can think of solving the task of drawing a line through a maze. If the maze formation is very simple, one can see the whole and quickly generate and execute the program for solving the task. If, however, it is a complex maze, then parts of the maze are taken in serial order while the planning functions of searching, comparing, hypothesizing, and verifying are carried out.

Based on this particular understanding of cognitive processing, the memory aids to promote retraining can be planned to activate simultaneous and successive processing. For example, capitalizing on the dimension of simultaneous processing, the person can be taught to recall family members using a photo album. The person is asked to repeat aloud several times the name of a given person in a picture. He or she will be seeing the entire face, speaking the name and hearing it at the same time. The name is then used in a meaningful statement. For example, "Aunt Louise is my mother's sister." The name is further associated with a characteristic obvious in the picture, such as "Aunt Louise has red hair."

A simple method of using successive processing to improve memory, is to have lists of words that the person repeats after the examiner. The list becomes increasingly long and is varied from words that are similar in some way to those that have no similarities. Another technique may be to have a deck of playing cards in which one card at a time is laid down in front of the person. The next card is taken off the deck and placed on top of it. The person is asked to identify the *card before the last card* on the stack when the care giver stops dealing. As the person's memory improves, the instructions can be made more difficult by having the person name the second card back or the third card back.

Simultaneous and successive processing practice (Roy 1989) can be used with a specific deficit such as recalling place names, as in an example of a person who cannot remember the name of the city in which he or she lives. This practice involves a set of simple exercises in which families can be involved. The simultaneous strategies described are used with a map as the stimulus to learn the name of the city. Then an additional strategy is to have the person color the area of the city on the map. Sometimes many rehearsals of the task are required. Pictures of readily familiar landmarks of the city that contain the city's name are obtained, then the name is placed on a 3 × 5 card. The patient learns to match the name card with the landmark and says the name of the landmark including the name of the city each time.

There is a rapidly growing literature on memory retraining. Many different perspectives are represented. The nurse can help families evaluate any particular programs they might be considering, especially when these would add great expense to the already heavy financial burden of illness. Computer programs have not yet proven effective and most professionals in the field caution that they will never replace the human being who sits with the patient and provides support as well as feedback on performance. By increasingly understanding how the brain is operating, and how memory functions, and how the person has been affected by brain damage, the nurse can creatively help design simple and useful strategies for both daily care of the person with memory deficits by compensating for these, and for improving memory function by stimulating simultaneous and successive processing in memory tasks.

Evaluation

To evaluate the effectiveness of her interventions related to neurological functioning, the nurse examines to what extent the goals established have been met. Since the goals include the behavior to be focused on, a change or level of stability expected, and a given time, these are the dimensions for judging effectiveness. In the goal stated earlier as: the intracranial pressure reading on the monitor will remain below 15 for the next 30 minutes before the patient is suctioned for tracheal secretions, the nurse notes the moniter reading over this time frame. If there are deviations at 15 or above, the nurse might need to take further action to reassess the increasing pressure. A revised plan could then make it safe for her to suction the patient.

Some goals related to memory deficits are particularly difficult to evaluate. The nurse will use the notion of short-term and long-term goals. Remembering that some neurological functions are intact or recovering and that some are functioning at a slower pace, can help care givers to be patient with the long process involved. The nurse recognizes, and helps the family to recognize that improvement may take place only subtly, over long periods of time, and not in steady progression, but with days of better and worse functioning.

SUMMARY

This chapter focused on neurological functioning and the Roy Adaptation Model. The structures and functions associated with neuro processes were briefly described and the principles of integrated cortical function and neural plasticity discussed. This background knowledge of the complexities of neurological functioning are key to understanding the regulator and cognator subsystems of the model, as well as to planning nursing care in this particular physiological mode component. The nursing process was then applied to this component, with particular emphasis on consciousness and memory.

EXERCISES FOR APPLICATION

1. Devise a brief assessment tool for the cranial nerves. Use this tool to assess normal function of a colleague. While doing the assessment, have an image of the neural pathways that are operating.

2. Write down at least five different sources of information that come to you each day and think about what it might feel like to be in this environment without the ability to process it selectively.
3. Describe how a person with severe memory deficits might be affected in each of the adaptive modes, physiological, self concept, role function, and interdependence.

ASSESSMENT OF UNDERSTANDING

1. Identify the two major parts of the nervous system and the major subdivisions of each.
   a. _____
      1) _____
      2) _____
   b. _____
      1) _____
      2) _____
2. Which of the following statements apply to integrated neural functioning?
   a. brain centers for many functions are distributed throughout the brain
   b. specific brain areas have reciprocally interconnected systems
   c. the brain functions as a whole
   d. the two sides of the brain have specific functions
3. List the three criterion behaviors observed when using the Glasgow Coma Scale.
   a. _____
   b. _____
   c. _____

Situation

An elderly patient has been moved from her home to a long-term care facility. Her son lives at a distance and will be able to visit only infrequently. The decision for the change in her living was made because of her increasing inability to move about and care for her own needs in the community. She has high blood pressure.

4. For this person, describe how at least two of the adaptive modes may affect her neurological functioning.
5. State a goal for this patient with interventions to meet this goal.

Feedback

1. a. Central nervous system
      1) brain
      2) spinal cord

    b. Periperal nervous system
       1) cranial and spinal nerves
       2) afferent and efferent systems

2. a, b, and c
3. eye opening, verbal response, and motor response
4. If she does not stay on a low-salt diet, which at home she managed in a palatable way, this may affect her blood pressure. Her secondary role may suffer in not seeing her son and neighbors (tertiary role). The resulting stress can affect her blood pressure, which could increase neurological symptoms such as headache and possible cardiovascular accident. The environmental change and unfamiliar belongings around her (losses in self-concept and interdependence) may cause some confusion.
5. During the week after admission, this patient will remain oriented to time, place, and person. The entire staff will use clocks, calendars, and frequent reminders of time. They talk with her about the facility and about her home. She will be shown brochures of the facility, with the picture on it. The staff will assist her to write letters to friends about her move and make arrangements for the son to call her each day for the first week.

REFERENCES

Anthony, J.C., L. LeResche, U. Niaz, M.R. Von Korff, and M.F. Folstein. Limits of the mini-mental state, a screening test for dementia and delirium among hospital patients, *Psycholocial Medicine,* 12:397, 1982.

Bach-Y-Rita, P. *Recovery of Function: Theoretical Considerations for Brain Injury Rehabilitation.* Toronto, Lewiston, NY, Bern, Stuttgart: Hans Huber Publishers, 1978.

Bignami, A. et al. *Central Nervous System Plastiscity and Repair.* New York: Raven Press. 1985.

Cammermeyer, M. Assessment of cognition, in *AANN's Neurological Nursing: Phenomena and Practice,* eds. Mitchell, P. et al. E. Norwalk: Appleton & Lange, pp. 155–169, 1988.

Das, J.P. Intelligence and information integration, in *Cognitive Strategies and Educational Performance,* ed. Kirby, J. New York: Academic Press, 13–31, 1984.

Das, J.P., J.R. Kirby, and F.R. Jarman. Simultaneous and succesive synthesis: An alternative model for cognitive abilities, *Psychological Bulletin,* 82: 87–103, 1975.

Das, J.P., J.R. Kirby, and R.F. Jarman. *Simultaneous and Successive Cognitive Processes.* New York: Academic Press, 1979.

Diamond, M.C., R.E. Johnson, and C.A. Ingham. Morphological changes in the young adult, and aging cerebral cortex, hippocampus, and diencephalon, *Behavioral Biology.* 14:163–174, 1975.

Folstein, M.F., S.E. Folstein, and P.R. McHugh. Mini-Mental State, a practical method for grading the cognitive state of patients for the clinician. *Journal of Psychiatric Research,* 12: 189, 1975.

Finger, S., and D. Stein. *Brain Damage and Recovery: Research and Clinical Perspectives.* New York: Academic Press, 1982.

Guyton, A. *Human Physiology and Mechanisms of Disease.* Philadelphia: W.B. Saunders, 1987.

Jennett, B. and G. Teasdale. Aspects of coma after severe head injury, in *Lancet,* pp. 878–81, 1977.

Luria, A.R. *Higher Cortical Function in Man.* New York: Basic Books, 1980.

Luria, A.R. *The Working Brain: An Introduction to Neuropsychology.* New York: Basic Books, 1973.

Mitchell, P. Consciousness: An overview, in *AANN's Neuroscience Nursing: Phenomena and Practice,* eds. Mitchell, P. et al. E. Norwalk: Appleton & Lange, pp. 57–66, 1988.

Mountcastle, V.B. An organizing principle for cerebral function: The unit module and the distributed system, in *The Neurosciences,* eds. Schmitt, F.O. and F.G. Worden. Cambridge: MIT Press, 1979.

Plum, F., and J. Posner. *The Diagnosis of Stupor and Coma.* Philadelphia: F.A. Davis Company, 1982

Roy, C. Altered cognition: An information processing approach, in *AANN's Neuroscience Nursing: Phenomena and Practice,* eds. Mitchell, P. et al. E. Norwalk, Conn.: Appleton & Lange, pp. 185–211, 1988.

Roy, C. Nursing care in theory and practice: Early interventions in brain injury, *Recovery from Brain Injury: Expectations Needs and Processes.* pp. 95–110. Northfield, South Australia: Institute for the Study of Learning Difficulties, South Australian College of Advanced Education, 1989.

Jelkurt, E.E. *Basic Physiology for the Health Sciences.* Boston: Little, Brown and Company, 1982.

Sisson, R. Alterations in memory, in *AANN's Neuroscience Nursing: Phenomena and Practice,* eds. Mitchell, P. et al. E. Norwalk: Appleton & Lange, pp. 171–183, 1986.

Talland, G.A. *Deranged Memory.* New York: Academic Press, 1965.

Willis, W. Jr., and R. Grossman. *Medical Neurobiology: Neuroanatomical and Neurophysiological Principles Basic to Clinical Neuroscience.* St. Louis: The C.V. Mosby Company, 1981.

Additional References

Brooks, N. *Closed Head Injury: Psychological, Social, and Family Consequences.* Oxford: Oxford University Press, 1984.

Pi Lamda Theta, San Jose Area Chapter. (1983). *Helping Head Injury and Stroke Patients at Home: A Handbook for Families.* San Jose, CA: Pi Lama Theta, 1983.

Taylor, J., and S. Bellenger. *Neurological Dysfunctions and Nursing Intervention.* New York: McGraw-Hill, 1980.

Chapter Twelve ———————————

Endocrine Function*

Zona Chalifoux

Endocrine function is the last of the complex processes identified in the Roy Adaptation Model. The endocrine system in conjunction with the nervous system integrates and controls all the body's physiological systems responsible for adaptive processes. In this dual regulatory system, nervous system actions that are rapid and of short duration are supplemented by slower and longer hormonal actions, permiting precise control of body function. Even minute changes are recognized immediately and effective adaptation can be accomplished. When all interrelated processes are running smoothly, adaptive behaviors can be observed. However, when one part is disrupted, other components of the endocrine system and the person as a whole may be affected.

This chapter briefly reviews the normal structure and function of the endocrine system. Emphasis is placed both on its functions as a single system and its interaction with other body processes, particularly the nervous system. Knowledge of endocrine structure and functioning serves as a basis for assessing the person's behavior and significant stimuli. Possible nursing diagnoses are identified and several appropriate goals and nursing interventions are discussed.

OBJECTIVES

After studying this chapter, the reader will be able to do the following:

1. Identify behaviors indicating dysfunction of the endocrine system.
2. State behaviors indicating activation of the neuroendocrine mechanisms in response to stimuli.

*This chapter is a revision and expansion of the chapter "Endocrine Function" Mary Howard and Sally Valentine in *Introduction to Nursing: An Adaptation Model* (2nd ed.) Sister Callista Roy pp. 238–252.

3. Identify focal, contextual and residual stimuli that may influence endocrine functioning.
4. Establish nursing diagnoses for a person exhibiting ineffective behaviors related to endocrine functioning.
5. Derive goals for a patient with endocrine dysfunction in a given situation.
6. Discuss common nursing interventions related to endocrine functioning.
7. Evaluate the effectiveness of nursing interventions in meeting previously determined goals in a given situation.

KEY CONCEPTS DEFINED

- *Stress:* the transaction between the environmental demands requiring adaptation and the individual's cognator and regulator coping mechanisms (Roy and McLeod 1981).
- *Stress response:* the process that results from any physical or psychological stimulus disturbing the adaptive state (Andrews and Roy 1986).
- *Stressor:* the focal stimulus confronting an individual. (Roy and McLeod 1981).
- *Adaptation level:* the changing point that represents the person's ability to respond positively in a situation (Andrews and Roy 1986).

STRUCTURES AND FUNCTIONS RELATED TO ENDOCRINE FUNCTION

This section provides an overview of the endocrine system and includes a description of the component glands of the endocrine system and their related functions. Consideration is given also to the interrelationship of the endocrine and nervous systems in maintaining physiological integration.

The endocrine system is composed of the endocrine glands: pituitary, thyroid, parathyroid, adrenal, pineal, and thymus glands; pancreatic islets of Langerham; ovaries; testes, and specialized endocrine cells located in parts of the gastrointestinal tract. Each endocrine gland secretes one or more hormones directly into the bloodstream where they influence other anatomical structures and physiological processes. The glands of the endocrine system and their principle sites of action are outlined in the first two columns of Table 12–1.

The endocrine glands perform the intricate functions of coordination and integration of body functions through the action of their hormones. Each hormone is unique; yet, all hormones have some characteristics in

TABLE 12–1. ENDOCRINE SYSTEM IN SUMMARY

Endocrine Gland And Hormones	Principal Site of Action	Principal Processes Affected by the Hormone
Pituitary Gland		
Anterior Lobe		
Growth Hormone (GH)	General	Growth of body cells, soft tissues, bone, and cartilage
Thyroid-stimulating Thyrotropin (TSH)	Thyroid	Growth and secretory activity of the thyroid gland
Adrenocorticotropin (ACTH)	Adrenal cortex	Growth and secretory activity of the adrenal glands
Follicle-stimulating (FSH)	Ovaries	Development of follicles and secretion of estrogen
	Testes	Development of seminiferous tubules, spermatogenesis
Luteinizing (LH) or Interstitial Cell Stimulating (ICSH)	Ovaries	Ovulation, formation of corpus luteum, secretion of progesterone
	Testes	Growth of male testes, secretion of testosterone
Prolactin (Lactogenic (LTH))	Mammary glands	Secretion of milk, maintenance of corpus luteum and progesterone secretion
Melanocyte (MSH)	Skin	Pigmentation
Posterior Lobe		
Antidiuretic (ADH) (Vasopressin)	Kidney	Reabsorption of water, regulator of osmolarity
	Arterioles	Blood pressure
Oxytocin (Pitocin)	Uterus	Contraction of uterine muscles, facilitates migration of sperm in uterus
	Breast	Milk secretion, promotes release of prolactin
Thyroid Gland		
Thyroxine (T4) and Triiodothyronine (T3)	General	Regulates catabolic phase of metabolism, metabolic rate of all cells and body heat production, influences growth and development, insulin antagonist
Thyrocalcitonin (Calcitonin)	Bone	Inhibits bone resorption, lowers blood level of calcium and phosphorous
Parathyroid Glands		
Parathyroid (PTH)	Bone	Regulates plasma calcium and phosphorous levels, promotes bone reabsorption, increases absorption of calcium
Thymus		
Thymosin	Lymph nodes	Lymphocyte development (?)
Pineal Gland		
Melatonin	Gonads	Sexual maturation (?)

(continued)

TABLE 12–1. (Continued)

Endocrine Gland And Hormones	Principal Site of Action	Principal Processes Affected by the Hormone
Adrenal Gland		
Cortex		
Mineralocorticoids (Aldosterone)	Kidney	Reabsorption of sodium, elimination of potassium, ammonium, and magnesium, maintains volume status
Glucocorticoids	General	Maintains blood glucose level by increasing gluconeogenesis and decreasing rate of glucose utilization by cells
Androgens	General (?)	Preadolescent growth spurt of secondary sexual characteristics
Medulla		
Epinephrine (Adrenalin)	Cardiac muscle Smooth muscle Glands	Stimulator of β receptors in physiological response to stress, emergency functions same as stimulation of sympathetic nervous system: increases blood pressure, cardiac output, blood glucose levels and myocardial contraction, dilates bronchioles
Norepinephrine	Organs innervated by the SNS	Most potent stimulator of the α-receptors in the physiological response to stress, increases peripheral resistance, increases blood pressure
Pancreas		
Islets of Langerham		
Insulin	General	Lowers blood glucose levels, decreases glycogenolysis, gluconeogenesis, and ketogenesis, increases glycogenesis, decreases protein catabolism
Glucagon	Liver	Mobilizes glycogen stores, raises blood sugar levels, glycogenolysis
Somatostatin	General	Lowers blood sugar by interfering with release of growth hormone and glucagon
Ovaries		
Estrogen	Reproductive system	Development of secondary sexual characteristics, repair of the endometrium after menstruation.
Progesterone		Development of breast tissue and endometrium. Maintains pregnancy. Competes with aldosterone at level of renal tubule.
Testes		
Testosterone	Reproductive system	Development of male secondary sexual characteristics, normal functioning of male reproductive system

common. The common characteristics of endocrine hormones are described in Table 12–2. In general, endocrine hormones are secreted in small amounts and are concerned with metabolic processes. Hormone levels are influenced by closed and open loop feedback systems and by normal rhythms.

The extent of hormonal action varies among hormones. One, such as thyrocalcitonin, may have only regional effects, while another, like thyroxine, might exert its effects pervasively over all metabolic processes in the body. The principal body processes affected by each endocrine hormone are listed in column 3 of Table 12–1.

Although each endocrine gland can be viewed as a separate unit with its own independent functions, the various glands also function interdependently. The release of hormones from one gland often influences hormonal release from other glands. Similarly, a disturbance in one endocrine gland is likely to incur a disturbance in others. For example, a decrease in release of thyroid stimulating hormone (TSH) by the anterior pituitary gland causes the thyroid gland to secrete less thyroxine and triiodothyronine.

A full discussion of the complex structures and functions related to endocrine functioning is beyond the parameters of this text. The reader is directed to basic anatomy and physiology and specialty nursing science textbooks for a more in-depth presentation.

Neuroendocrine Integration
Together, endocrine and neurological functioning play a critical role in adaptation and the body's response to stress. To fully appreciate their

---

TABLE 12–2. COMMON CHARACTERISTICS OF ENDOCRINE HORMONES

1. The hormones secreted are concerned primarily with metabolic processes, the physical and chemical changes occurring within cells.

2. Hormones are secreted in minute concentrations which affect greatly body structure and function.

3. The level of each hormone is influenced by a number of regulating mechanisms:

   a. the closed loop negative feedback system. For example, gland A (the anterior pituitary gland) produces a hormone (ACTH) which stimulates gland B (the adrenal cortex). In turn gland B produces a hormone (cortisol) which then inhibits secretion of gland A's hormone (ACTH). The negative feedback system redirects the organism back to an optimal state (Hadley, 1988, p.9).

   b. the open loop positive feedback system. For example, in a state of unrelenting stress the body continues to secrete stress hormones (catecholamines) until a state of exhaustion occurs or outside intervention allows the body to rest.

   c. several types of internal rhythms of secretion (circadian, ultradian and infradian). Hormones are secreted cyclically and in response to body and environmental rhythms. For example, blood levels of adrenocortical hormones are highest in the morning, drop down to lower levels in the evening and then rise again in the morning varying more than fourfold in a 24-hour period.

effects, one must have an understanding of the concept stress and the coping mechanisms as viewed from the perspective of the Roy Adaptation Model.

Stress and its relationship to the human being is widely recognized as an important aspect of nursing practice; yet, it is a concept about which there is little theoretical and practical agreement. Building on the theories of Helson (1964), Selye (1976), and Lazarus (1966), the Roy Adaptation Model assumes a holistic approach to the person and his or her relationship to stress.

Stress is viewed as a general term given to the transaction between the environmental demands for adaptation and the person's response. Both environmental demands and the person's responses can be of a psychological or physiological nature. All three components of the stress adaptation process (demands, stress, and coping) are dynamic processes, continually changing over time; and therefore, not entirely measurable or observable as a singular event. As a totality, they account for individual differences in the stress experience.

When conceptualized in this manner, stress is focal to the process of adaptation and possesses two dimensions. On the input side of the stress interaction, stressors or focal stimuli, mediated by contextual and residual factors, determine an individual's adaptation level. Cognitive appraisal is central in determining which stimuli constitute stress for each individual. Roy and McLeod (1981) described the *adaptation level* as a variable standard against which the pooled impact of new stimuli and feedback from prior responses is compared in order to direct further output from the system. The other half of the stress interaction, or output dimension, involves activation of one or more of the coping mechanisms (the cognator and regulator subsystems), which then produce adaptive or ineffective behaviors.

According to Roy and McLeod (1981), an individual will exhibit adaptive responses in two situations. The first situation is when the gradient difference between the focal stimuli and the adaptation level is small enough that the person's usual responses are adequate to cope with the situation. The second instance occurs when the individual's first responses are not adequate. Yet, the person retains the ability to further activate cognator and/or regulator subsystems, which ultimately prove to be adequate in coping with the situation. For example, a patient may respond to test results indicating an elevated cholesterol level by changing only his diet. When a subsequent test shows continued elevation, the person would be making an adaptive response to stress if his perception of the seriousness of the condition was altered and he undertook an exercise program. Figure 12–1 illustrates this stress adaptation process.

Although both the cognator and regulator subsystems determine the body's total response to stress, that part of the adaptation response associated with endocrine function is located within the regulator coping

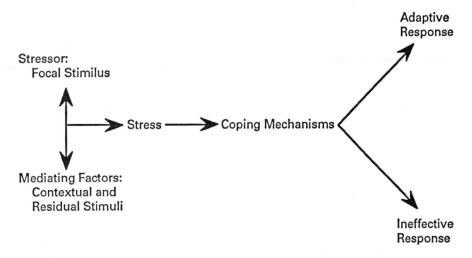

Figure 12–1. The Stress Adaptation Process (*Based on Roy Model of Stress Adaptation in Roy and McLeod, 1981.*)

mechanism. The major parts of the regulator subsystem are the neural, chemical, and endocrine, All three are activated in response to a major stimulus. The perception-psychomotor part is considered neural in nature and overlaps with the cognator coping mechanism. It serves to connect the two mechanisms; thereby, allowing physiological responses to influence cognitive responses and vice versa.[1] The remaining two components of the regulator coping mechanism, chemical and endocrine responses, act together to regulate the body's physiological response to stress.

Selye (1976) proposed that the body's physiological response can take two forms. The first response form, the Local Adaptation Syndrome (LAS), occurs when the body is confronted by a local stimuli and only one organ or part of the body reacts to a stimuli. One example of the LAS is the inflammatory response or immune response. The neuroendocrine mechanisms are not activated during this process. The second response pattern, the general adaptation syndrome (GAS), occurs whenever a collective of body systems is threatened and/or the person undergoes prolonged periods of stress. The GAS is a neuroendocrine response involving primarily the sympathetic branch of the autonomic nervous system, and the pituitary, adrenal, and thyroid glands. The body's neuroendocrine responses to stress (GAS) in which the hypothalmus and medulla oblongota are activated in response to a sensory stimuli, such as severe pain, is outlined in Figure 12–2.

[1]Discussion of the cognitive response to stress and anxiety as a common adaptation problem is included in chapter 15 on the personal self.

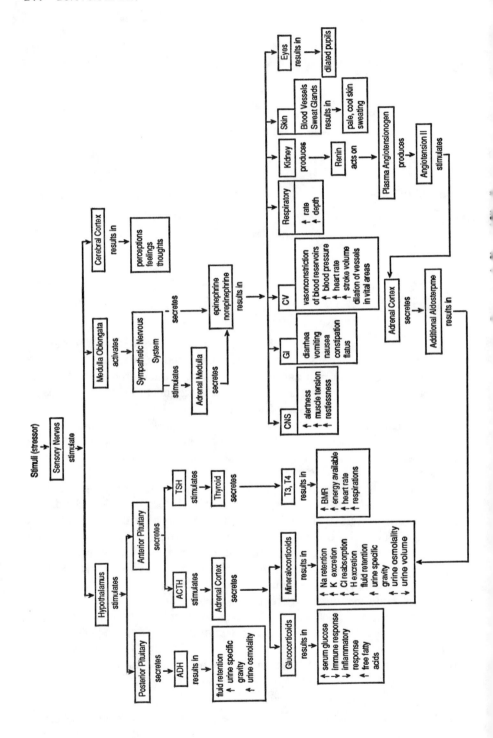

Selye (1976) suggested that both the GAS and the LAS develop in three distinct stages. First, the alarm reaction stage, when the whole body's neuroendocrine defenses against the stimulus, regardless of whether it is bacteria or verbal abuse, are alerted and mobilized to protect the body. Second, the stage of resistance, when the body attempts to cope by limiting the stimulus' effects to the smallest possible area. Lastly, the stage of exhaustion, in which the body's adaptive ability to resist the stressor becomes exhausted.

The phases vary in duration and intensity in relation to the strength of the stimuli that initiated the stress response (Howard and Valentine 1984). For example, a brief, sudden, unexpected noise may elicit only very brief unmeasurable responses reflective of the alarm phase; the stress response does not continue into the resistance or exhaustion phases. On the other hand, a major surgical operation may produce more measurable, prolonged responses of the second and third phases.

APPLICATION OF THE NURSING PROCESS

As was the case with neurological function, integrity of endocrine function, or lack thereof, has profound effects on physiological integrity as a whole and ultimate functioning of the individual in all of the other modes. In addition disruptions of the endocrine system are often long term in nature. The role of the nurse in assessment and supportive nursing interventions contributes to the promotion of integrity of the whole person over time.

Assessment of Behavior

As has been described, endocrine hormones affect the functioning of all the body's needs and processes inherent in physiological integrity. Therefore, the nurse must implement an overall appraisal of an individual's physiological integrity when carrying out a nursing assessment for adaptive and ineffective behaviors related to endocrine functioning. The nurse uses the skills of interviewing, inspection, and measurement of internal and external responses to gather both subjective and objective data in each of the areas of the physiological mode. The focus is not only on the patient's current status in each area but also on any changes over time noted by the patient. The person may exhibit behaviors reflective of endocrine dysfunction in one or more needs or processes. The behavior manifested depends upon the characteristics of the focal stimuli. The needs and complex processes identified in the Roy Adaptation Model provide the basis for assessment of behavior in relation to endocrine functioning.

Although the endocrine system consists of nine glands, sample behaviors related to seven are included in this chapter since the endocrine functions of the pineal and thymus glands are as yet poorly understood.

Oxygenation. In assessing oxygenation as related to endocrine functioning, the nurse considers the patient's mental status as well as respiratory and circulatory functioning. Particular areas of focus are temperature, pulse, respirations, blood pressure, predominant mood, memory, degree of alertness, and thought patterns. Abnormal behaviors, such as hypertension related to fluid retention, lability of moods, and irritability are associated with excessive ACTH. Endocrine functioning also affects a person's need for activity and rest. Areas to assess include energy level, sleep patterns, coordination and extent of body movements, and the presence of abnormal behaviors. Generalized weakness is a common complaint in patient's who have alterations in adrenocorticoid, thyroid, insulin, and pituitary hormonal levels.

Nutrition. The patient's appetite, amount and type of food intake, and weight changes are all indicators of endocrine functioning in the nutritional need. A decrease in body weight in the absence of voluntary caloric restriction or a marked general increase in exercise suggest the presence of underlying hormonal dysfunction.

Fluids and Electrolytes. Fluid and electrolyte balance often is altered in endocrine dysfunction. Assessment of this need area considers the patient's desire for fluid, status of the mucus membranes, and the presence of abnormal behaviors, such as diaphoresis and edema. Mineralocorticoids secreted by the adrenal glands play a major role in elimination and retention of body fluid through their influence on the kidney.

Elimination. Elimination, in terms of the amount, characteristics, and patterns of urinary and intestinal output, should be assessed relative to endocrine functioning. For example, the volume, timing, and frequency of urinary output is an important indicator of diabetes mellitus; while, the constituents of urine are important in diagnosing conditions of adrenocorticoid hormonal alteration.

Protection. Relative to the need for protection, assessment data reflecting endocrine functioning are integrity of the skin, hair, and nails and the body's ability to withstand and recover from infections. Areas of focus include skin characteristics (color, texture, moisture, turgor, and depth), pigmentation distribution, tanning ability, tendency to bruise, and rate of healing. The patient's hair is assessed for color, amount, texture, distribution over the body, and how easily it can be broken. Nail characteristics, such as growth, texture, and smoothness reflect endocrine functioning. For example, abnormal behaviors resulting from an elevation of thyroxine are warm, damp, soft textured skin, silky hair, loosening of the nail from the nail bed, and absence of forehead wrinkling.

The Senses. Endocrine functioning can also be assessed by looking at the status of a person's senses. The absence or alteration of ability in the senses of touch, vision, and smell may be indicative of endocrine dysfunction. Other behaviors to note are the presence of abnormal sensations such as pain and intolerance to temperature changes. Diminished sensory responses to stimuli in the lower extremities and neuropathies of the bladder and bowel are associated with decreased insulin production.

Physiological Structure. Other assessment areas to consider involve the structural development of the body's skeletal system, soft tissues, and organs. The body's skeletal structure is affected profoundly by levels of growth hormone, thyroxine, and triiodothyronine. Therefore, assessment of endocrine functioning considers the patient's actual skeletal and soft tissue development in relation to age-predicted growth and body proportions. For example, decreased linear bone growth is associated with decreased thyroxine levels. An increased rate of linear bone growth, with premature closure of the epiphyseal centers and altered body proportions can be related to decreased levels of androgen or growth hormone. An increase and redistribution of soft tissue is associated with high levels of adrenocorticoid hormones. In cases of increase in thyroid hormones, the thyroid gland is noted to be larger, tender, and sometimes asymmetrical in shape.

Similarly, the growth and development of the person's reproductive structures and their related functioning is dependent upon adequate endocrine hormones. Alterations in the size and shape of genitalia, libido, secondary sexual characteristics, onset of menarche and menopause, and penile erectile functioning are indicators of endocrine functioning. For example, reduced output of follicle stimulating hormone (FSH) and luteinizing (LH) hormones may result in breast and uterine atrophy in females and reduced beard and testes size in males.

Laboratory Tests. Because of the multiple functions of the endocrine system, various tests are used to determine whether disease of this regulating system is present and if so, to help in identifying the factors influencing the patient's ineffective behaviors. These tests are of two general types. First are those tests involving direct measurement of the concentration of various hormones or antibodies specific to chemical groups or conformations of hormones in the plasma, blood, or urine. Examples of these are bioassay of thyroid hormone and chemical assay of cortisol and PTH levels. Second, tests in which indirect methods of measuring hormonal concentration are used, such as the urine test for 17-ketogenic steroids and the thyroid stimulation test.

A careful analysis of the person's behavior in each of these areas is essential for the basis of a realistic, individualized nursing care plan. The nurse must decide if a particular behavior is adaptive, requiring supportive interventions, or ineffective, necessitating management of stimuli. This nursing judgement is made by considering each behavior in light of the indicators of effective adaptation. The same as the foundation of a house determines the quality of the home, the data gathered and decisions made at this stage determine the merit and success of the subsequent nursing care plan.

Assessment of Stimuli

The assessment of endocrine functioning is not complete until the nurse has also searched the person's internal and external environments for focal, contextual, and residual stimuli that are contributing to the behaviors. The most common stimuli influencing endocrine dysfunction can be grouped into those related to glandular dysfunction and those arising in the internal and external environment.

Glandular Dysfunctions.

Ineffective endocrine behaviors are most commonly caused by the focal stimulus of glandular dysfunction resulting from cellular damage or defective genetic endowment. The same as other cells of the body, those of endocrine glands are susceptible to trauma, vascular interference, autoimmune disorders, infection, and neoplasm. Disturbances in function also may result from a malfunction in the gland's regulating mechanism or from the failure of a gland's target cells to respond to the hormones being secreted. For example, diabetes mellitus is considered to be related to a loss of cell sensitivity to insulin.

The functional and structural changes in endocrine glands precipitated by these stimuli take similar forms regardless of the specific gland affected. Hormonal disturbances are characterized by either hyposecretion or hypersecretion of a hormone, or an imbalance between or among hormones. As Felig, Baxter, Broadus, and Frohman (1987) described, structural changes experienced can be hypoplasia (decrease in number of organ cells), hyperplasia (increase in number of organ cells), atrophy (shrinkage in organ or cell size), or hypertrophy (increase in cell or organ size). Discussions of specific glandular pathologies can be found in medical and other nursing science textbooks.

Environmental Conditions.

Contextual stimuli, such as external environmental conditions, frequently augment the effects of the focal stimuli. For example, the internal temperature changes noted in dysfunction of the thyroid gland may be increased by changes in environmental temperature and humidity. Similarly, the lassitude evident in hypothyroidism may be accentuated by a socially impoverished milieu.

Cognator Effectiveness.

Another important contextual stimulus relates to individuals' perception of their ability to control health-related outcomes in life, that is, their health locus of control (Wallston and Wallston 1978). There appear to be three distinctive belief patterns held by people regarding the responsibility for health care outcomes: powerful others (health care providers), chance or luck (one's predetermined fate), and oneself (own personal abilities). Since the process of perception links the regulator and cognator subsystems, the person's perception of the impact of glandular dysfunction on daily life and ability to control health state may have a profound effect upon the person's responses.

What is perceived as a minor occurrence (stimuli) by one person may be seen as extremely stressful by another (Lazarus and Folkman 1984). Similarly, a person's locus of control may change with the situation. A person may feel in control when in the home environment, but feel subject to the control of others or luck in the hospital. Cognitive appraisal of the demands of the situation, that is, the severity and extent of the stimuli, the number of stimuli to be coped with at one time and the duration of exposure to the stimuli, determines the manner in which an individual visualizes the stimuli.

Health Care Interventions. Medical and nursing interventions designed to assist the patient in adapting to a disease process contribute additional contextual stimuli. For example, medications are one group of stimuli that tend to compound difficulties of adapting. It is not unusual for a patient to be receiving an antibiotic, a corticosteroid, and an analgesic all at the same time for an endocrine related condition. Each of these drugs has a desired effect on the focal stimuli (glandular dysfunction) and associated adverse effects, which often affect other endocrine glands and neuroendocrine integrating mechanisms. Other interventions related to treatment of ineffective behaviors in another mode can have also a negative impact upon patients. These include diet, exercise, availability of fluids, and activity level.

Although less obvious, the nurse needs to assess for other common stimuli of the residual category. Sources for these are developmental stage, culture, climate, and past experience with similar stimuli.

Nursing Diagnosis

Identification of nursing diagnosis associated with endocrine regulation is accomplished in the same way as it is in the other areas of the physiological mode. First, the person's behaviors together with the influencing stimuli establish the nursing diagnoses (Andrews and Roy 1986). Nursing diagnoses may reflect either adaptive or ineffective behaviors. In the former case, the nursing diagnosis may state, "Effective hormonal regulation of metabolic and body processes due to adequate glandular functioning (with the specific behaviors, gland and hormones of concern stated)." In the case of ineffective behaviors, a multitude of nursing diagnoses may result.

The endocrine system is closely interrelated with other body systems; therefore, a disturbance in one endocrine regulating mechanism is likely to precipitate a disturbance in others. Problems commonly occur in one or several of the following areas: cardiac output, comfort, safety, nutrition, self concept, skin integrity, activity and rest, elimination, coping abilities, compliance, fluid volume balance, knowledge level, cognitive processing, and stress tolerance.

As has been described previously in this text, nursing diagnoses may be of three types according to the Roy Adaptation Model: (1) a statement of the behaviors within one mode with their most relevant influencing stimuli, (2) a summary label for behaviors in one mode with relevant stimuli, or (3) a label that summarizes a behavioral pattern when more than one mode is being affected by the same stimuli.

Using the first method, an example of a nursing diagnosis could be, "Intolerance to heat, increased appetite associated with weight loss, frequent diarrhea, fine hand tremors, weakness, clumsiness, fatigability and nervousness associated with thyroid hyperactivity."

More commonly and because of the interrelated nature of endocrine function, the nurse will be utilizing the second method. Here, the nursing diagnosis is a statement of behavior within one area along with the most relevant stimuli. The same behaviors and stimuli referred to previously could be written as, "Feelings of fatigue related to thyroid hyperactivity," or "Nervousness related to hyperactivity of the thyroid."

Finally, a cross-modal diagnosis can be made where a behavioral pattern relating to more than one mode is being affected by a stimulus. An example of this type of diagnosis is, "Decreased energy and decreased responsibility for self-care due to stress of illness."

Regardless of the method, a well written nursing diagnosis aids in setting priorities and establishing direction for the next step of the nursing process—goal setting.

Goal Setting

Many endocrine dysfunctions have a chronic as well as an acute phase. Thus, the goal setting process includes both long and short-term goals, stating the behavior to be changed, the desired change and the time frame for the change to occur.

The following statements provide examples of possible goals for a person with thyroid hyperactivity. "The person will gain one pound per week in weight." "Within one week the person will provide evidence of higher energy level." or "Within this day, the person will demonstrate an increased knowledge level of thyroid hormones and their actions by listing three hormones and one major action of each hormone." Each of these goals indicates the behavior to be changed, the change desired and the associated time frame.

Nursing Interventions

Given the chronic, long-term nature of many endocrine dysfunctions, the nurse, through her frequent and prolonged contact with these patients, plays an important role in their care. Through individualized, thoughtful interventions, the nurse can support patients' adaptive endocrine responses and aid in altering ineffective endocrine related behaviors toward an adaptive state. Many interventions which are diagnostic, pharmacological and treatment related require physician initiation. The nurse ensures that these are carried out in a supportive manner (Howard and Valentine 1984). Other interventions are initiated by the nurse. These include designing a coordinated individual plan of care with the patient based on assessment, nursing diagnosis, and behavioral goals. Although each patient will require a unique combination of interventions, there are basic approaches nurses take in assisting a patient with an endocrine imbalance. Several of these are discussed here.

Glandular dysfunction is the most common focal stimulus for patients experiencing endocrine dysfunction. Therefore, the nurse should direct actions toward promoting normal functioning of the body, especially in fluid and electrolyte balance, nutritional status, elimination, activity and rest, protection, and oxygenation. For example, nursing interventions in fluid and electrolytes may include maintaining intake and output records and recording losses by other routes such as perspiration and diarrhea. In promoting nutritional status, the nurse may ensure regular intake of the correct amount and type of food by giving emotional support and creating a controlled environment conducive to food intake and retention. Further discussion of nursing measures to promote adaptation in the specific physiological needs and complex processes can be found in Chapters 4 to 11.

A second approach relates to improving the patient's and his or her family's understanding of associated anatomical and structural changes. Research has shown that some people will have a more positive reaction to illness if they understand their disease process and anticipated course of illness (Harrigan 1987). Since illness adds additional burden to the patient experiencing endocrine dysfunction, the nurse includes health teaching in the plan of care. The principles of learning and teaching need to be observed closely during the health teaching process.

Learning is more likely to occur when the learner perceives a need to learn, sees a way to meet that need, is actively involved in the learning process and receives positive reinforcement for behavior changes. Teaching involves extensive planning giving consideration to the learning environment, complexity level and amount of information to be covered per session and the physical and emotional state of the learner. Health teaching is especially important in chronic illnesses where the person witnesses irreversible progressive changes in body appearance and function.

Obesity, decreased peripheral sensitivity, coarsening of facial features, hirsutism, loss of sexual functioning, and deepened voice are just a few overt disruptions that occur in endocrine imbalances.

The nurse also teaches the patient and his or her family about diagnostic tests, procedures, and treatment protocols. Many people with endocrine disorders face a lifelong program of therapeutic intervention. The person needs to know why the prescribed diagnostic procedures and treatment protocols are necessary, how they will affect bodily functions, what they can do to ensure successful completion of therapeutic measures, such as dietary regulation and hormone replacement therapy, and when signs and symptoms indicate a need to seek further medical attention. Some of the major complications arising from impaired endocrine regulatory mechanisms to which the nurse alerts the patient are: respiratory and genitourinary infections, fluctuations in energy level, alterations in vital signs and peripheral perfusion, decreased sensation and perception abilities, and complications arising from reproductive dysfunctions.

Since fatigue is a common component of endocrine imbalances, it is often necessary to aid the patient in acquiring an energy level which allows him or her to carry out the maximum activities of daily living. Careful planning and scheduling of activities to provide for rest are carried out with extensive patient input. Activity priorities are set daily based on planned diagnostic procedures and treatments. Short periods of activity followed by rest with the greatest activity periods in the morning are appropriate for some people.

The nurse assists the patient in developing a life plan which promotes freedom from avoidable stressors and minimizes the effects of those that are unavoidable. In order to focus on major unavoidable stimuli, the person's environment is freed from all avoidable ones. Consideration is given to the person's biological and psychological characteristics, socioeconomic environment and coping strategies in co-planning stress management and reduction with the patient. Since many endocrine imbalances are unavoidable and require permanent lifestyle changes, the nurse helps the person to be adequately prepared to regulate stress levels as these occur.

Sutterly (1982) and Smith and Selye (1979) have described six effective approaches: (1) proper nutrition, (2) regular exercise and recreation, (3) training in meditation, creative imagery, relaxation techniques, and biofeedback (Holden-Lund 1988, Moreno 1987), (4) lifestyle analysis to identify and remove from their environment unnecessary stressful stimuli such as noise and uncomfortable conditions, (5) counseling to replace ineffective coping mechanisms (eg alcohol intake) with more positive behavior (time management), (6) establishing support systems, and (7) self-reflection to neutralize the intensity of the stimuli by changing personal perspectives of the events or goals. The nurse's role is to assist patients in stress reduction efforts by helping them recognize the stress producing stimuli in their lifestyles, to gain insight as to why a particular stimuli is stressful, and to develop constructive coping mechanisms to deal with the stimuli.

The nurse facilitates the patient's achievement of role mastery in roles frequently disrupted by endocrine imbalance. Difficulties in fulfilling the roles of mother, father, wife, husband, or employee pose real threats to the person's self-concept. Some endocrine imbalances cause mood swings that may threaten all interpersonal relationships, while others induce impotency, affecting primarily sexual relationships and reproductive roles. These role disruptions are compounded often by periods of increased dependency. For example, periods of hospitalization and intensive therapy may require the spouse, relative, or friend to supply more manual, financial or emotional support. Interventions related to role function are discussed in Chapter 17.

Lastly, the nurse has an important role in promoting patient collaboration in the plan for therapy. The nurse can facilitate long-term participation by encouraging the person to undertake self-assessment of motivational factors. Some individuals will be motivated towards behavior change by feelings of control gained through greater knowledge and skills while others may respond to encouragement from supportive significant others. Once identified, positive motivators can be strengthened and avoidance motivators limited or altered (Armstrong 1987). One self-assessment session or teaching session will not ensure permanent cooperation; continued contact with the health care team for evaluative feedback and support is vital.

Evaluation

The nurse's role includes evaluation of whether or not the nursing interventions have been successful in altering stimuli and assisting the person to meet the behaviors outlined in the predefined goals. Modification of nursing approaches is planned and carried out based upon this evaluation.

To evaluate, the nurse focuses on the person's behavior using observation, measurement, interviewing and other interpersonal skills. For example, for the previous goal, "Within one week, the person will provide evidence of higher energy levels," the behavior of focus is the person's energy level. Evidence of this change may be statements by the person indicating feelings of "less tiredness" or "more energy." Such behavioral statements indicate that the person is achieving the preestablished goal.

If the goals were not being achieved, the nurse would revisit previous steps of the nursing process in an attempt to identify further assessment data or refine decisions made in the other steps of the process, such as diagnosis, goal setting, or selecting interventions.

SUMMARY

As part of the regulator coping mechanism, the endocrine system plays an important role in maintaining the body's adaptive processes and in the body's physiological response to stress. This chapter presented endocrine functioning from both perspectives. Assessment areas indicative of endocrine functioning were outlined, and possible stimuli influencing disruption in endocrine functioning were identified. Examples of goals, nursing diagnoses, and common adaptation problems related to functioning of endocrine processes were presented. Seven common types of nursing interventions were discussed. Within these basic principles and a broad knowledge base, the nurse recognizes that the complexity of endocrine functioning requires a unique plan for the care of each patient.

EXERCISES FOR APPLICATION

1. Recall a recent stressful situation in your life, perhaps an examination or a car accident. Using the behavioral assessment categories in this chapter, list the behaviors you exhibited which reflect activation of your neuroendocrine mechanisms (General Adaptation Syndrome responses).
2. Using the material in this chapter and the references at the end of this chapter, describe two methods you could use to reduce your stress response before encountering a similar situation again.

ASSESSMENT OF UNDERSTANDING

1. Which of the following behaviors may indicate activation of the stress response?
   a. patient's face appears as "white as a sheet"
   b. respiration rate of 30 per minute with an increase in depth of respiration
   c. pupil constriction
   d. periods of stuttering, muscle twitching
   e. bouts of nausea, vomiting or diarrhea
   f. blood pressure of 90/60
2. Which of the following behaviors indicate a need to completely assess a patient's endocrine functioning?
   a. amenorrhea in a twenty-four year old female
   b. patient states "I don't know what the matter is . . . I just don't have any pep"
   c. increase in facial hair in women
   d. weight loss in presence of caloric restriction or increased exercise

e. recent increase in pigmentation of elbows, palmar creases, scars and axilla

f. excessive sweating unrelated to environmental temperature

3. If an endocrine problem is suspected, the patient should be specifically questioned about

a. delays or excessive growth of their skeletal system

b. mood and memory status

c. tolerance to stressers

d. ability to feel sensations in their lower extremities

e. changes in their hair and nail characteristics

f. volume of urine output

4. List five categories of injury that commonly cause the focal stimulus of glandular dysfunction in the process of endocrine regulation.

5. Formulate nursing diagnosis for the following sets of information.

Behavior	**Stimuli**
Person A	
"I just can't seem to get myself out of bed in the morning and I feel so weak"	Uncontrolled Cushing's Syndrome for five years
Requires assistance of walker to ambulate	Patient's room is very small with lots of furniture
Weight of 200 lb, height 5 ft	Age, 50 years
Thin arms and legs with truncal obesity	
Osteoporosis of long bones on x-ray	
Left foot painful with an open sore on great toe	
Edema 2+ of ankles	
Cool feet, absence of pedal pulses	
Person B	
Rapid, deep respirations	Ate a large breakfast
Blood glucose level >400 mg/dL at 11 AM this morning and 120 mg/dL at 11 AM yesterday morning	Insulin dosage reduced yesterday
	Diabetes Mellitus Type II for 10 years controlled by insulin
Lassitude, drowsiness	Received notification from insurance company that coverage may be stopped
Urine output of 3500 cc in last 24 hours	
Weight loss of 5 lb in 2 weeks	
Dry mucus membranes	

6. Derive a goal related to one of the nursing diagnosis you developed in the previous item.
7. List four groups of nursing interventions that are commonly implemented when caring for a patient with endocrine dysfunction.
8. If the goal developed in item 6 was, "Person A will not show evidence of injury during hospitalization," or "Person will be better able to cope with stress within one week," how would you evaluate the effectiveness associated with the interventions?

Feedback

1. a, b, d, e.
2. a, b, c, e, f.
3. All
4. a. trauma
   b. vascular interferences
   c. autoimmune disorders
   d. infection
   e. neoplasms
   f. genetic defects
5. Person A. Examples of Nursing Diagnoses

Altered Skin Integrity (open sore on great toe)	related to	Cushing's Syndrome (increased susceptibility to infection and lowered resistance to stress)
Altered Tissue Perfusion (edema 2+, cool feet, absence of pedal pulses)	related to	Cushing's Syndrome (Na and H_2O retention)
Potential for Injury (left foot painful, obese, requires assistance)	related to	Cushing's Syndrome (muscle wasting, potassium depletion and hyperglycemia)
Fatigue (complaints of weakness)	related to	Cushing's Syndrome (poor muscle strength and electrolyte imbalance)

Person B. Examples of Nursing Diagnosis

Polyuria (urine output of 3500 cc the last 24 hours)	related to	Diabetes Mellitus (excretion of large in amounts of glucose, ketones and protein)

Thirst (intake of 3000 cc in last 24 hours)	related to	Diabetes Mellitus (loss of ECF)
Alteration in Nutrition: (more than body requirements of glucose) Ketoacidosis (thirst, polyuria, increased respiratory rate and blood sugar levels)	related to	Diabetes Mellitus (insulin deficiency)

6. Examples of Goals

Person A will not show evidence of injury during hospitalization. Person B will be better able to cope with stress within one week as shown by actively dealing with the insurance company.

7. a. promotion of adaptive behaviors in physiological mode
   b. teaching patient and patient's family about disease processes, diagnostic procedures and treatment regimes
   c. encouraging life style analysis to identify stressors and plan management of energy expenditure
   d. facilitating role mastery in affected roles
   e. promoting effective participation in treatment protocols

8. Examples of Evaluation

Observe and examine the patient, gather reports from the patient, and review the patient's records to see if all measures indicate that the patient did not sustain injury during hospitalization.

Discuss with the patient his subjective feelings of stress, and observe the patient's nonverbal behaviors and his interactions with others. All measures should indicate a reduction in stress levels within one week. The patient should state that he is experiencing less stress. He should appear more free of anxiety as evidenced by a relaxed facial expression, lack of restlessness, and appropriate interactions with staff and active attempts to deal with sources of stress such as dealing directly with the insurance company.

REFERENCES

Andrews, H., and Sr. C. Roy. *Essentials of the Roy Adaptative Model*. E. Norwalk, Conn.: Appleton-Century-Crofts, 1986.

Armstrong, N. Coping with diabetes mellitus: a full-time job. *Nursing Clinics of North America*, 22(3): 559–569, 1987.

Felig, P., J. Baxter, A. Broadus, and L. Frohman, *Endocrinology and Metabolism* (2nd ed.). New York: McGraw-Hill, 1987.

Hadley, M. *Endocrinology* (2nd ed.). Englewood Cliffs, N.J.: Prentice-Hall, 1988.

Harrigan, J. Application of locus of control to diabetes education in school aged children, *Journal of Pediatric Nursing,* 2(4): 236–243, 1987.

Helson, H. *Adaptation Level Theory,* New York: Harper and Row, 1964.

Holden-Lund, C. Effects of relaxation with guided imagery on surgical stress and wound healing. *Research in Nursing and Health,* 11: 235–244, 1988.

Howard, M., and S. Valentine. Endocrine Function, in *Introduction to Nursing: An Adaptation Model,* ed. Sr. C. Roy, pp. 238–252. Englewood Cliffs, N.J.: Prentice-Hall, 1984.

Lazarus, R., and S. Folkman. *Stress, Appraisal and Coping.* New York: Springer Publications, 1984.

Moreno, C. Concepts of stress management in cardiac rehabilitation. *Focus of Critical Care,* 13–14: 13–19, 1987.

Roy, Sr. C., and D. McLeod. Theory of the person as an adaptive system, in *Theory Construction in Nursing: An Adaptation Model,* Sr. C. Roy and S. L. Roberts, pp. 49–69. Englewood Cliffs, N.J.: Prentice-Hall, 1981.

Selye, H. *The Stress of Life* (2nd ed.). New York: McGraw-Hill, 1976.

Smith, M., and H. Selye. Reducing the Negative Effects of Stress, *American Journal of Nursing,* 79(11): 1953–1955, 1979.

Sutterly, D. Stress and health: A survey of self regulation modalities, in *Coping with Stress,* eds. D. Sutterly, and G. Donnelly, pp. 173–194. Rockville, Md.: Aspen Systems Corp., 1982.

Wallston, K., and B. Wallston. Development of multidimensional health locus of control scales, *Health Education Monographs,* 6(2): 160–170, 1978.

Additional References

Bille, D. Tailoring your diabetic patients care plan to fit his lifestyle, *Nursing,* 16(2): 54–57, 1986.

Clarke, M. Stress and coping: constructs for nursing, *Journal of Advanced Nursing,* 9: 3–13, 1984a.

Clarke, M. The constructs: "Stress" and "coping" as a rationale for nursing activities. *Journal of Advanced Nursing,* 9: 267–275, 1984b.

Guyton, A. *Textbook of Medical Physiology* (7th ed.). Philadelphia: W.B. Saunders, 1986.

Lanuza, D., and S. Marotta. Endocrine and psychologic responses of patients to cardiac pacemaker implantation, *Heart and Lung,* 16(5): 496–505, 1987.

Howe, J., E. Dickason, D. Jones, and M. Snider. *The Handbook of Nursing.* New York: J. Wiley and Sons, 1984.

Malasanos, L. et al. *Health Assessment* (3rd ed.). St. Louis: The C.V. Mosby Co., 1986.

Phipps, W., B. Long, and N. Woods. *Medical-Surgical Nursing: Concepts and Clinical Practice.* (3rd ed.). St. Louis: The C.V. Mosby Co., 1987.

Resler, M. Teaching strategies that promote adherence, *Nursing Clinics of North America,* 18: 799–811, 1983.

Riordan, J., P. Malan, and R. Gould. *Essentials of Endocrinology* (2nd ed.). Oxford: Blackwell Scientific Publications, 1988.

Rotter, J. Some problems and misconceptions related to the construct of internal versus external control of reinforcement, *Journal of Consulting and Clinical Psychology,* 43:(1), 56–67, 1975.

Rotter, J. Generalized expectancies for internal versus external control of reinforcement, *Psychological Monographs,* 80(1), 1966.

Shaver, J. A biopsychosocial view of human health, *Nursing Outlook,* 33(4): 186–191, 1985.

Vander, A. et al. *Human Physiology: The Mechanisms of Body Function.* New York: McGraw-Hill Co., 1980.

PART II: CONCLUSION

Part II has focused on the physiological mode as described in the Roy Adaptation Model for Nursing. As has been described, the physiological mode is associated with the way the person responds physically to stimuli from the environment. Behavior in this mode is a manifestation of the physiological activity of the cells, tissues, organs, and systems comprising the human body although the influence of the psychosocial aspects of the person on physiological processes also was pointed out.

Five needs were identified in the physiological mode relative to the basic need of physiological integrity: oxygenation, nutrition, elimination, activity and rest, and protection. Also described were four complex processes associated with physiological integrity: the senses, fluids and electrolytes, neurological function, and endocrine function. Each of these was the topic of an individual chapter in which associated structures and functions were described, the theoretical basis for the component was identified, and the application of the steps of the Roy Model nursing process was illustrated.

Part II concludes with a case study that illustrates application of the Roy Model to a patient care situation. The case study is structured using the six steps of the nursing process following a brief description of the patient situation.

The Physiological Model—Case Study
Donna M. Romyn

Using the nursing process, the nurse assists the individual to maintain biopsychosocial integrity. In this summary, a case study will be utilized to demonstrate application of the nursing process in the physiological mode. Data regarding a client's physiological behavior is documented and the focal, contextual and residual stimuli which influence that behavior are identified. A nursing diagnosis is formulated and client-centered goals are set to change ineffective physiological behavior to adaptive behavior. Nursing interventions are planned to assist the client to achieve the goals by managing the specific stimuli identified in the nursing diagnosis. The effectiveness of nursing intervention is evaluated by assessing client progress towards the preset goals.

CASE STUDY

Mr. K., 68-year-old retired farmer, was admitted to the hospital suffering obstructive urinary retention. A urinary drainage tube was inserted into his right kidney and Mr. K. subsequently was discharged to a palliative (hospice) care unit.

History
One year ago Mr. K. was admitted to hospital with a diagnosis of cancer of the rectum. Further investigation revealed metastasis to the liver and lymph nodes. Mr. K. refused treatment at that time. The reason for this decision is unknown.

Present Condition
During the past three months Mr. K. has experienced a weight loss of about 25 pounds. He has frequent episodes of nausea and vomiting and suffers severe intermittent abdominal pain.

Family History
Mr. K.'s father died of cardiovascular disease at the age of 76 and his mother died of a stroke at the age of 72. All other family members are alive and well.

ASSESSMENT OF BEHAVIORS—PHYSIOLOGICAL MODE

In assessing the physiological mode the nurse assesses behavior related to each of the physiological needs. Data is collected using observation, interview/interaction and measurement skills. Assessment of Mr. K.'s physiological behavior is summarized in Table II–1.

TABLE II–1. ASSESSMENT OF MR. K.'S PHYSIOLOGICAL BEHAVIOR

Oxygenation:	TPR: 97.5-88-22; BP: 110/72
	No adventitious breath sounds
Nutrition:	Able to tolerate fluid diet only
	Takes fluids frequently in small amounts; poor appetite
	5'9" tall; 120 pounds
Elimination:	Urine clear, concentrated
	Constipated stool from colostomy
Activity and Rest:	Stands to transfer; weak
	Tolerates being up short periods of time
	Tired but sleeps only a few minutes at a time
Protection:	Dehydrated
	Excoriated areas around colostomy and urinary drainage tube
	Skin pale, warm, dry to touch

Senses:	Hearing and vision within normal ranges
	Severe intermittent abdominal pain
Fluids and Electrolytes:	Poor fluid intake
	Minimal urinary output: Below 400 cc in 24 hours
	Electrolyte levels abnormal: Potassium 6.5 mEq/L
	Sodium 133 mEq/L
	Urine specific gravity: 1.01
Neurological Function:	Drowsy
	Oriented to person, place, time
	Basic reflexes and touch within normal limits
Endocrine Function:	No known endocrine abnormalities

On completion of the assessment of behaviors related to each of the physiological needs, the nurse considers each behavior to determine whether it is adaptive or ineffective in promoting physiological integrity. Behaviors of concern are identified and priorities are set for further assessment and intervention.

Mr. K. identified extreme fatigue as the problem which was most troublesome at this time. Thus, the remainder of this case study will focus primarily on his need for rest.

ASSESSMENT OF STIMULI

In addition to assessing the individual's behaviors related to each of the needs of the physiological mode, the nurse uses observation, interview, interaction and measurement skills to identify the focal, contextual and residual stimuli influencing the behaviors assessed. Recall that behaviors in one mode also may be stimuli to behaviors within that mode or another mode. In this case study, several of the physiological behaviors assessed were also factors which influenced or contributed to Mr. K.'s extreme fatigue. Table II-2 summarizes the assessment of stimuli influencing Mr. K.'s need for rest.

TABLE II–2. ASSESSMENT OF STIMULI RELATED MR. K.'S NEED FOR REST

	Stimuli		
Behaviors	**Focal**	**Contextual**	**Residual**
Extreme fatigue	Pain	Nausea	Fluid and electrolyte imbalance
Sleeps only a few minutes at a time	Vomiting		
Weakness	Anxiety Hospital routines		

NURSING DIAGNOSIS

A nursing diagnosis summarizes the behavioral and stimuli data collected. Two different formats could be utilized to establish a nursing diagnosis for Mr. K. The nurse could (1) formulate a statement which summarizes the physiological behaviors of concern and the most relevant influencing stimuli or (2) the nurse could select a label which most appropriately summarizes the behaviors from the typology of common adaptation problems presented in Chapter 2.

Nursing diagnoses for Mr. K. could be stated as: (1) extreme fatigue related to pain, nausea and vomiting, anxiety and hospital routines, or (2) inadequate pattern of rest. Based on the assessment data, the nurse also would establish nursing diagnoses related to other physiological behaviors of concern such as Mr. K.'s impaired skin integrity and his altered fluid and electrolyte levels.

GOAL SETTING

In setting goals, the nurse identifies the client-centered behavioral outcomes of nursing care that will promote adaptation for the person. Both long- and short-term goals may be set. In this case, the short-term goal is: "Mr. K. will sleep for a minimum of two hours at a time within one day." The long term goal for Mr. K. was stated as: "Mr. K. will sleep, without waking, a minimum of two hours in the afternoon and six hours at night within one week." Note that each goal includes the behavior to be observed, the manner in which the behavior will change and the time frame within which the goal is to be attained.

NURSING INTERVENTION

In planning and implementing nursing interventions within the physiological mode, the nurse manages the focal and contextual stimuli which influence the behaviors of concern identified in the nursing diagnosis. This approach to intervention is most likely to be effective because these stimuli directly influence the ineffective behavior identified in the first level of assessment. Thus, to intervene with Mr. K.'s extreme fatigue, the nurse would plan nursing interventions managing his pain, nausea and vomiting, anxiety, and hospital routines.

In an attempt to provide relief of pain, nausea, and vomiting, a variety of medications are administered on a regular schedule. Comfort measures, including back massage, positioning and providing a quiet environment are implemented to reduce pain and promote rest. As an adjunct to medication administration, a referral to the occupational therapist may be initiated for the purpose of teaching relaxation and imagery, with the nurse continuing to use these techniques with the patient. Mr. K. expressed an interest in trying "anything that might help, even if it was only for a little while."

In dealing with Mr. K.'s nausea, fruit juices and high-protein liquids are offered every hour. Mr. K's food preferences are considered in selecting his diet. Attention is given to providing frequent oral hygiene, rest periods before meals and an environment conducive to eating. Meal trays are provided for Mr. K's wife to encourage social interaction.

Energy conservation is an important measure in intervening with Mr. K.'s fatigue. Hospital routines are examined and activities important to Mr. K. are identified. Activities are scheduled to allow for periods of uninterrupted rest and a wheelchair is utilized to reduce energy expenditure in moving about the unit. Opportunities are provided to do those things important to him as a means of reducing anxiety and enhancing quality of life.

EVALUATION

Evaluation is a continuing process involving reassessment and modification. The nurse determines the effectiveness of nursing intervention by comparing client behavior following intervention to the expected behavioral outcomes identified in the goals. If the goals are not met, the stimuli influencing the behaviors of concern are reassessed and the nursing diagnosis, goals, and nursing interventions are modified as required.

The degree to which Mr. K. is able to meet the goals set varied from day to day. At times he is able to sleep for two hours but rarely does he sleep longer. The effectiveness of interventions to control his pain, nausea, vomiting, and anxiety also vary. He almost never speaks of his symptoms but comments that it is a "relief to be without the pain and nausea even if it is only for for a few minutes" and that it feels "good to sleep, even for a little while."

Based on a reassessment of his fatigue level and the influencing stimuli, it is determined that the short-term goal set for Mr. K. would be retained but that the long-term goal requires modification. The nursing diagnosis and planned nursing interventions are unchanged.

SUMMARY

In this section a case study was utilized to demonstrate application of the nursing process, as described by the Roy Adaptation Model in the physiological mode. This case study also is used at the end of Part III to demonstrate application of the nursing process in the self-concept mode.

In this case, behavioral data related to each of the physiological needs were collected and priorities for further assessment were identified. The focal, contextual and residual stimuli influencing selected physiological behaviors were identified and a nursing diagnosis was formulated. Goals to attain adaptive physiological behavior were set and nursing interventions were planned to manage the focal and contextual stimuli identified in the nursing diagnosis. The process of evaluation and the continuous nature of the nursing process were illustrated.

Part III

The Self-Concept Mode*

Inherent in the description of the person as an adaptive system and the philosophic assumptions associated with humanism and veritivity is the concept of holistic functioning. In viewing the person as an integrated whole, the nurse is concerned with the well being of the total person as well as the physiological concerns discussed in the previous section. Ineffective behavior in any area affects the person as a whole.

The self-concept mode is one of three psychosocial modes; it focuses specifically on the psychological and spiritual aspects of the person. The basic need underlying the self-concept mode has been identified as *psychic integrity*—the need to know who one is so that one can be or exist with a sense of unity. In the process of adaptation, a person strives to achieve this psychic integrity. Adaptation problems in this area may interfere with the person's ability to heal, to do what is necessary to maintain health and to be a healthy person. Thus it is important for the nurse to have knowledge about the self-concept mode in order to assess behaviors and stimuli influencing a person's self concept.

In this section, the self-concept mode and its components are addressed. Chapter 13 provides an overview of the mode while Chapters 14 and 15 deal with the physical self and the personal self, respectively. As a conclusion to Part III, the previous case study is developed to illustrate selected concepts associated with the self-concept mode.

*The material presented in this section was initially developed by Marie J. Driever in the first edition of *Introduction to Nursing: An Adaptation Model,* Sister Callista Roy, Englewood Cliffs, N.J.: Prentice-Hall, 1976: "Theory of Self-Concept," pp. 169–179, and "Development of the Self-Concept," pp. 180–191. The original literature review, including the development of this classification and the theory underlying the self-concept mode, was done by Marie J. Driever at Mount St. Mary's College under USPHS Grant No. 5T02MH06442 1969–70.

Chapter Thirteen

Overview of the Self-Concept Mode

Heather A. Andrews

The self-concept mode is one of three psychosocial modes focusing specifically on the psychological and spiritual aspects of the person. The need underlying the mode is termed *psychic integrity*. This mode is viewed in the Roy Adaptation Model as having two subareas: the physical self and the personal self. The subareas are divided further into five components.

In this chapter, the self-concept mode and its components are described. The theoretical basis providing direction for the assessment of behaviors and stimuli in the mode is identified and a general description of the nursing process as applied to the self-concept mode is provided. More thorough exploration of the components of the mode and their related adaptation problems is the focus of Chapters 14 and 15. The previous case study is expanded to illustrate the self-concept mode at the conclusion of the section.

OBJECTIVES

After studying this chapter, the reader will be able to do the following:

1. Define self concept.
2. Describe the self-concept mode together with its components.
3. Identify the theoretical bases of the self-concept mode.

KEY CONCEPTS DEFINED

- *Body image:* how one views oneself physically and one's view of his or her appearance.
- *Body sensation:* how one feels and experiences oneself as a physical being.

- *Moral-ethical-spiritual self:* that aspect of the personal self which functions as observer, standard-setter, dreamer, comparer, and most of all, evaluator of who this person says that he or she is (Buck 1984).
- *Personal self:* the individual's appraisal of one's own characteristics, expectations, values, and worth.
- *Physical self:* the person's appraisal of one's own physical being, including physical attributes, functioning, sexuality, health-illness states, and appearance.
- *Psychic integrity:* the basic need of the self-concept mode; the need to know who one is so that one can be or exist with a sense of unity.
- *Self concept:* the composite of beliefs and feelings that one holds about oneself at a given time, formed from internal perceptions and perceptions of others' reactions.
- *Self-consistency:* the part of the personal self component which strives to maintain a consistent self-organization and thus to avoid disequilibrium.
- *Self-esteem:* the individual's perception of self-worth.
- *Self-ideal/self-expectancy:* that aspect of the personal self component which relates to what the person expects to be and do.

DESCRIPTION OF THE SELF-CONCEPT MODE

Self concept was defined by Driever (1976) as the composite of beliefs and feelings that one holds about oneself at a given time. Formed from internal perceptions and perceptions of others' reactions, self concept is instrumental in directing one's behavior. Self concept addresses the question, "Who am I?"

Perception of self plays a major part in everything a person does. The self-concept mode is the manifestation of behavior and level of adaptation relative to a person's beliefs and feelings about himself or herself. It is one of three modes related to psychosocial adaptation and focuses specifically on the psychological and spiritual aspects of the person. The basic need of the self-concept mode is psychic integrity.

The self-concept mode is viewed in the Roy Adaptation Model as having two subareas: the physical self and the personal self. The physical self includes two components: body sensation and body image. Body sensation applies to the ability to feel and to experience oneself as a physical being. Statements such as "I feel sick," "I feel exhausted," or "I feel great!" are examples of body sensation behaviors. Body image applies to how one views oneself physically and one's appearance. "I need to lose some weight," "I feel I'm rather attractive," or "I'm not very physically fit," are all behavioral statements related to body image. Figure 13–1 is a diagram-

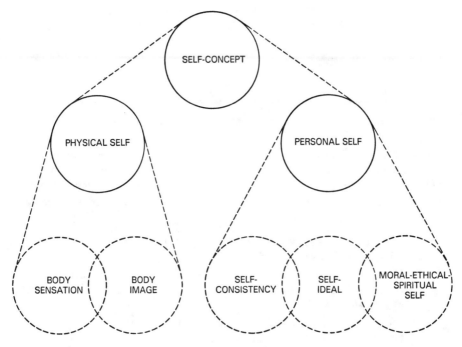

Figure 13–1. Self-concept mode with subareas and components

matic representation of the self-concept with its two subareas and their components. Body sensation and body image are depicted as the two component parts of the physical self.

The personal self is viewed as having three components: self-consistency, self-ideal, and moral-ethical-spiritual self. *Self-consistency,* a concept based on the work of Coombs and Snygg (1959), strives to maintain a consistent self-organization and thus avoid disequilibrium. Behavior relative to self-consistency can be observed in a person's response to a situation and his or her verbal statements: "I'm really anxious about my surgery," or "I'll be able to make a good grade in this exam." *Self-ideal* relates to what one would like to be or is capable of doing. "I want to be a nurse," or "I would like to be able to do better in this subject," are statements manifesting a person's self-ideal. One's *moral-ethical-spiritual self* includes one's belief system and an evaluation of who one is. It is evidenced by such statements as, "I believe that euthanasia is wrong," or "God will take care of me during this surgery."

The self concept with its related components addresses for the person the question, "Who am I?" The need to know who one is so that one can exist with a sense of unity is termed *psychic integrity.* This is the underlying need of the self-concept mode and the goal of the adaptation process. Inherent in each component of the self concept is *self-esteem,* the individual's perception of worth. One's level of self-esteem reflects the self concept and related behaviors give insight into adaptation in the self-concept mode.

THEORETICAL BASIS FOR THE SELF-CONCEPT MODE

The description of the self-concept mode is based on a number of specific psychological, biological, and social theories and principles, as synthesized by Driever (1976). These provide direction for the assessment of behavior and stimuli relative to the self concept and for each of the other steps of the nursing process. The following is an identification of the theoretical bases of the self-concept mode as described in the Roy Adaptation Model.[1]

- *Coombs and Snygg* (1959)—Theory of Self-Perception. Self is seen as a constellation of self-perceptions.
- *Cooley* (Epstein 1973)—Social Interactionist Theory. The person bases self-perception on the way he or she perceives the responses of others.
- *Mead* (1934)—Social Interactionist Theory. The person puts self in the position of others and assumes their attitude towards self.
- *Sullivan* (1953)—Social Interactionist Theory. Interaction with others is the key to development of self concept.
- *Jackins* (1974)—Sense of Self. The concept of the model, ideal and potential human being and the factors that contribute to the current sense of self.
- *Kubler-Ross* (1969)—Death and Dying. The five identified stages are (1) denial and isolation, (2) anger, (3) bargaining, (4) depression, and (5) acceptance.
- *Erikson* (1963)—Developmental Theory. The person encounters eight maturational crises throughout the life span:

  trust versus mistrust (birth to 1 year)
  autonomy versus shame and doubt (1 to 3 years)
  initiative versus guilt (3 to 6 years)
  industry versus inferiority (6 to 12 years)
  identity versus role confusion (12 to 18 years)
  intimacy versus isolation (18 to 35 years)
  generativity versus stagnation (35 to 60 years)
  ego integrity versus despair (60 years to death)

[1]It is important to refer to the works of the identified theorists in conjunction with the following chapters if a working knowledge of the use of these theories in the Roy Adaptation Model is sought.

APPLICATION OF THE NURSING PROCESS

Application of the nursing process to the self-concept mode is illustrated in a general manner in the diagrammatic conceptualization of the model in Figure 13–2. In the following two chapters on the physical self and the personal self, specific information about the application of the nursing process is presented. The following section takes a general look at how the six steps of the nursing process must be applied in consideration of the self-concept mode.

Assessment of Behavior
The five components of the self-concept mode form the basis for behavioral assessment of psychic integrity. Behavior is manifest through the person's appearance relative to such factors as grooming, posture, and facial expression and through statements the person makes about himself or herself. For example, a person may appear pale and drawn and make the comment, "I'm not feeling so good." Both appearance and statement are behaviors relating to the component of the physical self, body sensation. Similarly, a person who has brought a rosary into the hospital is telling something about the moral-ethical-spiritual self. At times, it may be necessary to purposefully question a person relative to his or her self concept. To do this effectively, the nurse must provide a comfortable and trusting environment for the person; she is asking the person to share some intimate feelings about self.

Consider the example of a girl who has been gaining weight progressively since she entered college. She wears clothes that are much too small for her and, although she was previously neatly groomed, her self care is becoming increasingly lax. In assessing behaviors relative to her self-concept mode, the following framework is suggested and illustrated:

1. *Body sensation* (How does she feel?)—States "I don't feel attractive to others"; "I seem to have so little energy"; "I feel so fat."
2. *Body image* (How does she view herself?)—States "I'm probably a little heavy for my height"; "I don't look as good as I could just now."
3. *Self-consistency* (What is her response to the situation?)—She is slouching and appears rather dejected. Grooming has been neglected and clothes are too small. States "I'm plain and ugly."
4. *Self-ideal* (What would she like to be?)—States "I wouldn't mind losing about 70 pounds"; "I'd sure like to be able to wear the size dress my sister does."
5. *Moral-ethical-spiritual self* (In what does she believe?)—States "I was probably meant to be fat"; "If I weren't fat, fate would give me some other problem."

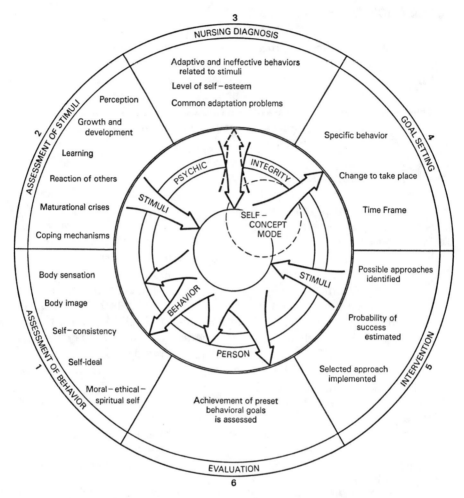

Figure 13–2. The nursing process applied to the self-concept mode

Assessment of Stimuli

In assessing the stimuli influencing the person's behavior in the self-concept mode, the nurse again relies heavily on the theoretical basis of the self concept as identified in the Roy Adaptation Model. To facilitate this process, six general categories of stimuli have been identified (Buck 1984). These are listed here and explored further in the next chapters.

1. *Growth and development*—Age and degree of physical development affect one's self concept as abilities change and control of bodily functions change. Known standards of growth and development provide the basis for assessment of this factor. (Havinghurst 1954).

2. *Learning*—Based on an identified theory of learning, this concept incorporates such stimuli as societal expectations and values as well as those of significant others.
3. *Reactions of others*—This concept is based on the work of interactionists such as Cooley [Epstein (1973)], Mead (1934), and Sullivan (1953) and focuses on the influence of significant others on the person's self-concept. Montagu (1986) is used as a basis for the responses of infants to touching and nurturing.
4. *Perception*—This concept is based primarily on the self-perception theory of Coombs and Snygg (1959) and on the work of Sanford (1982) in relation to self-perception. The individual's perception of self influences the development and maintenance of a self concept.
5. *Maturational crises*—Based on the developmental crises identified by Erikson (1963), the age-defined developmental stage and associated maturational tasks suggest confronting challenges, achievement of which affects the person's self concept.
6. *Coping strategies*—The manner in which the person characteristically functions on a day-to-day basis and in times of stress is an important stimulus influencing self concept.

There also may be other stimuli relevant in an individual's situation and these should be included in the second level of assessment, as well. Once the stimuli influencing the person's self-concept behaviors have been identified, the behaviors, in light of the theoretical bases, are evaluated as adaptive or ineffective in maintaining psychic integrity; stimuli are identified as focal, contextual, or residual and are labeled as to whether they are exerting a positive or negative influence on the person.

Thinking again of the example of the overweight girl, assessment information relative to stimuli may be as follows:

1. *Perception*—All statements related to how the girl sees herself apply here: "I have to work hard for my grades at school"; "My concentration span is short"; "In one word, 'fat.'"
2. *Growth and development*—She's 18 years of age, 5 feet 4 inches tall, weighs 200 pounds.
3. *Learning*—Past experiences and rewards related to learning apply: "I had top grades in secondary school and received a scholarship to this college."
4. *Reactions of others*—"I think my sister feels uncomfortable when she's in public with me"; "My parents say that 'fat' runs in the family."
5. *Maturational crises*—Identity versus role confusion is Erikson's crisis stage for an 18-year-old. The girl is studying to become a nurse: "I spend three hours each night studying."
6. *Coping strategies*—How does she normally deal with stressful situations? "I find I'm constantly eating when I study."

Nursing Diagnosis

As in the other modes, nursing diagnosis in the self-concept mode involves relating the assessment data obtained in the first two steps of the nursing process. The label can take the form of identification of adaptive or ineffective behaviors related to the specific stimulus. An example of this from the previous illustration might be "Negative comments about self related to reaction of sister and compulsive eating habits." Diagnosis in the self-concept mode also may be related to the person's level of self-esteem—his or her perception of self-worth. Using this method, a diagnosis for the overweight girl is, "Low self-esteem related to the individual's perception of her appearance."

A major concept of adaptation of the physical self concept is life closure. Life closure is viewed in the Roy Adaptation Model as a normal part of the human life cycle—a process through which a person resolves the issue of the meaning of one's life and accepts the reality of one's own eventual death. This concept is addressed in further detail in Chapter 4.

In addition, common adaptation problems have been identified related to the physical self and the personal self.

1. *Physical self*—Problems include body image disturbance, sexual dysfunction, rape trauma syndrome, and loss.
2. *Personal self*—Problems include anxiety, powerlessness, guilt, and low self-esteem.

Goal Setting

Goals must be set in collaboration with the person. Such involvement is the essence of the self-concept mode and includes the ability to deal with and be in control of the situation. The focus of the goal is on the behavior and how it will change in a given time frame, for example, "By tomorrow, the girl will make a verbal commitment to begin a diet in order to improve her sense of body image." This goal contains as a behavior "the verbal commitment to begin a diet"; the time frame is "by tomorrow" and the change is related to her commitment. Obviously, for this goal to be achieved, the person must be involved in its formulation in order to be committed to its achievement.

Assisting the person with the achievement of integrity in the self-concept mode may be the key to enabling the person to deal with ineffective adaptation in other modes. In fact, the adaptation problems of the self-concept mode may constitute primary problems that must be resolved for adaptation to be effective in other modes. An accurate assessment of the components of self concept assists the nurse in working with the person to formulate realistic goals. Knowledge of the self-concept mode and the related theoretical bases direct the nurse as goals are considered.

Intervention

Interventions always focus on the stimuli that are influencing the behaviors being observed. Stimuli having a positive effect on the person will be maintained or enhanced while stimuli having a negative force are altered, decreased, or eliminated. In the example, the person's coping mechanism of compulsive eating needs some attention. Also, her sister's reaction seems important to her; it may be possible to incorporate both influencing factors in an intervention approach. The approach chosen out of the possible alternatives is the one with the highest probability of succeeding.

Possible nursing interventions for any given adaptation problem form a large body of knowledge in the scientific discipline of nursing. The study of nursing involves detailed analysis of such approaches.

Evaluation

Evaluation of the self-concept mode, as with any other mode, involves behavioral assessment to determine if behavioral goals have been met. In this manner, direction is provided for nursing activity.

Consider this long-term goal related to the physical self: "Within two weeks, the patient will have lost 3 pounds in weight." The behavior that is the focus of the goal is the person's weight and that factor is also the key to evaluation. If the person is to achieve the goal, she will have lost 3 pounds in the two-week period. If the goal is not achieved, the patient and the nurse must determine what interfered. To do so, the process must be repeated.

SUMMARY

The self-concept mode with its underlying need for psychic integrity has as its basis many psychological, biological, and social theories that provide direction throughout each aspect of the nursing process to promote adaptation. This chapter described the self-concept mode, its two subareas and their components, and demonstrated the application of the nursing process to the mode.

Chapters 14 and 15 focus, respectively, on the physical self and the personal self and explore indicators of effective adaptation and adaptation problems associated with these two subareas.

EXERCISES FOR APPLICATION

1. Formulate questions for each component of the self-concept mode (body sensation, body image, self-consistency, self-ideal, moral-ethical-spiritual self) that would be appropriate for a nurse to ask

a given patient in order to elicit assessment data relative to behaviors and stimuli.
2. Interview a family member or friend to assess their self concept and note behaviors and stimuli. Write a nursing diagnosis for each of the five components of the self-concept mode.

ASSESSMENT OF UNDERSTANDING

Questions

1. Which of the following statements apply to the *self concept* as defined in the Roy Model?
   a. It focuses on social aspects of one's behavior.
   b. It is a composite of beliefs and feelings about self.
   c. It is influenced by perceptions of others' reactions.
   d. It is one's perception of oneself.
   e. It directs one's behavior.
2. Match the descriptions on the left with the components of the self-concept on the right. More than one description may apply.

1.	Strives to avoid disequilibrium	(a) _____ Body sensation
2.	What one would like to be	(b) _____ Body image
3.	Evaluation of who one is	(c) _____ Self-consistency
4.	The ability to feel	(d) _____ Self-ideal
5.	What one is capable of doing	(e) _____ Moral-ethical-spiritual self
6.	The ability to experience oneself as a human being	
7.	How one views one's appearance	
8.	Belief system	

3. Match the theorist in column A with the description of the theory provided in column B.

Column A	Column B
1. Kubler-Ross	(a) ____ interaction as the key to development of self-concept
2. Cooley	
3. Coombs and Snygg	(b) ____ model, ideal, and potential being
4. Sullivan	(c) ____ five stages of death and dying

5. Jackins
6. Erikson

(d) ＿＿ self-perception based on others' responses
(e) ＿＿ maturational crises
(f) ＿＿ theory of self-perception

Feedback

1. b, c, d, e
2. (a) 4, 6
   (b) 7
   (c) 1
   (d) 2, 5
   (e) 3, 8
3. (a) 4, (b) 5, (c) 1, (d) 2, (e) 6, (f) 3.

REFERENCES

Buck, M.H. Self-concept: Theory and development, in *Introduction to Nursing: Adaptation Model* (2nd ed.) Sr. C. Roy, pp. 255–282. Englewood Cliffs, N.J.: Prentice-Hall, 1984.

Coombs, A., and D. Snygg. *Individual Behavior—A Perceptual Approach to Behavior.* New York: Harper Brothers, 1959.

Driever, M.J. Theory of self-concept, in *Introduction to Nursing: An Adaptation Model,* Sister Callista Roy, pp. 255–283. Englewood Cliffs, N.J.: Prentice-Hall, 1976.

Epstein, S. The self-concept revisited or a theory of a theory, *American Psychologist,* 28, no. 5 (May 1973): 404–416.

Erikson, E.H. *Childhood and Society* (2nd ed.). New York: W.W. Norton & Co., Inc., 1963.

Havinghurst, R.J. *Development Tasks and Education.* New York: David McKay Company, 1952.

Jackins, H. *The Human Side of Human Beings.* Seattle: Rational Island Publishers, 1974.

Kubler-Ross, E. *On Death and Dying.* New York: Macmillan, 1969.

Mead, G.H. *Mind, Self and Society.* Chicago: University of Chicago Press, 1934.

Montague, A. *Touching: The Human Significance of the Skin* (3rd. ed.). New York: Harper and Row, 1986.

Roy, Sr. C. *Introduction to Nursing: An Adaptation Model* (2nd ed.). Englewood Cliffs, N.J.: Prentice Hall, 1984.

Sanford, John. *Between People: Communicating One-to-One.* New York: Ramsey Paulist, 1982.

Sullivan, H.S. *The Interpersonal Theory of Psychiatry.* New York: W.W. Norton & Co., Inc., 1953.

Additional References
See Chapters 14 and 15.

Chapter Fourteen

The Physical Self

Marjorie H. Buck

The physical self is one of the two components of the self-concept mode. This chapter will describe how to apply the Roy Adaptation Model nursing process to the physical self component. Positive adaptation of the physical self in terms of physical sensations, body image and sexual self will be identified. Life closure will be discussed as a normal part of the life cycle. Adaptation problems of sexual dysfunction, rape trauma syndrome, body image disturbance, and loss will be examined.

OBJECTIVES

After studying this chapter, the reader will be able to do the following:

1. Describe the physical self component of the self-concept mode.
2. Identify behaviors related to the physical self and their effect on the person.
3. List the six common stimuli associated with the physical self.
4. Derive nursing diagnosis conveying positive adaptation and adaptation problems related to the physical self.
5. Given a situation, state a goal for a specified adaptation problem.
6. Identify possible nursing interventions for a specified goal for the physical self.
7. Describe evaluative behaviors relevant to a given situation.

KEY CONCEPTS DEFINED

- *Body image disturbance:* negative feelings about one's body, its characteristics, functions, or limits which interfere with the person's ability to function.

- *Grief:* the series of emotional responses that occur following the perception of or anticipation of a loss of valued object(s).
- *Life closure:* the process of resolving the issue of the meaning of one's life and accepting the reality of one's eventual death.
- *Loss:* any situation which renders a valued object inaccessible or altered in such a way that it no longer has the qualities that made it valuable.
- *Physical self:* the person's appraisal of own physical being including attributes, appearance, functioning, sensations, sexuality, and wellness-illness status.
- *Rape trauma syndrome:* the sequela, immediate and long term, of a forced sexual activity.
- *Sexual dysfunction:* ineffective sexual behavior caused by physiological and/or psychological factors.

DESCRIPTION OF THE PHYSICAL SELF

The human being is a complex creature made up of many interacting parts. Mysteriously the whole is greater than the sum of the parts. The Roy Adaptation Model for nursing recognizes the four adaptive modes of the person: physiological, self concept, role function, and interdependence, for ease of learning and applying the nursing process. This chapter focuses on the physical self aspects of the self-concept mode. Just as the person is an integrated whole, nurses using the model focus on integrating the parts into a view of the whole.

The adaptation model for nursing defines the physical self as the individual's appraisal of one's physical attributes, appearance, functioning, sensations, sexuality, and wellness-illness status. It includes two components: (1) body sensation—how one's body feels personally, and (2) body image—how one views and feels about the appearance and function of one's body. The first impressions of the self and the world are experienced physically through body sensations. Throughout the stages of life, each person is challenged to integrate the changing physical (as well as emotional, spiritual, and social) aspects of being human. Mastering the first stage of maturational development, trust versus mistrust (Erikson 1963), is dependent upon how body sensations are managed by the nurturing person and the kind of touch the infant receives.

Physical self experiences at this age lay the ground work for the person's sense of self throughout life. Sexuality is included in the assessment and management of the physical self. As human beings we all share the fact of sexual functioning (Calderone and Ramey 1982). Human sexuality involves far more than the sex act and reproduction. "It involves who and what we are as male and female, how we get that way, how we feel about it and how we deal with each other about it. It also involves dreams, fantasies and ideals, and gives us pleasure, even laughter. And it involves learning, thinking, planning, postponing, developing moral values, and decision-making."[1] The nurse uses sensitive awareness and observational, interviewing, interactional, and physical assessment skills to assess behaviors and stimuli in each component of the physical self.

APPLICATION OF THE NURSING PROCESS

Consideration of the person's physical self in the promotion of adaptation is of primary importance. Adaptation problems in the area of the self-concept mode and specifically the physical self component may interfere with the person's ability to heal and to do what is necessary to maintain health. The two components of the physical self, body image and body sensation, represent categories of behaviors that suggest to the nurse the effectiveness with which the patient will be able to adapt in the situation at hand.

In addressing the self-concept component of physical self with the patient, it is important that the nurse understand and be comfortable with his or her own physical self and the related body image and body sensation. Not only is an adaptive physical self required by the patient in dealing with other adaptation problems, it is a personal requirement for the nurse attempting to assist the patient towards effective adaptation in the self-concept mode.

Assessment of Behavior

The first prerequisite for assessing a person's physical self-concept is an awareness of and comfort with one's own physical self-concept including sexuality. The nurse will not be able to discuss physical self issues comfortably, honestly, and without judgment otherwise. The nurse takes the necessary steps to meet this first prerequisite. An optimal situation for carrying out the assessment is the second necessary condition. This is established by explaining the purpose of the interview to the person receiving care. The nurse also provides for privacy and meets the person's immediate needs. Confidentiality is discussed. The nurse tells the client who else, if anyone, will have access to the information. The patient may wish to keep certain aspects of the interview strictly between the nurse and self. The nurse tells the patient whether that is possible in advance and honors the agreement. The nurse, being aware of and comfortable with own physical self-behaviors, does not impose judgments or stereotypes on the person receiving care. Good communication skills including open-ended questions, use

[1]Mary Calderone and James W. Ramey, *Talking With Your Child About Sex, Questions and Answers for Children from Birth to Puberty.* New York, N.Y.: Ballantine Books, 1982, p. ix.

of silence, and reflection are used. Questions are related to the individual's current health care situation and placed in the realm of common concern. For example, the nurse could say, "Many people are concerned about their sexual activity following colostomy surgery." Campsey (1985) viewed sexuality as a human experience that needs to be explored, experienced, and shared. The person receiving care, however, often is hesitant to bring up the subject. The nurse has the responsibility to show a willingness to deal with sexuality issues.

Body Sensations. The nurse assesses the pre- or nonverbal person's body sensation component by observing or obtaining a report from the nurturing person of facial expressions, body posture, physical tensions, level of relaxation, ease of feeding and eliminating and depth of sleep. The neurophysiology for orgasm is intact at birth. The person experiences pleasurable sexual sensations from the time of birth or possibly before. Self-stimulation to achieve orgasm is not unusual in the first year of life (Calderone 1982). The genital expression of sexuality for males stays fairly constant throughout adult life until the seventh decade. Thereafter a decrease in interest is often experienced.

Once the young person has become fairly verbal the nurse can add questions to the assessment of body sensations. Examples of such questions are listed in Table 14–1. The nurse changes the questions into her own words. The person's developmental level and personal communication style are also taken into consideration. The nurse uses accurate terminology and checks with the person receiving care for mutual understanding of terms being used by each. The body sensation behaviors are the observations listed as are the individual's responses to the questions. For example, the person may state, "I feel _____ (strong, weak, sexually responsive, faint, pained)." The nurse validates any hunches drawn from observation. For instance the nurse might say, "I see your brow is furrowed and your jaw is clenched. What are you feeling now?"

Body Image. Body image behaviors, how one's body looks to oneself and how one feels about how one's body looks and functions, is assessed next. Part of sexual self body image is identifying self as male or female. The adaptation model deals with sex identification in the role function mode—primary role. Sex role identification is discussed here as related to self-concept. The nurse makes direct observations of the person's posture, carriage, and level of personal hygiene, and grooming. A complete physical assessment including pelvic, Pap, and breast examinations for women and genitourinary examination for men is included, when relevant or appropriate. The nurse may perform this examination or obtain the information from the written record. Detailed information on how to do the physical assessment can be found in a textbook of physical examination.

TABLE 14–1. ASSESSMENT OF BEHAVIOR OF THE PHYSICAL SELF COMPONENT[1]

Characteristics	How to Elicit Behavior	How Behavior is Manifested
Body sensation: how one's own body feels to self: sensations allow one to experience own body:	How do you you feel physically? What physical sensations are you experiencing?	"I feel _____" (strong, weak, tired, rested, etc.) "I feel _____" (cold, warm, pained, sexy, etc.) Facial expression. Muscular tension.
sensations allow one to experience self as a sexual being.	How often do you have sexual feelings?[2] How do you usually deal with your sexual feelings? How satisfied are you with your methods of dealing with your sexual feelings?	"I have sexual feelings _____" (daily, weekly, never, etc.) "I usually _____" (ignore them, masturbate, make love, etc.) "I am _____" (fairly satisfied, not satisfied at all, etc.)
Body image: how one feels about own body: how one's body looks to self: level of satisfaction with appearance.	How do your feel about your appearance? Describe how your see yourself physically. What aspects of your physical appearance do you like? What, if anything, would you like to change about your appearance?	"I feel _____" (pretty good, upset since this surgery, etc.) "I am _____" (slim, fat, tall, well built, pretty, ugly, etc.) "I like _____" (my height, my hair, my smile, etc.) "I would like to change _____" (my weight, my teeth, etc.)

[1]Content of Table 14–1 is based in part the unpublished work of Joan Cho, Department of Nursing, Mount Saint Mary's College, Los Angeles, 1979–1980.
[2]When the person does not bring up the subject of sexuality, the nurse decides if specific questions are indicated. Questions are asked in the context of the person's health situation.

During the physical exam the nurse has the opportunity to talk with the person about any concerns and questions and to teach about sexuality and self care (Weinberg 1982). Based on these observations and the list of questions in Table 14–1, the nurse asks open-ended questions to identify body image behaviors. Taking into consideration the person's health care situation and cues from the person, the nurse decides whether or not to carry out a detailed sexuality assessment. The person's responses as well as the nurse's observations are the body image behaviors.

The identified behaviors can be judged to be adaptive or ineffective. Adaptive behaviors contribute to the person's psychic integrity. Ineffective behaviors detract from or prevent formation and maintenance of the person's psychic integrity. On completion of the assessment of physical self behaviors the nurse is ready to assess the factors influencing those behaviors.

Assessment of Stimuli

The following discussion of stimuli will be divided into the six categories of common influencing factors for the self-concept mode identified by adaptation nursing theory. See Table 14–2 for a summary of those categories and suggested ways to elicit the information.

Growth and Development. All the normal changes of growth and development are stimuli for the physical self behaviors. The human body is continually changing and demands accompanying alterations in the sense of physical self. As the nervous system matures, the infant learns to roll over, sit, crawl, stand, and walk. Further growth leads to the physical changes of puberty. Continuing growth brings on the initially subtle and then blatant changes of aging. All of these events affect the person's concept of self. The nurse is aware of normal growth and development theory and applies it when identifying physical self stimuli.

In addition, one reviews the physiological behaviors assessed. These provide important stimuli for the physical self component of the self-concept mode. The applicable physiological mode behaviors are considered stimuli for the physical self component. For example, the person's height, weight, color and distribution of hair, muscular strength, skin condition, ability to control bodily functions, neurological function all influence how the person perceives and feels about the body. The nurse using the adaptation model for nursing completes the physiological mode assessment using direct observation, physical assessment skills, and review of the written record. The information gained in that assessment is applied to the physical self component as stimuli.

Learning. The person's past experiences with rewards or absence of rewards for having certain physical characteristics, abilities, and sensation strongly influence the formation of physical self behaviors. From the moment of birth and even before, societal standards are applied to the individual. The pregnant woman might say, "The baby kicks so hard, I know he's a boy." Comments at the delivery of a newborn might include statements such as, "Too bad you had another girl" or "He's so tiny he'll never make a football player." Each society and culture values certain physical attributes. The values are communicated through myths, legends, fairy tales, books, television, movies, magazines, and advertising. The individual who inherits the desirable physical characteristics is rewarded while the person who does not, lacks rewards and often receives negative input. The North American culture values the young, slim, firm, well proportioned female body and the tall, muscular, male body. The ideal is infrequently the reality. The nurse is aware of the cultural norms and uses open-ended questions to obtain information from the individual about how such norms have influenced that person's sense of physical self.

Religions teach certain attitudes about body image, function, and sexu-

TABLE 14–2. ASSESSMENT OF STIMULI OF THE SELF-CONCEPT MODE

General Categories of Stimuli	How to Obtain Data
1. Growth and development (Gardner and Havighurst) Age, physical characteristics and abilities, ability to use tools, ability to control bodily functions.	Collect these data from direct observation, the behavioral assessment of physiological mode, the written record, and growth and development charts.
2. Learning Past experiences in relation to presence or absence of rewards for having certain characteristics. Standards by which specific characteristics are valued vary according to social class, culture and religion.	Collect these data by interviewing the person receiving care and significant other. Sample questions: (of the parents of the child receiving care) "What physical and/or personal characteristics do you particularly like to see in your child? How do you bring out these characteristics?" (of the child receiving care) "How do you think your parent(s) want you to look? How do you think your parent(s) like you to feel? What do your parents like best about you? What kind of person do your parents want you to be? What is it like when you are that way? What happens when you are not that way?" (of the adult receiving care) "What physical characteristics do you feel you are supposed to have? What personal characteristics do you feel you are supposed to have? What specific pressures do you feel to be that way? Who gave you information about your sexuality? What were you taught? What does your religion teach about sexuality?
3. Reactions of others The response of others Looking glass self—how the person perceives the responses of others to self.	Collect these data by observing the interaction between the young person receiving care and the significant other and by interviewing the person. Observe the manner in which the significant other cares for the infant. Is the touch firm, gentle and reassuring? Do the responses of the significant other meet the needs of the infant? Is there a sense of relaxed confidence on the part of the care giver? Is the care needed for bodily functions done matter-of-factly or with a sense of disgust? Sample questions of the person receiving care are: "What do you know about how your parents reacted to you when you were a baby? a young child? an adolescent? What kind of person do you think _____ (a specific significant other) sees you as? When you are with that person, how do you feel about yourself?"

(continued)

TABLE 14–2. (Continued)

General Categories of Stimuli	How to Obtain Data
4. Perception How the person generally sees self. *Inner cell*: the most vital, fundamental, and important views one holds about self—the inner voice. *Phenomenal self*: all perceptions of self regardless of their importance. *Perceptual field*: all perceptions of self and nonself.	Collect these data by interviewing the person Sample question: "When faced with important change in your life (e.g., surgery, graduation, etc.) what particular personal qualities do you use to help you through the transition?" (Inner cell) *Phenomenal self*: all statements the person makes about self during the interview; look at those statements that relate to the person's current situation in particular.
5. Maturational crisis Stage of life according to Erikson. Tasks of current stage: individual's level of mastery of the tasks of the previous stages.	Collect these data by listing the tasks according to Erikson for the person's stage of development: compare the person's current functioning (role, interdependence, and self-concept behaviors) to the tasks for that stage of development: ask questions based on the tasks to collect further data as necessary.
6. Coping mechanisms How the person habitually responds to maintain a state of adaptation.	Collect these data by interviewing the person. Sample questions: "What activities do you do regularly to help you feel positive about yourself? (eg exercise, diet, prayer, sports, talk with a friend, have sexual relationship). In the past when faced with a situation similar to this one, how have you handled it?"
7. Other: any factors that do not fit in the categories above that influence self-concept behaviors.	Collect these data by direct observation, interview of the person and the significant others, from the chart, from report of other health care professionals, and from theory.

Source: Based on content in Chapter 14 Self-Concept: Theory and Development by Marjorie H. Buck in *Introduction to Nursing An Adaptation Model*, (2nd ed.) by Sister Callista Roy (Englewood Cliffs, N.J.: Prentice-Hall, Inc., 1984) pp. 255–283.

ality. For example, masturbation, abortion, and homosexuality are forbidden in the religious teachings of the Orthodox Jews, Roman Catholics, and traditional Protestants. Intercourse is reserved only for marriage. Some liberal branches of Protestants may sanction any activity or behavior that is necessary for the maintenance of health and does not harm another person. The nurse assesses the person's religious beliefs as stimuli for physical self behaviors.

The primary view of the human body in Western societies is as an object, a machine which should perform to the "owner's" wishes. A level of mistrust, annoyance, and ignorance about bodily functions pervades the culture. Advertising promises that taking certain over-the-counter drugs will let the individual complete a full day's activities despite a cold or flu. Professional athletes take drugs to kill the pain of injury and continue playing. The message is "Don't feel sick and you won't be sick," in fact don't feel. A study by Amann-Gainotti (1986) demonstrated the lack of knowledge about body structure and function. She found that many adolescent girls do not know the source of menstrual blood. Western culture teaches individuals to be cut off from true awareness and understanding of their own body sensations and functions (Johnson 1983).

In light of this cultural situation, the nurse may need to be very sensitive and patient when interviewing the person concerning physical self-behaviors and stimuli. The person may have limited ability to discuss physical self data due to lack of information. The interview may be a rare instance of someone truly wanting to know how the body feels to and suits the person.

Reactions of Others. The formation and maintenance of a sense of physical self is influenced profoundly by the reactions of significant others. The infant gains information about self through body sensations (Montagu, 1986). Perception of touch from the nurturing person(s) as gentle, warm, and physically supportive leads to a sense of security in the infant. Consistent response by the care givers to the child's sensations of hunger and discomfort of position, need for touch, fatigue, and wet or dirty diapers also leads to a sense of security within one's body. The nurse observes interactions between the young person and the primary care giver when possible to gain information in this category. Questions are used to gather this information from adults. For example, the nurse might ask, "What do you know about how your parents reacted to you when you were a baby?" An overweight, unemployed adult stated, "My father never held me during my first year of life. Mother told me he was so disappointed I wasn't a boy he could hardly look at me. He still calls me Sam, never Samantha."

The young child's sense of physical self is influenced by the care givers providing names and values to the parts, sensations and functions of the body. Mothers play the age-old game of touching and naming body parts with the growing infant. Comments such as, "Is your nasty gut hurting you again?" or "Are you feeling pressure in your gut? Maybe you will go to the bathroom soon," help shape how the person feels about body sensations and functions. Studies have shown that the physiological arousal is the same for fear, joy, anger, and emotional attraction. It has been suggested that the interpretation of these sensations as distinct feelings of fear, joy, anger, or emotional attraction is due to in-put provided by others (Kleinke, 1978). The values and feeling the primary care givers have about their own body sensations and images are communicated to the child. Some people simply never talk about physical sensations and functions. Other people talk about them indirectly using euphemisms. Some people are able to talk openly and frankly about their bodily functions. The child's developing sense of physical self is influenced by the verbal and nonverbal—what is said as well as what is not said—messages of the significant others. The nurse gathers data in this category by direct observation when possible. Questions also are used to gather this data from the person and significant others.

Perception. Over time a perception of self results from the individual's interpretation of all the various interactions with others and the environment. According to Coombs and Snygg (1959) a *core* or *inner cell* of self-concept is formed of perceptions about self which are the most vital, fundamental aspects of the individual. The *phenomenal* self includes the inner cell plus all the other perceptions held about self regardless of their significance. The rewards, sanctions, and responses of others have been internalized. The person has developed an inner voice (Sanford 1982). Sometimes this "inner voice" gives an accurate appraisal of the true self; other times it gives an inaccurate appraisal of the true self. For example, an adult measuring 5 feet 7 inches tall and weighing 118 pounds may perceive self as fat. The nurse asks questions to elicit the person's perception of physical self and compares the responses to observable data.

Maturational Crisis. Erikson (1963) described eight psychosocial stages of development human beings go through from birth to death in old age (see Chapter 13). Each stage challenges the individual to resolve a maturational *crises*. A person moves through the stages at an individual rate. No crisis ever is completely resolved. As life events confront the person opportunity for reworking of each crisis is afforded. The nurse uses knowledge of Erikson's theory and direct questions to assess this category of stimuli.

Coping Strategies. *Coping strategies* are defined as the person's habitual responses used to maintain a state of adaptation. When assessing the physical self component the nurse seeks information from the individual regarding usual practices for maintaining a positive sense of physical self. For example, many people do regular physical work outs. Some poeple have grooming routines such as hair dresser appointments that help maintain a positive sense of self. Eating a specific diet and taking certain nutritional supplements and vitamins may give the person a sense of well being. Disruption of any of these and other routines might threaten the person's sense of physical self.

The six categories of influencing factors are not all inclusive. The nurse uses other applicable theories and information for determining stimuli for physical self behaviors. Behaviors in the other three adaptive modes can serve as stimuli for personal self behaviors.

Stimuli exert a positive or negative effect on the person's process of adapting the physical self. In preparation for the following steps in the nursing process, the nurse may wish to label the identified stimuli as positive (+) or negative (−). During the intervention phase, positive stimuli will be reinforced and negative stimuli will be altered or eliminated when possible.

Nursing Diagnosis

Formulation of the nursing diagnosis is the next step of the nursing process. The nurse using the adaptation model makes the diagnosis based on the assessed behaviors and stimuli. A beginning diagnosis involves making an evaluation about whether behaviors in each subcomponent of the physical self are effective or ineffective. For example, the nurse can state, "Adaptive body sensation," or "Ineffective body sensation." The second half of this beginning-level diagnosis lists the specific focal stimulus plus the most relevant contextual and residual stimuli. The focal and contextual stimuli listed in the diagnosis are the ones the nurse will manage when intervening. "Adaptive body sensations due to an intact neurological system (focal), regular exercise regimen and perception of self as a healthy, sexual person (contextual)," is an example of a beginning-level diagnosis.

The person with an adaptive physical self will be in touch with body sensations and take cues from those sensations. For example, when feeling tired the person will find a way to rest. When feeling ill or pained the person will seek help, not ignoring symptoms until the condition has reached an advanced stage. An adaptive physical self also is indicated by the person being aware of sexual needs and taking appropriate steps to meet them. Practicing "safe sex" is another indication of adaptive physical self-concept. The sexually transmitted disruptions of the physiological mode component of protection were noted in Chapter 8. These are relevant to integrity of physical self. Goedert (1987) suggested specific guidelines for safe sex. Doing monthly self-breast exams indicates an adaptive physical self for the adult woman. Ability to participate socially and to be seen by others without discomfort or shame indicates an adaptive body image. Acknowledging and integrating the physical changes of aging also indicates adaptive physical self, as does adequate compensation for bodily changes.

Life Closure. In the process of life, the work of mastering the tasks of previous stage(s) prepares the ground for the work of the next stage. The tasks of a stage are never achieved completely. Until the end, life affords another opportunity to resolve the tasks at yet a higher level. The process of life closure gives the person the opportunity to rework the tasks of the previous stages again.

Life closure, the process through which a person resolves the issue of the meaning of one's life and accepts the reality of one's own eventual death, is a normal part of the human life cycle. Erikson (1963) conceptualized the crises of this last stage to be ego integrity versus despair. Ego integrity is displayed by a personal assurance of one's life having order and meaning, a love of human beings in the context of some world order and spiritual sense, an acceptance of one's life just the way it has been, and a new and different love of one's parents. Despair is displayed by a fear of death, the feeling that time is too short, that one's life should have been lived differently. The despairing person may cover over the feeling with the expression of many small dissatisfactions and disgusts. Despair is the true feeling nonetheless.

Behaviors that indicate the person is working on the tasks of ego integrity versus despair include life review and mirror gazing (Kimmel 1974). The individual reminisces about self, previous experiences and their meanings. The person might contact old friends and relatives who have not been contacted in years. Mirror gazing is spending time looking at self in the mirror. Having formed a stable physical self-image in adulthood, the aging person may hardly recognize the image in the mirror as self. These behaviors generally begin in late middle age and are brought on by various life events or conditions that confront the person with the inevitability of one's own death. The person near death generally avoids introspection. Behaviors indicating the person is moving towards accepting the inevitability of death include making and legalizing a will, discussing the level of medical intervention desired for serious illness occurring late in life, and specifying funeral and burial wishes.

The stimulus for starting the process of life closure is often the aging and death of one's own parents. Interacting with parents in the last months of their lives forces the person to confront personal feelings about aging and death. Parents are a strong link to the individual's past. Death of the parents marks the end of a segment of life and leaves the individual next in line for death (Silverstone and Hyman 1976). Death of siblings, spouse, or other peers are other stimuli for the behaviors of life closure.

The physical changes of aging also serve as stimuli for the behaviors of the process of life closure. The relatively constant adult physical self-image is challenged by changes in appearance, function and stamina brought on by aging. Cultural views and the individual's perceptions of aging influence the behaviors of life closure. Illness is another stimulus for the behaviors of life closure. Pain, disability, infirmity in late middle age and old age years cause the person to stop and rethink their view of life and self.

The taboo against talking about death has been a negative stimulus for the individual's behaviors of life closure. In Western society, death still is talked about infrequently. Actual death often occurs in institutions away from family and friends. It is often difficult for the aging person to find someone to listen to personal feelings and views of the last stage of life and death. For example, statements like, "Don't talk that way; you're going to live a long time," discourage the person from expressing feelings honestly. Kubler-Ross (1969) found dying people in her study overwhelmingly grateful to have someone listen to their thoughts and feelings. Nursing approaches for promoting adaptive life closure behaviors will be presented in the intervention section. Adaptation problems of the physical self component will be discussed next.

Body Image Disturbance. *Body image disturbance* is an adaptation problem of the physical self component and is also an accepted nursing diagnosis (Gordon 1987). It is defined as negative feelings or perceptions about characteristics, functions, or limits of the body or a body part. Expected behaviors of body image disturbance are listed in Table 14–3. The focal stimulus for these behaviors is often the lack of integration of some bodily change resulting from accident, illness, surgery, or normal growth. The degree of emotional response to an altered body image has been found to be directly related to the intensity of the emotional struggle through which the person is going (Rubin 1968). The person's perception of the event rather than the actual event more strongly influences body image disturbance (Schawlb and Zahr 1985). Another common stimulus is the person's perceptions of self. Negative perceptions of one's physical self, whether based on the observable reality or not, serve to disrupt the person's body image. For example, the person mentioned weighing 118 pounds and measuring 5 feet 7 inches tall, may have weighed 165 pounds four years before. Even though the weight has changed, the person's perception of self has not adjusted to incorporate the new physical reality. Incorporation of the ideal body image defined by society as the standard for personal evaluation also can contribute to a body image disturbance. Responses of significant others is another category of factors influencing the person's ability to successfully integrate body changes.

Sexual Dysfunction. *Sexual dysfunction,* another adaptation problem of the physical self component, is defined as ineffective sexual behavior related to physical or psychological factors.[2] This diagnosis is accepted by the

---

[2]The material on sexuality in this chapter is based in part on Chapter 17 "Sexuality," Marsha Keiko Sato in *Introduction to Nursing: An Adaptation Model* 2nd. ed., Sister Callista Roy, Prentice-Hall, Inc., Englewood Cliffs, 1984, pp. 325–336.

TABLE 14–3. EXPECTED BEHAVIORS FOR PHYSICAL SELF ADAPTATION PROBLEMS[1]

Sexual Dysfunction[2]

Aggressive Sexual Behavior of the Hospitalized Person
    Asking the nurse personal and sexual questions
    Attempting to hold, fondle or kiss parts of the nurse's body
    Exposing private parts to the nurse
    Making seductive comments and jokes
Decreased Sense of Sexual Self
    Verbalized decreased or absent sexual desire
    Verbalized dissatisfaction during coitus
    Absence of orgasm
    Premature or incomplete ejaculation
    Verbalized fear of future limitations on sexual performance

Body Image Disturbance

Verbalized negative feeling about the body
Verbalized fear of rejection or reaction by others due to body appearance or function
Decreased social interactions
Lack of eye contact
Inability to acknowledge actual change in body or body part
Expression of preoccupation with change in body or loss of part
Self mutilating of body
Hiding or overexposing body
Not looking at body part
Refusal to do self care procedures
Verbalized misperceptions about body appearance and/or function
Verbalized feelings of guilt

Rape Trauma Syndrome

Acute Phase
    Physical trauma—traumatized genital area, bruises, edema, bleeding
    Report of pains in various parts of the body
    Expression of anger—may be displaced to police, health care workers, spouse
    Expression of shock—inability to talk
    Muscle tension and/or spasms
    Crying
    Expression of embarrassment
    Gastrointestinal irritability and discomfort
    Sleep pattern disturbance
    Expression of fears
    Expression of panic on seeing scene of attack or assailant
    Changes in sexual behavior
    Verbalized feelings of guilt and shame
Long-Term Phase
    Continuation of any of the behaviors from the acute phase
    Mentally reliving the event
    Changes in life style
    Behaviors of anxiety
    Recurring nightmares
    Changes in relationship with opposite sex
    Behaviors of decreased self-confidence
    Behaviors of depression

[1]Data for all three adaptation problems were drawn from the following three sources: Carpenito (1985), pp. 26–28, 53–54, 64–66; Gordon (1987), pp. 192–194, 200–204, 238, 240–244; and Kelly (1985), pp. 213–216, 227–230, 249–252, 253–257.
[2]In addition to the sources listed in footnote 1, data was drawn from Chapter 17 "Sexuality" by Marsha Keiko Sato in *Introduction to Nursing an Adaptation Model,* (2nd ed.) bv Sister Callista Roy (Englewood Cliffs, N.J.: Prentice-Hall. Inc., 1984), pp. 325–336.

North American Nursing Diagnoses Association and is used when the person identifies a problem with sexuality or when antisocial sexual behavior results in harm to others (Kelly 1985). The hospitalized person may demonstrate a sexual dysfunction problem in one of two ways—aggressive sexual behavior or verbalization of decreased sense of sexual self. Asking for the nurse's first name, address, telephone number, and personal information about the nurse's social and sexual life is considered aggressive sexual behavior. Attempts to hold, fondle, or kiss parts of the nurse's body are other aggressive sexual behaviors. The person with this problem might make seductive comments and jokes or expose the genitals inappropriately.

The focal stimulus for aggressive sexual behavior of the hospitalized person is often fear regarding the outcome of illness. Feelings of helplessness to control one's life in the face of a major illness are another stimulus for sexually aggressive behavior. Lack of information about sexuality and the effects of the illness or surgery upon sexual functioning are other stimuli for aggressive sexual behaviors.

Decreased sense of sexual self is revealed by the person's comments. Several factors inherent in the hospital experience contribute to these behaviors. The disease process, medications or chemotherapy may compromise directly the physiological sexual response. Other stimuli include the asexual hospital gown, hospital routines, and procedures which invade and assault the person's body, lack of privacy, and the interruption of one's regular routine of work, hobbies, recreation, and social interactions. Misinformation or lack of knowledge are other factors influencing the behaviors of decreased sense of sexual self.

Rape Trauma Syndrome. *Rape trauma syndrome,* the immediate and long sequela of a forced sexual activity, is another adaptation problem of the physical self and an accepted nursing diagnosis (Gordon 1987). The expected behaviors of rape trauma syndrome are listed in Table 14–3. The focal stimulus is the forced sexual event. The responses of significant others, police and health care workers are contextual stimuli. Cultural and religious factors also influence the person's response to a sexual assault. The person's previous sense of physical self and perception of self are stimuli for the behaviors of rape trauma syndrome. Stewart et al. (1987) found knowing the perpetrator, the trial, and withdrawal of family support over time all have a negative effect on the victim.

Loss. *Loss,* as it applies to the physical self component, is any situation, either actual or potential, in which part of the body or a body function is altered in such a way that it no longer has the qualities that render it valuable.[3] Loss is considered an adaptation problem of the physical self

[3]The material on loss in this chapter is based in part on Chapter 18 "Loss," Marjorie H. Buck in *Introduction to Nursing: An Adaptation Model,* 2nd ed., Sister Callista Roy, Prentice-Hall, Inc., Englewood Cliffs, 1984, pp. 337–352.

component. The series of emotional responses that occur following the perception of or anticipation of a loss is grief.

Grieving is an accepted nursing diagnosis (Carpenito 1985). In its broadest sense the diagnosis of grieving can be applied to any situation in which loss is involved. Loss is often a part of other adaptation problems, for example, body image disturbance and rape trauma syndrome. The nurse will decide if interventions for promoting grieving need to be applied prior to or in conjunction with other interventions dealing with the primary adaptation problem. The influencing factors cross-modes and include loss of physical function, loss of role function, loss of interpersonal relationship, or loss of sense of self. Aspects of loss relating to separation anxiety are discussed in Chapter 19. The ultimate loss, death of self, was examined in the life closure section of this chapter.

Life is filled with losses and grieving is the natural response. It should not be viewed as pathological. It is, in fact, the process that brings healing and a higher level of integrity when completed. The process of grieving can be viewed as consisting of four stages: (1) shock and disbelief, (2) apprehending the loss, (3) attempting to deal with the loss, and (4) final restitution and resolution. Behaviors listed according to the stages of grief are in Table 14–4.

Stimuli for the behaviors of grieving related to physical self include the physical changes of normal growth, including pregnancy and aging, and accidents or illnesses affecting body appearance and function. Past experiences with loss, level of success of grieving past losses and stress level also serve as stimuli. The six common stimuli for self-concept influence grieving behaviors. The nurse identifies the focal stimulus by her sensitivity to the meaning of the situation in interviewing the person and validating hunches gathered from theory and observation.

Goal Setting

The next step in the nursing process is goal setting. Goal setting is carried out with the person receiving care. The goal states a specific behavior, how it will change, and a time frame. The goal is realistic and attainable, agreeable to the person receiving care, and stated in measurable terms. A series of goals may be set starting with short term ones and moving toward the long-term goals as the preceding ones are met. An example of a goal for a person with the medical diagnosis of multiple sclerosis displaying inattention to personal appearance (behaviors of body image disturbance) is, "The person will wear clean, pressed clothes and have hair washed and combed at the next regular clinic visit."

Examples of goals for physical self problems follow. A goal for a person with a colostomy experiencing sexual dysfunction behaviors is, "The person will resume a sexual relationship that is satisfying to both partners as reported by the individual at the next monthly check up." For a person demonstrating behavior of inability to fall asleep at night following an

TABLE 14–4. STAGES OF GRIEVING A LOSS

Expected Behaviors	Common Stimuli	Common Nursing Approaches
Stage 1 Shock and Disbelief (lasts minutes to days) Statements indicating fact of the loss has not been apprehended: "Oh, I can't believe it's true." Verbal report of stunned numb feeling Blank facial expression Sitting motionless and dazed Little or no attention to the surroundings Automatic carrying out of routine Verbal expression of intellectual acceptance and making plans for dealing with the loss Inability to look at part of the body effected by the loss	Focal Need to protect self from being overwhelmed by painful feelings Contextual Suddenness of the news of the loss Residual Other circumstances surrounding the loss— eg. physical illness, need to support others affected by the loss	Be present—use touch to communicate caring and presence Tell the person you are there to help Refrain from making judgments Provide for privacy Allow denial—don't agree or refute it Ask the person to talk about current feelings Provide for contact with significant others Provide for physiological needs
Stage 2 Apprehending the Loss Sighing Verbal report of slight sense of unreality Verbal report of intense subjective distress Expression of anger at the circumstances and desire not to be bothered Crying Behaviors of fear and anxiety: Report of loss of strength Report of emptiness in chest or epigastrium Report of tightness in throat Appetite changes Weight loss Report of inability to sleep Inability to engage in organized activity Report of a sense of emotional distance from others	Focal Mention or thought of the lost object Contexual Presence of other people Importance of the lost object Degree of ambivalence towards the lost object Ability to tolerate and express painful feelings Response of significant others Residual Cultural norms of how to grieve	Be present and listen Gently remind person of reality Provide for privacy Tell person the responses of this stage are normal and expected Reflect, paraphrase, use silence to encourage expression of feelings Use all the above approaches with significant others Notify clergy of person's choice

(continued)

TABLE 14–4. (Continued)

Expected Behaviors	Common Stimuli	Common Nursing Approaches
Feeling of emptiness		
Seaching for lost object		
Feelings of guilt and shame		
Beginning ability to talk about the reality of the loss: "I guess it's really happening."		
Beginning ability to look at and touch the part of the body effected by loss		
Stage 3—Attempting to Deal with the Loss (the main work occurs intrapsychically and takes months to years)	Focal Contemplation of future without the lost object	Be present and listen Tell person it is normal to feel sorrow, guilt, anger, helplessness
Report of preoccupation with lost object or function	Contextual Importance of the lost object	Use open-ended questions to elicit expression of feelings
Waves of sadness and crying	Degree of ambivalence toward the lost object	Refrain from making judgments
Feelings of despair	Spiritual beliefs	Ask the person to talk about the meaning of lost object
Talk about the lost object and experiences with it prior to the loss	Number of and degree of resolution of past losses	Ask person to talk about past losses—how it felt, what helped, how it was resolved
Expression of feelings of loss of intactness and wholeness of self	Degree of preparation for the loss	Remind person it takes time to go through grieving process
Report of altered body sensations—itching feeling in a leg that has been amputated	Physical and psychological health of the person	Use touch to communicate presence and caring
Development of physical illness	Ability to tolerate and express painful feelings	Ask person about spiritual beliefs
Carrying out of self care routine—looking at and touching the effected part of the body	Amount of guilt felt Age of the person Residual Cultural prescription of how to grieve Contemplation of the unexpected experience of grief itself	Involve clergy person as requested by person Apply above approaches to significant others
Stage 4—Final Restitution and Resolution	Focal Level of success of completion of previous stages of grief	Active listening techniques Help person problem-solve how to form new patterns of functioning and relating
Expression of interest in alternatives for the lost object or function	Contextual All stimuli listed above	Refrain from judging
Ability to talk about the loss experience with out bitterness and guilt	Residual All stimuli listed above	Point out person's strengths and gains

Source: data drawn in part from the three books on nursing diagnosis—Carpenito 1985, Gordon 1985, Kelly 1985, and from Chapter 18 "Loss" by Marjorie H. Buck in *Introduction to Nursing an Adaptation Model,* (2nd ed.) by Sister Callista Roy (Englewood Cliffs, N.J.: Prentice-Hall, Inc., 1984), pp.337–352.

experience of forced sexual encounter, the goal could be, "The person will report having fallen asleep within a half hour of going to bed at the next clinic visit." The goals for the person who has the problem of loss should reflect the stage of grief currently occupied by the person. For the person with multiple sclerosis in the shock and disbelief stage due to loss of bladder control, the goal might be, "The person will begin to verbalize recognition of the loss of bladder control in three to five days."

In keeping with the model's overall goal of promoting adaptation of the individual throughout the life cycle, the nurse can state two main goals for the person in the last stage of life as determined by age or physical condition indicating nearness of death. "The person will demonstrate behaviors of integrity and acceptance of the inevitability of death," is the first goal. This goal is long term. Achieving it is a process that takes months or years and builds on a lifetime of experiences. "The person will demonstrate the behaviors of the stages of dying and achieve acceptance of death," is the goal for the person in the terminal stages of life.

In summary, the goals deal with the behaviors in a realistic way specifying a time frame for the quantity and direction of change. The person receiving care helps plan, understands and agrees to the goals. Current theory regarding the particular adaptation problem is reflected in the goal.

Intervention

Interventions are carried out to achieve the stated goal. Since the focal stimulus is the prime initiator of the behavior under consideration, the nurse will alter it to effect change or to stabilize adaptation whenever possible. The nurse works with the contextual and residual stimuli to broaden the adaptation level when the focal stimulus cannot be altered. The nurse reinforces stimuli that promote adaptive behaviors and alters stimuli that contribute to ineffective behaviors. The following discussion will outline common nursing approaches for promoting adaptation in the physical self component. Examples of approaches that manage stimuli in each of the six categories of common stimuli will be presented. Problems of the physical self are complex involving cross-modal diagnoses with stimuli affecting more than one mode. The nurse will decide which stimulus is the focal and how to best bring about adaptive responses. Interventions may be aimed at role, interpersonal, or physiological behaviors (acting as stimuli within this mode) first to broaden the adaptation level and thereby promote adaptive behaviors in the physical self component.

Growth and Development. The nurse can manage the stimulus of normal growth and development by assisting the person to obtain adequate nutrition, rest, and activity. Helping the person learn control of bodily functions also manages the stimulus of growth and development. The specific actions will vary with the age, physical ability, and health status of the person. Teaching the person and significant others the facts of normal growth and development, including sexuality, also falls in this category.

The normal physical changes of puberty, pregnancy, menopause, and old age can be the focal stimuli for the adaptation problem of **body image disturbance**. The nurse can provide information about expected physical changes and how to care for the body. The nurse provides the pregnant woman information on where to obtain attractive clothes that she can afford, and what to expect in terms of body appearance and function following delivery of the baby. The nurse uses purposeful communication techniques to help the individual identify and explore feelings about the body changes.

The normal physical changes of aging can be the focal stimulus for the adaptation problem of **loss**. These changes generally cannot be managed directly. The nurse works with other stimuli to promote adaptation. Table 14–4 lists approaches for helping the person through the grieving process. Nursing interventions for working with the grieving person are very similar to the approaches used with the dying person. In fact, the person's past experiences with loss are the ground work for the dying process.

Learning. The person's past experiences with rewards and lack of rewards or punishments influence the adaptation problems of the physical self discussed in this chapter. The nurse uses purposeful communication techniques to elicit information from the person receiving care about the presence or absence of rewards and to explore new ways of obtaining rewards in light of the current situation. For example, the person experiencing the adaptation problem of **sexual dysfunction** following ostomy surgery can be guided to explore ways of receiving and giving sensual pleasure in addition to coitus (Shipes 1987).

Interventions can be aimed at changing societal trends. As a member of the community the nurse works to broaden the spectrum of acceptable body and personality traits. "Once the standard of acceptable body image is changed to include more persons on the basis of their existence alone, the emotional stress that accompanies an altered body image would probably be much less severe or devastating" (Schawlb and Zahr 1985).

In the case of the adaptation problem of **loss** in the physical self component, the nurse assists the person to grieve the loss. (See Table 14–4.) Once the person has progressed to the third stage, attempting to deal with the loss, the nurse uses active listening, open-ended questions, reflection and silence to assist the person to find new value and rewards for the current physical self condition. Attempts to intervene in this manner before the person reaches the third stage of grief would be counter productive.

Nursing interventions managing the learning category of stimuli may focus on helping the client verbalize and analyze religious/moral teachings that affect the current physical self behaviors. For instance, the person experiencing the adaptation problem of **rape trauma syndrome—long-**

term phase may demonstrate behaviors of shame and guilt resulting from religious/moral teachings concerning female "purity, virginity, and chastity." Through use of purposeful communication, the nurse can help the person express the teachings learned in childhood and evaluate them consciously in terms of the rape experience. The nurse is careful to listen without judging the person or the beliefs. The process of verbalizing allows the individual to become aware of the influence of the beliefs and to decide what makes sense personally in the current situation. If the behaviors of shame and guilt are severe and prolonged the nurse will refer the person to a professional therapist or clergy person.

Reactions of Others. The nurse using the adaptation model will work with the significant others in the person's life to broaden the adaptation level and thereby assist the person achieve the goal. The nurse takes the necessary steps to establish trust and rapport with the significant other. Next the nurse explains the influence of the significant others' responses on the person receiving care. The nurse uses open-ended questions, reflection, and silence to facilitate expression of feelings. The nurse also gives information, answers questions, and provides anticipatory guidance to help the significant other have a positive influence on the person's behavior. For example, in the case of a 28-year-old person with no children who has the adaptation problem of **loss** following a hysterectomy, the nurse gives the significant other information about the grief process, what to expect and how long each stage might last. The nurse also listens to the significant other's expression of grief regarding the woman's lost ability to reproduce.

In the case of **body image disturbance** following ostomy surgery, the nurse informs the significant other of the appearance and care of the ostomy. Next the nurse listens to the significant other's responses and answers questions to prepare that person to be supportive to the person with the new ostomy. The nurse also intervenes by referring the significant other and the person to a support group when appropriate.

When the adaptation problem is **rape trauma syndrome** the nurse can intervene to broaden the person's adaptation level by teaching emergency room personnel and police officers the value and skill of using open-ended questions. The use of closed questions with implied values contributes to the person's behaviors of embarrassment and guilt. For example, the officer can ask, "What did you do when attacked?" rather than, "Did you do anything to defend yourself?"

For some individuals the responses of significant others have been internalized and continue to influence behavior even in the absence of the original responses. For example, a person with the adaptation problem of **sexual dysfunction** might have been told that sex is dirty and disgusting by a parent with a sexual dysfunction problem. Perhaps the parent prevented the young child from touching and exploring the genitals. In addition, the parent looked disgusted whenever cleaning and diapering the child. As an adult the person reports feeling unclean and degraded when having coitus with her spouse even though he is gentle and respectful of her. During the sexual self assessment, the person remembers the pronouncements of the parent. When intervening, the nurse uses therapeutic communication techniques to allow the person to identify and ventilate the feelings connected with the parent's reaction to sexuality. As the person releases the tension of those old feelings, she will be able to reassess her attitudes about sexuality and incorporate new information. The nurse allows sufficient time for the person to ventilate the feelings before attempting to give information. The nurse refers the individual to a professional counselor if necessary.

Perception. When the individual is experiencing an adaptation problem resulting primarily from the influence of perceptions of self, the nurse may use perception alteration as an approach.[4] To carry out this approach the nurse interviews the person seeking details about the events surrounding the perceptions which are having a negative effect on the person's self-concept. As the individual recalls more and more details, he or she frequently will come to see that current thoughts and feelings about self are based on misunderstood past events, incomplete information, and stereotypes. As the result of these realizations and ventilation of accompanying feelings, the person may be able to relinquish certain negative perceptions of self, thus clearing the way for a more positive self-view.

For example, a man with the adaptation problem of body image distrubance states that he feels fat and therefore ugly. He relates that he was 50 to 60 pounds overweight from the ages of 19 to 26. Six years ago he lost the extra weight and has maintained his current weight, which is within the normal range. He tells the nurse that he knows that he is not overweight but that he sees himself as fat in his mind's eye. He holds a perception of his body that is incongruent with the present reality. By exploring in detail the events around the inclusion of his perception of self as fat, and the events of his weight loss, he may be able to let go of the old perception and incorporate his actual body appearance into his body image.

Schawlb and Zahr (1985) discuss altered body image of people with multiple sclerosis. They conclude that an alteration in body image is more related to how the person perceives the disturbance than to the actual disturbance taking place. By exploring the person's perceptions of self and encouraging the expression of feelings about the perceived changes in body image, the nurse can assist the person to have a broader adaptation level.

---

[4]This discussion of perception alteration is based on the unpublished work of Betty Dambacker, School of Nursing, University of California at Los Angeles, 1972.

Jourard (1964) proposed that everyone is capable of disclosing the content of their phenomenal self unless its content conflicts with the person's "public self" or conscience. Subby (1987) observed that the person's private self (phenomenal self) becomes less accessible compared to the public self over time as the result of experiences of neglect, abuse, and enmeshment. The content of the phenomenal self is repressed to protect the person from chronic feelings of anxiety, shame and/or low self-esteem. The nurse applies interventions aimed at diminishing the behaviors of those adaptation problems first (see Chapter 15 for further discussion of these problems).

According to Jourard (1964), the second reason a person does not disclose phenomenal self content is the impression that no one is truly interested. The nurse purposefully conveys a sincere interest in what is on the person's mind as it relates to the person's current health situation. Sincere interest is expressed by making eye contact with the person and by reflecting and paraphrasing the person's statements. The nurse avoids responses such as, "You shouldn't feel that way," or "I'm surprised to hear you feel that way." The processes of assessment and intervention often overlap when working in the self-concept mode. Talking about self during assessment may naturally bring the ventilation of feelings and reevaluation of the past experiences that allow a more adaptive response.

Perception of self functions as an influencing factor for the behaviors of body image disturbance, sexual dysfunction, rape trauma syndrome, and loss. Accordingly, perception alteration can be used as the nursing approach for any of these physical self problems. Discussion of perception alteration as an intervention for personal self problems is presented in Chapter 15.

Maturational Crises. The nurse manages the stimulus of maturational crisis to promote integrity in each stage of development. Chapter 15 includes a discussion of nursing approaches applicable to each stage of development. Nursing interventions to promote mastery of the last stage, integrity versus despair will be discused here as related to life closure. The rationale for including this discussion in the physical self content is that the last stage ends with death, loss of self.[5] The nurse works directly with the person and through others to promote mastery of this stage of development. Nursing approaches are organized according to the two goals for this stage stated above.

The nurse must be comfortable with the subject of death and dying to intervene effectively. Reading the literature, attending classes and seminars, discussing personal feelings with family and friends helps the nurse

---

[5]The discussion of life closure is based in part on Chapter 28 "Life Closure," Marjorie Clowry Dobratz in *Introduction to Nursing: An Adaptation Model*, 2nd ed., Sister Callista Roy, Prentice-Hall, Inc., Englewood Cliffs, New Jersey, 1984, pp.497–518.

be prepared to assist the person with life closure. The nurse who has not attempted to deal with death on a personal level and who has unresolved grief will have great difficulty interacting effectively with the person in the last stage of life.

Butler (1963) proposed life review to be a universal, naturally occurring process brought on by realization of personal vulnerability to death. To promote achievement of the first goal, that the person will demonstrate behaviors of integrity and acceptance of the inevitability of death, the nurse encourages the process of life review by use of purposeful communication techniques—reflecting, paraphrasing, asking open-ended questions, and active use of silence. The nursing approach of asking the person to identify the things in life, past and present, for which he or she is thankful further contributes to the attainment of the goal (Linn et al. 1988).

After listening carefully to the person's life review, the nurse can provide anticipatory guidance by making a comment such as, "Some people in your situation take steps to _____ (what ever the next logical step in planning for the future might be, for example, write down memories for their children, write a will, plan for needs of a spouse)." The desired positive outcome of the process of life review is a sense of integrity as well as the possibility of personality reorganization, serenity, wisdom, and increased self-awareness (Kimmel, 1974).

Linn et al. (1988) proposed another approach for helping the person achieve integrity and accept the reality of one's own death without despair. In this approach, the nurse asks the person to answer the question, "Who are the most alive elderly people you have known or heard of?" Identifying and discussing a model of someone who embraced life to its last breath can inspire the person and help take the fear out of facing one's own death. The nurse uses the purposeful communication techniques listed throughout this process.

Erikson (1982) pointed out that the person in the last stage of development needs to maintain a "grand-generative" function. Doing so is often a challenge in the face of not being near grandchildren and other young people. The nurse uses approaches to reinforce the person's usual way of coping. In addition, the nurse can intervene by supporting community programs for senior citizens and referring the person to those programs when applicable. Examples of possible referrals are senior citizen centers and volunteer programs in hospitals to read to children and rock babies.

The nurse applies these approaches as often as needed with the person in the final stage of life and teaches them to the significant others. Mastery of the crisis of this stage, just as in all the others, is a continuing, never-completed process. Erikson (1982) pointed out that the historical change of the lengthening of the average life span may call for a more active anticipation of dying.

When terminal illness occurs, the nurse intervenes to help the person achieve the second goal, the person will demonstrate the behaviors of the stages of dying and achieve acceptance of death. Kubler-Ross (1969) identified five stages of dying: (1) denial and isolation, (2) anger, (3) bargaining, (4) depression, and (5) acceptance. As with the grief process, the dying process does not necessarily progress smoothly from stage to stage. The person may demonstrate behaviors in more than one stage at once and may move back and forth between stages. Not everyone will complete the dying process before actual death occurs. The person may become stuck at any stage. The nurse respects each individual and the method that fits the individual's needs and style. Kubler-Ross (1969) advised that the best approach is to take time to sit, listen and share. She pointed out that the person needs to be in charge of the timing of discussions. The dying person does not want to talk about dying day after day. The person will return to denial as a coping mechanism. Yet the person will want to talk about dying at other times. The nurse and significant others take cues from the person, allowing the person to function in the current stage until the person is ready to move on to the next stage. The nurse continues to convey the willingness to listen by making eye contact, sitting down, reflecting comments from past conversations, and asking open-ended questions. These approaches assist the person to progress to the next stage.

The nurse uses listening skills to allow the person to express behaviors in each of the stages of dying. Behaviors that would be considered ineffective in other situations are viewed as adaptive in the dying process.

The behaviors of significant others are important stimuli for the dying person's behaviors. The nurse assists the family members and friends to deal with their grief so they can assist the person through the stages of dying. The nurse uses interventions for loss to help the significant others deal with their feelings about the impending death of the person (see Table 14–4). The nurse also intervenes by giving the family members information about the dying process and what to expect from the person.

Kubler-Ross (1969) found hope to be an underlying aspect of each stage of dying. The people in her study expressed hope until the end. When an individual expressed hopelessness, death generally followed within 24 hours. The nurse intervenes by allowing the person to maintain hope without lying about the seriousness of the illness. "Yes, remission is a possibility," is an example of an honest and hopeful response. It is true that the exact moment of death cannot be predicted. Once the person stops expressing hope, the nurse, other health care workers and significant others need to allow the hopelessness. The individual will have difficulty accepting death if significant others and health care workers attempt to maintain hope at this point. The nurse and significant others must take cues from the dying person and help maintain hope until the person signals it is time to let go of hope.

Adaptive life closure is indicated by the individual demonstrating integrity throughout the process. Relationships with significant others have been maintained and brought to closure. In terms of the Roy Adaptation Model, the integration of the four adaptive modes is evident. Adaptive behaviors in each stage of dying have been expressed. Acceptance is indicated by the person surrendering to the internal self and turning away from life. It is a time almost devoid of feelings, a detached existence without fear or despair. The nurse supports this increasing detachment from the external into the internal. Nonverbal communication is often the best intervention—a quiet sitting with a touch of the hand, making the person as comfortable as possible. The person wants no demands placed on them. The family members need help at this point. They may not be ready to let the loved one go. The nurse intervenes by listening to their thoughts and feelings and by referring them to a clergy person when indicated.

Coping Strategies. The sixth category of common stimuli for physical self behaviors is coping strategies. The nurse intervenes by promoting use of usual ways of coping whenever reasonable and possible. For example, the nurse might help the person obtain special foods eaten routinely to help promote a sense of physical strength. At times coping mechanisms are no longer adaptive and the person needs assistance developing new ones. For instance, a person who eats a high-fat diet and leaves out necessary nutrients might state, "I don't eat fruits and vegetables since I am getting extra calories from potato chips." This person is demonstrating an ineffective mode of coping. The nurse intervenes with purposeful communication techniques to elicit expression of feelings around the issue and then supply information and guidance when the person is ready.

In summary, the nurse manages all impinging stimuli as appropriate. In addition to managing stimuli in the six categories of common stimuli, therapeutic measures to promote healing of physical illness and injury are carried out. Rehabilitative measures to help restore function and establish new functions are implemented. Health promotion interventions are carried out. All of these nursing approaches are used to facilitate adaptation in the physical self component.

Evaluation
Once the interventions have been carried out, the nurse reassesses the behaviors targeted in the goal. If the behaviors are present as stated, the goal has been met. The nurse then reapplies the nursing process focusing on the next priority. When the behaviors as stated in the goal are not present, the nurse reworks the nursing process in that problem area. First the behaviors and stimuli are reassessed. Some important aspects may have been missed or behaviors and stimuli may have changed in the time period since the first assessment. In the case of the dying process, the behaviors change constantly, necessitating ongoing reassessment.

Next the nurse looks at the goal to see if it was stated in realistic, measurable terms. Perhaps the goal itself needs to be altered. Without the person's involvement with the goal, the nursing interventions will be ineffective. The nurse checks with the person to see that both share the same understanding of the goal and that it is in keeping with the person's desires. Underlying issues may exist that must be dealt with before the behavior originally identified can become adaptive. For example, if the unmet goal dealt with the person learning self care of an ostomy, approaches to resolve the underlying issue of body image disturbance may be the step needed to pave the way for attaining the self care goal.

Finally, the nurse considers the interventions to see if they were carried out properly. Perhaps the intervention did not actually manage the identified stimulus. The interventions may not have been tried for long enough or possibly the timing was not correct. The physical needs for nutrition, rest and pain relief need to be met prior to carrying out physical self interventions. After the nurse determines aspects requiring reconsideration, the nursing process is reapplied reflecting the changes needed.

SUMMARY

This chapter has provided information on how to assess physical self behaviors and stimuli. Physical self behaviors are viewed in two categories— body sensations and body image. Sexuality is a part of the physical self displaying behaviors in both categories. The six common stimuli for self-concept behaviors were discussed in terms of the physical self component. Adaptive physical self behaviors were identified. Four adaptation problems, body image disturbance, sexual dysfuntion, rape trauma syndrome, and loss were presented briefly. Goal setting and interventions were presented. Life closure, the normal process of resolving the issue of the meaning of one's life and accepting the reality of one's death, was discussed in some detail. Finally, the evaluation of goals was examined.

EXERCISES FOR APPLICATION

1. Select a character from your favorite television show and complete a physical self assessment. Identify behaviors related to the physical self and the stimuli present which may have an influence on the assessed behaviors. Identify any problems encountered in completing your assessment. Do you think that similar problems might be encountered in completing a real-life physical self assessment? How would you overcome these problems.

2. Select a peer and complete a physical self assessment. Identify behaviors and stimuli. Establish a nursing diagnosis, set goals and plan nursing interventions for the individual. Describe how you would evaluate the effectiveness of the planned nursing inter-

ventions. Discuss your assessment, nursing diagnosis, goals and nursing interventions with your peer. Identify any modifications which you would make following this discussion.

ASSESSMENT OF UNDERSTANDING

1. Describe the importance of the physical self to adaptation nursing.
2. Identify the following behaviors as either adaptive or ineffective in promoting integrity of physical self.
   a. _____ "I can't go swimming because I look horrible in a swim suit."
   b. _____ At the six-week post-partum check up, a woman touches the stretch marks on her abdomen and states, "I know they'll fade in time."
   c. _____ The person in the first stage of grief states, "I just can't believe this is happening to me."
3. Write "S" before the physical self stimuli listed below.
   a _____ grimace and tense neck and arm muscles
   b. _____ trust versus mistrust stage of development
   c. _____ "I feel it is important to always be neat, clean, and well dressed."
   d. _____ Person's height is 4 feet, 9 inches.
4. Formulate a nursing diagnosis for the following set of assessment information.

Behaviors	Stimuli
Neatly dressed in worn, but carefully mended and pressed outfit	20-year old female, average height, and weight
Appears confident	"I am confident in my abilities."
"Some people might consider me attractive"	"My family is proud of me."
"I normally feel good about myself."	Intimacy versus isolation.
"I fancy myself as an independent thinker."	

5. Write a physical self goal for a ten-year old girl in good physical health who is showing signs of the onset of puberty.
6. Propose three nursing interventions to promote the first goal of life closure, that is, the person will demonstrate behaviors of integrity and acceptance of the inevitability of death.
7. Consider the goal: "The person will wear clean, pressed clothes and

have hair washed and combed at the next regular clinic visit." How would the nurse evaluate whether the goal had been achieved when the patient next visits the clinic?

Feedback

1. The first impressions of the self and the world are experienced physically through body sensations. Throughout the life cycle the individual receives and interprets information through body sensations. The body image influences a person's behaviors in all the adaptive modes: physiological, self concept, role function, and interdependence. Adaptation nursing views and promotes integrity of the individual as a whole.
2. a. ineffective
   b. adaptive
   c. adaptive
3. b, c, and d are stimuli for the physical self
4. Adaptive self-concept of body image due to realistic self-perception and positive reaction from others.
5. The girl will verbally express a positive feeling about her own body at the next clinic visit.
6. a. The nurse will use purposeful communication techniques to encourage life review.
   b. The nurse will refer the person to an agency where she or he can contribute in a meaningful and personally appropriate way.
   c. The nurse will give information to significant others about the life closure process and teach them ways of assisting the person to achieve integrity and accept the inevitability of death.
7. The nurse would evaluate the person's behavior in terms of their appearance. The person would be expected to be dressed neatly in clean clothes and have clean and orderly hair.

REFERENCES

Amann-Gainotti, M. Sexual socialization during early adolescence: The menarche, *Adolescence,* 21 (Fall 1986): 703–710.

Buck, M. Loss, in Sister Callista Roy, *Introduction to Nursing: An Adaptation Model* (2nd. ed.). Englewood Cliffs, N.J.: Prentice-Hall, 1984.

Butler, R. The life review: An interpretation of reminiscence in the aged, *Psychiatry* 26 (1): 65–76, 1963.

Calderone, M., and J. Ramey. *Talking With Your Child About Sex.* New York: Ballantine Books, 1982.

Campsey, J. The sexual dimension of patient care, *Nursing Forum,* 22 (2): 69–71, 1985.

Carpenito, L. *Handbook of Nursing Diagnosis.* Philadelphia: J.B. Lippincott, 1985.

Coombs, A., and D. Snygg. *Individual Behavior—A Perceptual Approach to Behavior.* New York: Harper Brothers, 1959.

Dobratz, M. Life closure, in Sister Callista Roy, *Introduction to Nursing: An Adaptation Model* (2nd. ed.). Englewood Cliffs, NJ: Prentice-Hall, 1984.

Erikson, E. *Childhood and Society* (2nd. ed.). New York: W.W. Norton, 1963.

———————. *The Life Cycle Completed: A Review.* New York: W.W. Norton, 1982.

Goedert, J. What is safe sex? Suggested standards linked to testing for human immunodeficiency virus, *The New England Journal of Medicine,* 316 (21): 1339–1342, 1987.

Gordon, M. *Manual of Nursing Diagnosis.* New York: McGraw-Hill, 1987.

Johnson, D. *Body.* Boston: Beacon Press, 1983.

Jourard, S. *The Transparent Self.* Princeton, N.J.: D. Van Nostrand, 1964.

Kelly, M.A. *Nursing Diagnosis Source Book: Guidelines for Clinical Application.* E. Norwalk, Conn: Appleton-Century-Crofts, 1985.

Kimmel, D. *Adulthood and Aging.* New York: John Wiley & Sons, 1974.

Kleinke, C. *Self-Perception: The Psychology of Personal Awareness.* San Francisco: W.H. Freeman, 1978.

Kubler-Ross, E. *On Death and Dying.* New York: Macmillan, 1969.

Linn, M., S. Fabricant, and D. Linn. *Healing the Eight Stages of Life.* New York: Paulist, 1988.

Montagu, A. *Touching: The Human Significance of the Skin* (3rd. ed.). New York: Harper & Row, 1986.

Sanford, John. *Between People: Communicating One-to-One.* New York/Ramsey: Paulist Press, 1982.

Sato, M. Sexuality, in Sister Callista Roy, *Introduction to Nursing: An Adaptation Model* (2nd. ed.). Englewood Cliffs, NJ: Prentice-Hall, 1984.

Schawlb, D. and L. Zahr. Nursing care of patients with an altered body image due to multiple sclerosis, *Nursing Forum* 22 (2): 72–76, 1985.

Shipes, E. Sexual function following ostomy surgery, *Nursing Clinics of North America.* 22 (2): 303–310, 1987.

Silverstone, B., and H. Hyman. *You and Your Aging Parent.* New York: Pantheon Books, 1976.

Stewart, B., C. Hughes, E. Frank, B. Anderson, K. Kendall, and D. West. The aftermath of rape: Profiles of immediate and delayed treatment seekers, *The Journal of Nervous and Mental Disease,* 175 (2): 90–94, 1987.

Subby, R. *Lost in the Shuffle: The Co-dependent Reality.* Deerfield Beach, Fl.: Health Communication, 1987.

Weinberg, J. *Sexuality Human Needs and Nursing Practice.* Philadelphia: W. B. Saunders, 1982.

Additional Reference

Rubin, R. Body image and self esteem, *Nursing Outlook,* 6: 20–23, 1968.

Chapter Fifteen ─────────

The Personal Self

Marjorie H. Buck

The personal self is one of two components of the self-concept mode. In the Roy Adaptation Model, the personal self is described in terms of self-consistency, self-ideal, and the moral-ethical-spiritual self as they relate to psychic integrity. Application of the Roy Adaptation Model nursing process to the personal self component will be illustrated. Positive adaptation within this component will be identified. The adaptation problems of anxiety, powerlessness, guilt, and low self-esteem will be discussed.

OBJECTIVES

After studying this chapter, the reader will be able to do the following:

1. Describe the personal self component of the self-concept mode.
2. Identify behaviors related to the personal self and their effect on the person.
3. List the six common stimuli associated with the personal self.
4. Derive nursing diagnoses conveying effective adaptation and ineffective adaptation related to the personal self.
5. Given a situation, state a goal for a specified adaptation problem.
6. Identify possible nursing interventions for a specified personal self goal.
7. Describe evaluative behaviors relevant to a given situation in this mode component.

KEY CONCEPTS DEFINED

- *Anxiety:* a painful uneasiness of mind due to a vague, nonspecific threat.

- *Guilt:* the judgement a person makes about his or her personal transgression.
- *Moral-ethical-spiritual self:* that aspect of the personal self component which functions as observer, standard-setter, dreamer, comparer, and most of all, evaluator of who this person says she or he is.
- *Powerlessness:* perception of a lack of internal or personal control over events.
- *Self-consistency:* the part of the personal self component which strives to maintain a consistent self-organization and thus to avoid disequilibrium.
- *Self-esteem:* the individual's overall perception of self-worth.
- *Self-ideal/self-expectancy:* that aspect of personal self component which relates to what the person expects to be and do.

DESCRIPTION OF THE PERSONAL SELF

Each human being must have some sense of self to be able to function as an individual in the world. "Who am I? What are my special and unique characteristics? What are my aspirations in life and how close am I to attaining those aspirations? In what do I really believe? For what am I willing to put my life on the line?" These are the philosophical questions of being that elicit the behaviors of the personal self component.

The personal self is divided into three subareas: self-consistency, self-ideal/self-expectancy, and the moral-ethical-spiritual self. *Self-consistency* is one's actual performance, one's response to a situation, and one's "personality traits." *Self-ideal/self-expectancy* is what one would like to be, related to what one is capable of being. Examples of self-ideal behaviors include statements as, "I would like to be (less jumpy, calm in all settings, a caring person)." The *moral-ethical-spiritual self* is the person's belief system, morals, and the evaluator of who one is. Examples of behaviors include such statements as "I believe in (being honest at all costs, taking care of me first, a just and kind God)" and "I believe I am (doing the best I can, a lousy person)."

Several sociological and psychological theories contribute to the theoretical basis of the personal self. These have been outlined in Chapter 13 and are identified as relevant throughout in this chapter. Those specifically relevant to the personal self are the Coombs and Snygg (1959) theory of self perception; the social interactionist theories of Cooley (Epstein 1973), Mead (1934), and Sullivan (1953); the developmental theories of Erikson (1963) and Gardner (1964); and Jackins' (1974) ideas on the sense of self.[1]

[1]The original literature review, including the development of this classification and the theory underlying the self-concept mode was done by Marie J. Driever at Mount St. Mary's College under USPHS Grant No. 5T02MH06442, 1969–70.

APPLICATION OF THE NURSING PROCESS

Consideration of the individual's personal self in the promotion of adaptation is of primary importance. Adaptation problems in the area of the self-concept mode and specifically the personal self component may interfere with the person's ability to heal and to do what is necessary to maintain health. The three components of the personal self, self-consistency, self-ideal/self-expectancy, and the moral-ethical-spiritual self, represent categories of behaviors that suggest to the nurse the effectiveness with which the patient will be able to adapt to the situation at hand.

In addressing the self-concept component of personal self with the patient, it is important that the nurse understand and be comfortable with his or her own personal self and the related subareas. Not only is an adaptive personal self required by the patient in dealing with other adaptation problems, it is a requirement for the nurse attempting to assist the patient towards effective adaptation in the self-concept mode.

Assessment of Behavior

Personal self behaviors are expressed in the verbalization of thoughts and feelings as well as in actions. An individual's view of self cannot be inferred from observing a few behaviors. A thorough assessment is done before a nursing diagnosis can be made. To obtain the assessment data, the nurse creates an atmosphere in which the person feels safe to express thoughts and feelings. The attitude of the nurse does much to set the tone of safety or lack thereof. Since feelings are the subjective response of the individual, there are no good, bad, right or wrong feelings. Laughing, crying, raging, shaking, and talking are expressions of feelings. The tension of unexpressed feelings is contained within the person. It is possible to feel very angry, for example, without raging or even talking about it. Such suppression of feelings, however, ties up psychic energy and interferes with the ability to do other things, such as thinking clearly and healing. In terms of the Roy Model, this is cognator ineffectiveness.

The nurse who conveys an accepting, nonjudgmental attitude can facilitate the expression of feelings. The nurse needs to be in touch with his or her own personal feelings and have an appropriate outlet for them. When this is the case, the nurse will be able to listen to the expression of feelings by the other person without imposing personal feelings.

Another aspect in creating a safe environment for the person is the ability to state clearly and directly the purpose of an interaction. For example, the nurse might say, "I am going to spend some time talking with you about your thoughts and feelings about yourself. Since each person is different and responds differently to (giving birth, surgery, cancer, for example) it is important for me to understand how you are feeling now. That way I can plan care based on your needs and wishes." The actual wording will vary for the individual situation.

The time and place of an interview and other nurse/patient interactions will be planned appropriately. The person who is in pain, for example, cannot attend to questions relating to the personal self. The person whose room is filled with other people also may be unable to attend to a nursing interview. The immediate physiological needs and the need for privacy must be met prior to beginning a personal self assessment.

Table 15–1 lists the subcomponents of personal self, how to elicit behaviors and how the behaviors may be manifested. The nurse will find the words that are appropriate to the actual setting and communication style of those involved. Nonverbal behaviors of posture, facial expression, tone of voice, eye contact are noted.

Once the personal self behaviors are identified, the nurse makes an initial judgment as to whether each behavior is effective or ineffective. Adaptive behaviors promote survival, growth, reproduction, and mastery.

TABLE 15–1. ASSESSMENT OF BEHAVIOR OF THE PERSONAL SELF COMPONENT

Characteristics	How to Elicit Behavior	How Behavior is Manifested
Self-consistency: personality traits; how one views self in relation to actual performance or response to situation	How would you describe yourself as a person? What are your personal characteristics?	"I am _____" (a smart person, a person of strong will, like a child, not worthwhile, etc)
Self-ideal: what one would like to be or do—related to what one is capable of being or doing	What are your aspirations for yourself as a person? What would you change about yourself if you could?	"I would like to be _____" (someone who makes a difference, famous, a strong person, etc.) "I would change _____" (how I loose my temper, my inability to do math, my sense of not belonging anywhere, etc)
Moral-ethical-spiritual self: one's sense of self in relation to one's sacred, ethical beliefs; how self is viewed in relation to one's value system, beliefs about "rightness" or "wrongness"; evaluator of "who I am"	How would you describe your spiritual beliefs? How do your spiritual beliefs affect your view of self? How do you measure up to your own standards of right living? How do you evaluate yourself?	"I believe in _____" (God, a higher being, natural order, etc) "I go to _____" (church, AA meetings, the mountains, etc) "I like to _____" (read certain books, meditate, practice yoga, etc.) "I am _____" (pretty consistent, a long way from doing as I believe, etc) "I tend to be _____" (hard on myself, patient with myself, pretty happy with myself, etc)

Source: Based on the unpublished work of Joan Cho, Department of Nursing, Mount Saint Mary's College, Los Angeles, 1979–80.

Another criterion for judging behaviors as adaptive or ineffective is the extent to which the behaviors lead to the realization of the individual's goals relative to development. Andrews and Roy (1986) have identified three indicators of effective adaptation: (1) norms—normal values and guidelines for expected behaviors are applied to the assessed behaviors; (2) coping mechanism activity—levels of regulator activity and cognator effectiveness are looked at in terms of the assessed behaviors; and (3) person's perception—how realistic is the person's perception of his or her own behavior as adaptive or ineffective? Through the application of these indicators, the nurse can identify the behaviors as adaptive (A) or ineffective (I). Priorities for the next step of the nursing process, assessment of stimuli, are based on the judgment of how effectively the person is coping with changes in the internal and external environments.

Assessment of Stimuli

After the personal self behaviors have been assessed, the second level of assessment, which identifies the influencing factors or stimuli, is done. The theories related to self-concept discussed in Chapter 13 provide the categories to be covered in the second level of assessment. Table 14–2 listed the general categories of influencing factors, gave a brief discussion of each and provided examples of how to collect data in each category. The order in which the categories are assessed will vary according to the individual situation. For a young child, growth and development, learning, and reactions of others factors may be more prominent than perception factors, for example.

Self perception. Content related to the perception of self is based primarily on the theory of Coombs and Snygg (1959). According to their theory, the individual's perception of "what is self" and "what is not self" influences the formation and maintenance of a concept of personal self. For example, if one perceives ones self as weak willed and easily controlled, the person may agree to tests and procedures that really are not wanted. Data in this category are obtained from interviewing the person and observing nonverbal cues.

Growth and Development. When assessing stimuli in the category of growth and development, the nurse using an adaptation approach considers the physiological mode behavioral assessment as influencing factors for the personal self behaviors. The person's age and degree of physical development are taken into consideration. For example, the physiological behavior of inability to control excretion of urine will have a different effect on the self-concept of a 1-year-old person than on that of a 16-year-old person. The nurse also applies norms of growth and development, such as height and weight charts, in this category. Data in this category are obtained from interviewing the person, reviewing the physiological assessment and written records, and from knowledge of growth and development standards.

Learning. Learning is another category to consider in the assessment of stimuli for personal self behaviors. The concept of the model, ideal or potential human being is applicable here (Jackins 1974). The very young child has a sense of self as all-powerful, very intelligent, loving and joyful. Over time the effects of receiving positive or negative input for personal characteristics affects this original sense of self. Which personal characteristics are valued is determined by cultural and social norms. Race, sex, class, religion, and other societal discriminations affect the individual's concept of self. By assessing what the significant people in an individual's life expect, what an individual has learned is expected of her or him, and what the social values are, the nurse will discover how the person's current sense of self differs from that original ideal self. Data in this category are obtained by interviewing the person and significant others and by reviewing the literature on social discrimination.

Reactions of Others. The reactions of others is another category of stimuli. The work of the interactionist theorists Cooley, Mead, and Sullivan, as identified in Chapter 13, forms the basis of this division of stimuli. In essence, these theories state that the individual starts to think of self in the ways in which he or she perceives that others view him or her. For example, the person who is repeatedly told, "You are thoughtless of others," may incorporate a sense of being a selfish person. The family members of an individual have a significant impact on the formation of self-concept. The nurse assesses the family's influence on the person's self concept in this category. Sample questions are: Who are the family members? What is the family's value of the individual? Who does the person receiving care feel particularly close to in the family? What are the levels of self-esteem of the various members? Of course, not all this data will be available for some people. Once a person reaches adulthood, the messages significant others gave regarding that person's personal value have been incorporated into the self concept. Therefore, interviewing the individual can provide this data. When possible the nurse will also interview any significant others available and observe interactions.

Developmental Stage. Next the nurse considers the person's stage of development according to Erikson (1963). Knowledge of developmental tasks gives the nurse an understanding of the challenges facing the person. Major threats to the self-concept, be they physical, emotional, or social may cause the person to regress to an earlier stage of development. The nurse identifies the stage of development in which the person is exhibiting behaviors and compares these with behaviors of the stage defined by the person's age. Data in this category are obtained by observing and interviewing the person and from knowledge of Erikson's theory. In addition Gardner's (1964) developmental tasks of selfhood are considered, including physical learning to live with tools and personal learning to live with self.

Coping Mechanisms. Another category of stimuli the nurse will consider is the person's coping mechanisms. *Coping mechanisms* are the habitual ways the person functions to maintain integrity in everday life and in times of stress. It is important to find out if the person has previously faced an experience similar to the current one and how the experience was dealt with then. Data in this category are obtained by interviewing the person and significant others.

There are other factors that influence an individual's personal self-concept. As the nurse interviews and interacts with the person receiving care, data may arise that do not fit in the specified six categories but which do influence the person's personal self. These additional data are included in the assessment as well and used to plan nursing interventions.

When obtaining stimuli assessment data, the nurse refers back to the information obtained in the behavioral assessment as much as possible. For example the nurse might say, "You mentioned earlier that you feel you are a strong and capable person (self-consistency behavior). How have people important to you helped you feel that way about yourself?" Such a question will probably elicit stimuli assessment data under the category "reactions of others." The nurse phrases the questions specifically to help keep the person focus on the current situation. In that manner, the nurse obtains the data needed to plan the nursing approaches.

The focal stimulus will be the factor in the immediate situation which is responsible primarily for the individual's personal self-concept. The contextual stimuli are all other factors influencing the person's behavior that can be identified by the person or through theory. The focal stimulus also must be validated with the person. All other factors that the nurse suspects are influencing the personal self-concept but which have not been validated are residual stimuli.

In general, the nurse will find a common group of contextual and residual stimuli for all of the self-concept components and a separate focal stimulus for each component. The importance of the response of others has been emphasized. In an actual assessment, the nurse may find one person's reaction to be focal and the reactions of others to be contextual. The situation of illness itself will be a stimulus for changes in the personal self, especially self-consistency and self-ideal. The person's development of self-concept will be a pervading residual factor for the current view of self.

Influencing factors exert either a positive influence, one that promotes adaptation, or a negative influence on the person's behavior. It may be helpful to identify whether each stimulus has a positive or negative effect on the person. The benefit of doing so will become evident when the step of planning interventions is reached.

Nursing Diagnosis

The next step of the nursing process is formulation of the nursing diagnosis. The nurse using the adaptation model bases a diagnosis on the assessed behaviors and stimuli. A beginning diagnosis involves making a nursing judgement of whether behaviors in each subarea of the personal self are adaptive or ineffective. For example, the diagnosis may state, "stable pattern of self-consistency." The second half of the diagnosis states the specific focal stimulus plus the most relevant contextual stimuli. The nurse will manage these influencing factors when intervening. A complete beginning-level diagnosis for an adolescent might be: "Stable pattern of self-consistency related to positive feedback from peers (reaction of others)—focal, height above the norm for his age (growth and development), star of his high school basketball team (other), and positive input from parents (reaction of others)—contextual.

Another example of a beginning-level diagnosis is one based on the person's level of self-esteem. *Self-esteem* is that pervasive aspect of the personal self component which relates to the overall worth or value the person holds of self. The person experiences self-esteem in the form of a feeling. Self-esteem is a part of every emotional response of the person. Since the person experiences self-esteem so totally and continually, it may be difficult for the person to isolate and identify it in words. The nurse evaluates the level of self-esteem based on the assessment of self-concept behaviors.

High self-esteem is indicated by active involvement in the world, a balance between participating and listening, eagerness to express one's opinions regardless of the possibility of disagreement, ability to listen to criticism without becoming overly defensive or hurt, confidence that efforts will be successful, ability to handle anxiety effectively, success in work and social settings, expectations of being received well by others, and infrequent psychosomatic difficulties. Moderate self-esteem is indicated by ready compliance with norms, dependence on social acceptance, active seeking of social approval, and uncertainty of one's own capabilities and worth. Both high and moderate self-esteem may be functional. Low self-esteem is considered an adaptation problem and will be discussed in the following section.

The adaptation problems of the personal self component may be the primary problems to be resolved for adaptation to be regained or they may be secondary problems that will resolve when the primary problem is brought into an adaptive range. Anxiety, powerlessness, guilt, and low self-esteem are four adaptation problems of personal self.

Anxiety. *Anxiety* is the result of anything that threatens a person's sense of self-consistency[2] and is defined as a painful uneasiness of mind due to a vague, nonspecific threat. Anxiety has been identified as a nursing diagnosis by the North American Nursing Diagnosis Association (Gordon 1987). A mild to moderate anxiety response can activate the person to confront and cope with a threatening event in an adaptive way. A severe anxiety response, on the other hand, may hinder the individual's attempt to adapt to the environment. A thorough assessment of behaviors and stimuli is made before the conclusion of anxiety as an adaptation problem can be reached. The behaviors indicative of anxiety are complex, individualistic and diverse. They often mimic behaviors of other adaptation problems. Some of the behavioral reactions that can be associated with anxiety are listed in the first column of Table 15–2.

The focal stimulus for anxious behaviors will be the perceived threat. Common stimuli include experiences of loss—actual or anticipated, sudden changes in life-style—positive or negative, assault, invasive procedures, disease, unknown or fatal prognosis in illness, rapid or extreme changes in role function, disruptive family life, history of past anxiety states, unconscious conflict, unmet needs, and transmission of another person's anxiety to the individual.

Powerlessness. *Powerlessness,* another problem of the personal self, is defined as the individual's perception of lack of internal or personal control over events.[3] Powerlessness has also been identified as a nursing diagnosis by the North American Nursing Diagnosis Association (Gordon 1987). Since it implies a lack of control over one's being, it is a problem in this mode component. The nurse looks for a pattern of actions and statements indicating a sense of low control. Behaviors associated with powerlessness are listed in Table 15–2.

The focal stimulus for powerlessness will be the immediate situation impinging upon the person's sense of control. Illness is often the focal stimulus. Other common factors include hospitalization, sensory function loss, physical immobility, major changes in life style, loss of financial independence, lack of knowledge, growth and development transitions, challenge of taking on new roles, and general life philosophy of low control.

[2]The material on anxiety in this chapter is based in part on Chapter 19 "Anxiety," Nancy Zewen Perley in *Introduction to Nursing: An Adaptation Model* (2nd. ed.), Sister Callista Roy, Englewood Cliffs, N.J.: Prentice-Hall, pp. 353–367, 1984.

[3]The material in this chapter on powerlessness is based in part on Chapter 20 "Powerlessness," Sister Callista Roy in *Introduction to Nursing: An Adaptation Model,* (2nd. ed.) by Sister Callista Roy, pp. 368–375, 1984.

TABLE 15–2. EXPECTED BEHAVIORS[1]

	Anxiety	Powerlessness	Guilt	Low Self-Esteem
Physiological Mode				
Activity and Rest				
Foot shuffling				
Arm movements				
Aimless wondering		x		x
Sleep disturbances		x	x	x
Over sleeping		x		x
Complaints of fatigue		x		x
Poor posture		x	x	x
Withdrawal from activity		x	x	x
Hesitency to initiate activity		x		
Skin Integrity				
Cold clammy skin				
Rashes and acne				
Alopecia				
The Senses				
Complaints of aches and pains				x
Fluids and Electrolytes				
Dry mouth				
Pseudo-Cushing's disease				
Neurological				
Dilated pupils				
Voice tremors/pitch changes				
Shakiness, trembling, hand tremor				
Difficulty concentrating				
Narrowed perceptual field				
Inability to relate parts to the whole				
Scattered attention				
Conversion reactions			Compulsive hand washing	

Endocrine			
Amenorrhea			
Pseudocyesis			
Oxygenation			
Breathing disturbance		x	
Pale appearance			
Tachycardia			
Palpitations			
Premature ventricular contractions			x
Cardiac neurosis			x
Nutrition			
Heartburn			
Loss of appetite		x	x
Over eating			
Nausea and vomiting		x	x
Gastrointestinal disease conditions		x	x
Psychogenic polydipsia			
Elimination			
Flatus and eructation			
Constipation or diarrhea		x	x
Polyuria			
Increased perspiration			
Self Concept Mode			
Physical Self			
Changes in sex drive and performance	x	x	x
Expression of disgust with body		x	x
Decrease in self-care, hygiene	Substance abuse	x	x
Personal Self			
Appearance of sadness/crying	x	x	x

(continued)

TABLE 15–2. (Continued)

Self Concept Mode (continued)

Anxiety	Powerlessness	Guilt	Low Self-Esteem
Pseudo-cheerfulness			x
Difficulty expressing feelings			x
Preoccupied with inner problems		x	x
Self degrading talk		x	x
Rumination about problems		x	x
Angry actions/talk	x		x
Expression of fear, apprehension, worry			x
	Feeling that what ever one does will fail	Expression of loss/sorrow	
	Expression of feeling unable to confront and overcome difficulties	Expression of culpability	
		Expression of apology, amend remorse	
		Expression of feelings of badness	x
		Expression of feelings of worthlessness, inadequacy	x
		Seeing self as burden to others	x
			Tendency to stay in background
			Behaviors of self-consciousness
			Inability to express self
			Fear of angering others
			Avoidance of situations of self disclosure/notice of any kind

Role Function Mode

Behavior	Complaints of being boxed in	Sensitive to criticism	Denial of past success/accomplishments
Inability to make decisions	x		x
Difficulty doing simple tasks	x	x	x
Difficulty meeting responsibilities	x	x	x
Decrease in interest, motivation, concentration	x		x
Complaints of being boxed in			x
Tendency to be a listener not a participant			
Lack of direction			x
Feeling that anything one does will fail			x
Becoming pregnant in teen years			x
Sensitive to criticism			x

Interdependence Mode

Behavior	Expression of feeling unlovable	Denial of past success/accomplishments
Expression of feelings of isolation		
Expression of feeling victimized		x
Temper tantrums		x
Expression of feeling unlovable		

[1]Read down the column for the expected behaviors in that category. An x in the column indicates that the behavior to the left applies to that adaptation problem also.

Guilt. *Guilt,* the third adaptation problem of the personal self, results from a disruption of the moral-ethical-spiritual self.[4] For purposes of this discussion of the personal self, guilt is defined as the judgment a person makes about his or her personal transgression. The transgression can be of social, moral or ethical codes, laws or rules. Guilt has not been identified as a nursing diagnosis by the North American Nursing Diagnosis Association at this time. The list of accepted nursing diagnoses, however, is still being developed and expanded. The adaptation problem of guilt has some aspects in common with those of the accepted diagnosis of spiritual distress. (Kelly 1985)

The experience of guilt is part of being human. Guilt can be divided into two types: (1) Real guilt occurs when the individual consciously violates a moral-ethical code. This type of guilt arises from a real transgression and calls the individual to personal growth. One is challenged to face, accept and rectify the guilt-producing action. (2) False guilt arises from an inner accusing voice that makes negative comments about the self at the slightest provocation. False guilt is destructive, leads one to feel worthless and ties up psychic energy needed for dealing with stressful situations and healing. Expected behaviors of guilt are listed in the third column of Table 15–2.

Common influencing factors for the behaviors of guilt include the individual's perception of the guilt-producing incident, beliefs about self and level of control, value system, level of self-esteem, the presence of peer pressure or support, and reactions of significant others.

Low Self-Esteem. *Low self-esteem,* which is another adaptation problem, is indicated by a pattern of discouragement and depression, feelings of isolation and unworthiness, extreme difficulty in expressing or defending oneself, feelings of helplessness and lack of ability to change, asserting self over others to prove or elevate one's self, fear of angering others, fear of self-exposure, and a persistent pattern of listening as opposed to participating.[5] Disturbance in self-concept is an approved nursing diagnosis (Gordon 1987). Norris and Kunes-Connell (1985) have recommended that the nursing diagnosis of self-esteem disturbance be further delineated into three problem categories. Low self-esteem (basic level) includes long-standing self-esteem problems stemming from childhood experiences. Low self-esteem (functional level) includes self-esteem disturbances resulting from a current situation. The defensive self-esteem category includes persons who present with verbalizations indicating moderate to high self-esteem, but whose histories show marked problems such as be-

[4]The material in this chapter on guilt is based in part on Chapter 21 "Guilt," Joyce Van Landingham in *Introduction to Nursing: An Adaptation Model* (2nd. ed.), Sister Callista Roy, pp. 376–393, 1984.

[5]The material on low self-esteem in this chapter is based in part on chapter 33 "Self-Esteem," Marie J. Driever in *Introduction to Nursing: An Adaptation Model* (2nd. ed.), Sister Callista Roy, pp. 394–404, 1984.

ing fired from several jobs, substance abuse, court referral for treatment and claiming false accomplishments. The beginning student or inexperienced nurse can be expected to identify and intervene in the second type of low self-esteem (functional level). People manifesting the other two categories of low self-esteem are referred to psychiatric clinical nurse specialists or other professional therapists for treatment. Expected behaviors of low self-esteem are listed in the final column of Table 15–2.

Common influencing factors for low self-esteem include any situation leading the person to question and/or decrease the value of self, loss experiences, bodily changes, maturational crises, feedback of significant others, self evaluation, feeling of lack of control over positive feedback from the environment, and the current life situation.

Goal Setting

Following formulation of the nursing diagnosis or adaptation problem, the nurse and the patient set goals for any desired change in the person's behavior. Mutual goal setting with the person is important. The individual's participation in setting a goal is vital to the success of the nursing approaches and to maintaning the person's integrity. The goal states a specific behavior, how it will change, and a time frame. The goal must be measurable. Stating, "The person will have an improved sense of personal self" is not sufficient. "The person will be able to verbally identify some area of satisfaction with her or his self-consistency by noon today" is a more clearly stated goal. Goals must be realistic and attainable. Sample goals for the personal self adaptation problems follow.

Perley (1984) identified three sequential goals for the person displaying anxious behaviors. (1) The person will be able to verbalize that he or she is anxious, (2) the person will be able to verbalize insight into the anxiety, and (3) the person will be able to demonstrate the ability to cope with the anxiety in more constructive ways. When working with an actual situation, the goals would include the time frame for attainment. A beginning goal for the person experiencing powerlessness is: the person will be able to verbally express an increased sense of power in the immediate situation.

Van Landingham (1984) identified an overall goal for the person experiencing the problem of guilt: the person will resolve the guilt experience and regain coping energy in order to reestablish conscious adaptive functioning and increased self-esteem. The nurse identifies subgoals specific to the unique behavior and stimuli associated with the individual's situation.

Driever (1984) suggested the following goal for the person experiencing the problem of low self-esteem: the person will be able to verbalize an understanding of the focal stimulus as having a positive valuing influence, rather than as being another negative devaluing experience.

Nursing Intervention

Once the goals are set, the nurse plans and carries out the nursing approaches. The interventions manage the identified influencing stimuli to allow the person to make an adaptive response. Stimuli having a positive effect will be reinforced. Factors having a negative effect will be altered, eliminated, or countered whenever possible. When intervening in the psychosocial modes, the nurse uses self in a therapeutic way. Therefore, self-awareness and a solid sense of self are called for on the part of the nurse. The steps to create a trusting nurse-client relationship discussed in the first section of this chapter will be continued throughout the use of the nursing process. The following discussion will cover some possible ways of managing the categories of stimuli identified in Table 14–2 in the previous chapter.

When the individual is experiencing a problem in the personal self component resulting primarily from the influence of **perceptions of self,** the nurse may use perception alteration as an approach.[6] To carry out this approach the nurse interviews the person seeking details about the events surrounding the perceptions that are having a negative effect on the person's self concept. As the individual recalls more details, he or she frequently will come to see that current thoughts and feelings about self are based on misunderstood past events, incomplete information, and stereotypes. Through such realizations and ventilation of accompanying feelings, the person becomes able to relinquish certain negative perceptions of self, thus clearing the way for a more positive self-view.

The following is an example of using perception alteration as an approach. A nursing student states she feels stupid and incapable of writing her term paper (self-consistency behavior). She relates that as a child she had great difficulty learning to read and actually failed the second grade (learning). Classmates teased her and called her stupid (reaction of others). Her parents had her tested and she was found to have dyslexia (growth and development). After receiving treatment she learned to read and made Bs and an occasional A in school (learning). The student currently holds an incorrect perception of herself. By exploring the details of how that misperception came about, the student may be able to let go of the incorrect perception and incorporate the current reality into her self concept.

Growth and development, the second category of influencing factors, includes the ability to control bodily functions. The nurse intervenes by providing the individual with materials and instructions for use of needed tools. For example, an individual may be exhibiting behaviors related to self-consistency manifested as feeling incompetent and incapable. The factors influencing these behaviors are, for example, the need to self-administer insulin injections to control diabetes, the lack of information about how to give injections, and feeling that it will be too difficult a skill to learn (growth and development factors—inability to use needed tools). The goal of having the person express feeling competent and capa-

---

[6]This discussion of perception changes is based on the unpublished work of Betty Dambacker, School of Nursing, University of California at Los Angeles, 1972.

ble can be met by providing the person with the necessary tools, instructions, and learning trials to master the skill of giving an insulin injection to one's self.

In another situation a person's self-consistency is affected by the stimulus of loss of control of bodily function. Consider the example of loss of ability to speak resulting from a laryngectomy. The nursing approach for reestablishing the person's self concept would be taking steps that lead to the person's regaining control over the lost function. (See a current textbook of medical-surgical nursing for specific steps to take.)

One nursing approach that manages the stimulus of **learning** is interviewing the person to allow reexamination of past experiences in terms of presence or absence of rewards. The effect of adult role models on establishing which personal characteristics are valued is discussed, as well. The nurse then helps the person devise current means of obtaining rewards for personally valued characteristics. The current rewards may be obtained externally or from within. For example, a man in his midforties may come to view himself as unable to express his true feelings (self consistency behavior) and acknowledges the inability as a problem. The assessment of stimuli reveals that, as a child, he was expected to be "the man of the family" after his father and mother divorced. He was told, "Men are tough and can handle anything: men don't cry" (Learning). His mother would leave the room if he tried to tell her about his feelings (Learning). Despite changing norms, the image of men as rugged, unfeeling tough guys is still presented in books and by the media (Learning). The mutually set goal for this man might be to express how he is feeling to his wife at least once a day. The wife stated she had been longing to know how her husband was feeling. Together they decided to spend 15 minutes every afternoon before dinner sharing about their day's experiences and how they were feeling. The wife's enthusiasm about listening and her willingness to share her own feelings provided the reward for the man's new behavior.

Since the individual's self concept is greatly affected by societal norms, the nurse intervenes at the group and social level as well as the individual level. For example, a school nurse may work with groups of students to help them understand how the oppression of racism works and how to relate to each other outside those stereotypes. Another approach that manages social stimuli is to work for legislation that guarantees access to health care for all regardless of sex, age, or income.

Approaches that manage **reactions of others** as an influencing factor include working directly with significant others and working with the person to alter the perceptions of the responses of others. In the first case, the nurse uses purposeful communication techniques to establish trust with the significant other and to encourage expression of feelings, thoughts and questions about the current situation of the person receiving care. The nurse then answers questions and gives feedback. Applying this process may help the significant other respond more positively to the individual. For example, an individual with a skin condition that greatly changes the appearance is struggling to maintain a sense of self worth. The responses of significant others who can hardly look at the person without showing disgust are having a negative effect on the person's self-concept behaviors. Sitting down with the others, allowing them to ventilate their feelings about the person's appearance and then giving them information about what kind of response the person needs is one way to manage this category of influencing factor. Sometimes the response of others cannot be altered. In that case, the nurse applies the perception alteration approach described above to help the individual change how the reaction of others is interpreted.

Nursing approaches to promote mastery of Erikson's *stages of development* are specific to the task to be mastered. Nursing interventions for each developmental stage will be discussed next.

To help promote mastery of the task of developing trust in the infant, the nurse provides classes to give parents information and support. The parents need to have a sense of conviction on which to base their actions. Organized religion has often served that purpose. Child development theories and books also contribute. For example, a popular phrase for years was, "Dr. Spock says————." In the hospital setting, the nurse models touch and responsiveness to needs in the infant that promote a sense of trust. Open visiting hours and rooming-in allow the parents to maintain the contact needed to establish trust with the infant. Consistent staff assignment also helps to promote a sense of trust in the infant.

The nurse can help promote mastery of autonomy in the toddler years by informing parents of the child's need for firm, reassuring outer controls and suggesting ways to provide them. The nurse provides the parent with information about safety issues related to toddlers, so that parents can allow the child to explore the environment without undue risk of harm. Modeling respect for the child's "no" whenever possible is another nursing approach for this stage of development. Parents can be taught to pick their battles with the toddler carefully. When the child does not actually have a choice, statements, not questions are used. For example the nurse might say, "It is time to go to bed," rather than, "Are you ready to go to bed?" The child is more likely to achieve a sense of autonomy if shaming is not used for training or punishment. The nurse teaches parents alternative approaches. The nurse also provides anticipatory guidance for and listens to expression of feelings of "I'm losing my baby" on the part of the parenting people. Referrals to community agencies are made when needed.

The parenting figures continue to play a primary role with the preschool child and the nurse helps promote mastery of initiative by supporting the parenting efforts. Parenting classes provide needed information and support. When interacting with the child, the nurse promotes initiative by answering the child's questions, being a moral and work role model, making sure words and actions are congruent, setting reasonable limits, providing for vigorous activities, and making clear that thoughts and wishes do not cause serious harm to others. Avoiding use of shame- and guilt-inducing approaches continues to be important. In today's society, a large number of children in this age range are in day-care centers for a significant number of hours each week. Therefore, the nurse may find it necessary to intervene on a social level.

The nurse supports normal self-concept development and mastery of the tasks of industry in the school-aged child by facilitating adjustment to school and providing preventive health measures (for example, immunizations and vision and dental screenings). During this stage the nurse continues to intervene by working with the parenting people. The nurse helps parents to provide firm, reasonable limits while allowing the child to take on more responsibility. The nurse suggests activities that allow the child to gain recognition. The parents may need support to be able to listen to the child expound on what the hero or heroine does and says. Parents may feel that their authority and influence over the child is being threatened by that "other" person. The nurse promotes industry in the hospitalized child by encouraging self-care and maintenance of control of bodily functions and whenever possible, involving the child in decision making and facilitating continuing contact with peers.

To help the adolescent master the task of identity as it relates to self concept, the nurse provides accurate information about how the body works (that is, health, nutrition, sexuality). The nurse also conveys a warm, nonjudgmental attitude that encourages the young person to express feelings and ask questions. Appropriate limits are set as needed. Use of peer pressure to limit behavior is often the most effective during this stage of development. The nurse can facilitate school programs that make use of peer pressure (for example "Just say no to drugs" and conflict resolution programs). Classes for parents continue to be an effective nursing intervention. The nurse models use of direct communication for the young person and the parents. The nurse is aware that adolescents frequently set up situations that lead adults to disagree and argue. The nurse teaches parents that the best way to avoid unnecessary arguments is to reserve judgment until all the information can be obtained. Good communication between the parents is vital during this stage of the child's development. For example, an adolescent tells his mother, "Dad said I could go to the beach with my friends over the spring break." The mother feels angry when she hears this statement. She had hoped to go on a family vacation but realized they do not have enough money to go. She wants the family to be together even if they stay home. She also feels uneasy about letting her son go off with his friends without adult supervision. Angrily she confronts her husband as soon as he gets home. Depending on how he responds, a huge family argument may result. Perhaps he never said the son could go. He may not have thought of his wife's concerns. He may be unaware of the financial situation. If the father takes the bait, the son successfully plays the parents against each other.

The nurse supports the parents of adolescents by providing nonjudgmental listening as well as information. Often the parents simply need someone to listen to their thoughts and feelings. At the community level, the nurse is aware of various programs and activities available to adolescents and their families. The nurse makes referrals when indicated.

The two primary nursing approaches to facilitate mastery of the task of intimacy for the young adult are nonjudgmental listening and information sharing. The young adult needs accurate information on family planning, sexually transmitted diseases, pregnancy, birthing, and parenting. The young adult also needs an environment free of judgment in which to ventilate frustrations and goals of vocational, social and family situations. Some people at this stage need assistance in finding meaning in the choice to remain single and/or childless. Again the nurse is familiar with community agencies that provide services for this age group and makes needed referrals.

Other interventions are specific for the adaptation problem diagnosed. When intervening with the person experiencing the problem of **anxiety** the nurse will open discussion of the problem by reviewing with the person the current situation. The nurse makes a mental note of the signs of anxiety displayed. A suggestion that the person may be feeling anxious may be offered. If the person is able to validate that suggestion, the first goal for the problem of anxiety has been met. If the person reacts strongly against the suggestion, the nurse will not pursue the discussion at that time. To do so would serve only to increase the person's anxiety.

Once the person has been able to acknowledge the anxious feelings, the nurse starts working towards goal two: the person will gain insight into the anxiety. The nurse can open discussion in this area by noting to the person some of the assessed stimuli for validation and further exploration. For example, "You seemed particularly upset when you returned from x-ray today." As the person begins to identify the source of the uneasy feeling, a greater understanding of the limitations of the threat can be gained. At the same time, some of the energy associated with it can be dispelled leading to a more realistic view of the situation.

After the person has gained some insight into the anxiety the nurse will use the perception alteration approach discussed above to facilitate the person's reassessment of the severity of the threat. Nursing management of other relevant stimuli is carried out to increase the person's adaptive range. The person then will demonstrate either the ability to reduce the threat or the ability to respond to it differently.

With the problem of **powerlessness,** the focal stimulus is often illness or hospitalization. As the nurse carries out the therapeutic measures to promote an increased level of wellness, an increased sense of power will often be attained. In addition, the nurse informs the person of the routines and schedules and allows the individual control and involvement in decision making whenever possible. Helping the person set realistic goals and expectations for self is another approach that the nurse uses with the person experiencing powerlessness.

Van Landingham (1984) developed detailed interactional steps for helping the person resolve **guilt** feelings. The beginning nurse will use therapeutic communication skills to establish trust and rapport with the person and to facilitate the person's exploration of identified stimuli. Nonjudgmental listening, expression of interest in and acceptance of the person, and offering information are approaches the nurse uses with the person experiencing the problem of guilt. When the problem of guilt is severe, the nurse will make the appropriate referral to clergy or a professional therapist.

Nursing approaches for the problem of **low self-esteem** are based on the use of therapeutic communication skills to help the person deal with the identified stimuli. Special attention is given to helping the client learn to identify and deal with feelings. The nurse gives the person permission and encouragement to verbalize all types of feelings. Crisis intervention approaches are used when the threat to self-esteem is related to a maturational or situational crisis. Olds (1987) described a technique for enhancing self-esteem in adolescents. This approach involves using classroom time to give each student a turn (three minutes) to share autobiographical information with the class. The facilitator starts the sharing by modeling the behavior desired from the students. After the autobiographical sharing has been completed the facilitator can suggest other topics for sharing concerns such as smoking, illicit drug use, sexuality. The key step in this approach is the facilitator's modeling. As the students share their own life stories, including feelings and reactions to events, they come to see how each person has struggles and hardships. The students can gain a sense of support and acceptance for who they are. This approach can be used with hospitalized adolescents as well as with those in out-patient settings. The perception alteration approach presented will also be used when the person's low self-esteem is influenced primarily by perceptions.

This discussion briefly illustrated how the nurse can use various theories, principles, and approaches within the Roy Adaptation Model to bring about adaptation in the personal self component. The nurse using this model considers all of the assessment data and carries out approaches designed to alter the person's behavior. Nursing interventions manage the stimuli specific to that person. The nurse often uses a combination of approaches, managing several factors to reach a specific goal. Interventions in the personal self component frequently involve working through and with family members, significant others, peers, other hospital staff, and community agencies, as well as with the individual directly.

Evaluation

The final step of the nursing process is evaluation of the behaviors to see if the goals were met. Further planning or revision of approaches is done based on the evaluation. The nurse reassesses the behavior defined in the goal to see if it is present. If the behavior is present, the goal has been met and the nurse and the person receiving care can decide if a new goal should be set. If the behavior is not present, the nurse reworks the entire process to discover aspects requiring further consideration. The nurse asks the following questions: Were the behavioral and stimuli assessment data accurate and complete? Was the goal realistic and acceptable to the person? Were the approaches carried out properly? The answers to these questions provide the basis for a revised plan of care.

SUMMARY

This chapter presented the application of the nursing process to the personal self component of the self-concept mode. Assessment of behaviors and stimuli, description of nursing diagnoses and adaptation problems, statement of goals, nursing approaches to manage the identified stimuli, and evaluation of the outcome of the approaches were discussed. The adaptation problems of anxiety, powerlessness, guilt and low self-esteem were also examined in terms of the Roy Adaptation Model for Nursing.

EXERCISES FOR APPLICATION

1. Assess yourself or a classmate in the personal self component. List behaviors and stimuli, write a diagnosis and goal, and propose nursing approaches.
2. Assess a person focusing on the individual's stage of development. Compare actual behaviors with expected behaviors for that particular stage of development. Identify factors influencing achievement of the tasks. Write nursing interventions for the goal: "the person will achieve mastery of the developmental tasks."

ASSESSMENT OF UNDERSTANDING

1. Personal self behaviors are classified into which three categories?
   a. body image
   b. moral-ethical-spiritual self
   c. self-consistency
   d. self-esteem
   e. self-ideal

2. Label each of the following personal self behaviors as adaptive (A) or ineffective (I).
   a. "I feel really good about myself and I'm proud I don't use drugs like so many kids at school do."
   b. "Why should I go to the assertiveness training class? I can't change anything in my life anyway."
   c. "I pray and meditate every morning to get my day off to a good start."
   d. "I plan to make all the money I can when I finish school and I don't care what I have to do to reach my goal."
   e. "Even though I'm 86-years-old and can see my body failing, I still feel like the same me I've always been."
3. Label the following personal self stimuli according to the following categories: growth and development (G), learning (L), and reaction of others (R).
   a. "I never saw my father cry."
   b. "My friends always tell me I'm smart."
   c. "All of a sudden my clothes don't fit, my feet are always in my way and my face is breaking out."
   d. "When I was a child, people laughed whenever I fell down or tripped."
   e. "When Jill sits quietly through dinner, she gets dessert."
4. Which of the following personal self diagnoses are stated in terms of the Roy Adaptation Model?
   a. Anxiety due to an unspecified threat.
   b. Stable pattern of self-consistency due to presence of rewards and positive feed-back from peers.
   c. Powerlessness due to being laid off of the job.
   d. Guilt
5. List three goals for a person experiencing anxiety.
6. Discuss nursing approaches that manage the focal stimuli of hospitalization and illness for the diagnosis of powerlessness.
7. Consider goal related to anxiety: "The person will be able to demonstrate the ability to cope with anxiety in more constructive ways." Suggest two behaviors that would indicate to the nurse that the person was achieving this goal.

Feedback

1. b, c, e
2. a—A, b—I, c—A, d—I, e—A
3. a—L, b—R, c—G, d—R, e—L
4. a, b, c
5. 1. the person will be able to verbalize recognition of being anxious by tonight,

2. the person will be able to verbalize insight into his or her anxiety, within two days,
3. the person will demonstrate an increased ability to cope with the anxiety, within one week.

6. The therapeutic measures to promote a higher level of wellness will also lead to an increased sense of power. Explaining routines and schedules and allowing the person choices and decision making whenever possible will promote further a sense of power.

7. Examples:
1. The person verbalizes that he is anxious.
2. The person identifies what it is that is making him feel anxious.
3. The person describes what he is doing to deal with the anxiety.

REFERENCES

Andrews, H., and Sr. C. Roy. *Essentials of the Roy Adaptation Model*. E Norwalk, Conn.: Appleton-Century-Crofts, 1986.

Coombs, A., and D. Syngg. *Individual Behavior—A Perceptual Approach to Behavior*. New York: Harper Brothers, 1959.

Driever, M.J. Self-esteem, in Sister Callista Roy, *Introduction to Nursing: An Adaptation Model* (2nd ed.). Englewood Cliffs, NJ.: Prentice-Hall, Inc., 1984.

Erikson, E.H. *Childhood and Society* (2nd ed.). New York: W.W. Norton & Company, Inc., London: Hogarth Press Ltd., 1963.

Epstein, S. The self-concept revisited or a theory of a theory, *American Psychologist*, 28, (5); 404–416, 1973.

Gardner, B.D. *Development in Early Childhood*. New York: Harper & Row, Publishers, 1964.

Gordon, M. *Manual of Nursing Diagnosis*. New York: McGraw-Hill Book Company, 1987.

Jackins, H. *The Human Side of Human Beings*. Seattle: Rational Island Publishers, 1974.

Kelly, M.A. *Nursing Diagnosis Source Book: Guidelines for Clinical Application*. E. Norwalk, Conn.: Appleton-Century-Crofts, 1985.

Mead, G.H. *Mind, Self, and Society*. Chicago: University of Chicago Press, 1934.

Norris, J., and M. Kunes-Connell. Self-esteem disturbance, *Nursing Clinics of North America*, 20, no. 4, December 1985.

Olds, R.S. Enhancing self-esteem through mutual self-disclosure, *Journal of School Health*, 57, no. 4: 160–61, April 1987.

Perley, N.Z. Anxiety, in Sr. C. Roy, *Introduction to Nursing: An Adaptation Model*, (2nd ed.). Englewood Cliffs, N.J.: Prentice-Hall, Inc., 1984.

Roy, Sr. C. Powerlessness, in Sr. C. Roy, *Introduction to Nursing: An Adaptation Model*, (2nd ed.) Englewood Cliffs, N.J.: Prentice-Hall, 1984.

Sullivan, H.S. *The Interpersonal Theory of Psychiatry*. New York: W.W. Norton & Company, Inc., 1953.

Van Landingham. Guilt, in Sr. C. Roy, *Introduction to Nursing: An Adaptation Model* (2nd ed.). Englewood Cliffs, N.J.: Prentice-Hall, 1984.

Additional References

Aguilera, D.C. et al. *Crisis Intervention*. St. Louis: The C. V. Mosby Company, 1970.

Anxiety—recognition and intervention, *American Journal of Nursing*, 64(9): 135–136, 1965.

Branch, M.F., and P.P. Phyllis. (eds.) *Providing Safe Nursing Care for Ethnic People of Color*. New York: Appelton-Century-Crofts, 1976.

Coopersmith, S. *The Antecedents of Self-Esteem*. San Francisco: W.H. Freeman and Company, Publishers, 1967.

Coopersmith, S. Studies in self-esteem, *Scientific American*, 218 (2):96–106, 1968.

Dean, D. G. Alienation: Its meaning and measurements, *American Sociological Review*, 24 (October): 753–758, 1961.

Fitts, W. et al. *The Self Concept and Self Actualization*. Monograph III. Nashville, Tenn.: Dede Wallace Center, July 1971.

Gould, R. The phases of adult life: A study of developmental psychology, *American Journal of Psychiatry*, 129 (5): 521–531, 1972.

Holderby, R.A., and E. McNulty. Feelings . . . feelings: How to make a rational response to emotional behavior, *Nursing*, October, pp. 39–43, 1979.

Johnson, D.E. Powerlessness: A significant determinant in patient behavior? *Journal of Nursing Education*, 6 (2): 39–44, 1967.

Jungman, L.B. When your feelings get in the way, *American Journal of Nursing*, 6: 1074–1075, 1979.

Kritek, P.B. Patient power and powerlessness, *Supervisor Nurse*, June 1981, pp. 26–34.

Lyon, G.G. Limit setting as a therapeutic tool, *Journal of Psychiatric and Mental Health Services*, November/December 1970, pp. 17–24.

Reasoner, R.W. Enhancement of self-esteem in children and adults, *Family Community Health*, 6: 51–64, 1983.

Satir, V. *Peoplemaking*. Palo Alto, Calif.: Science & Behavior Books, Inc., 1972.

Satir, V. *Self-Esteem*. Milbrae, California: Celestial Arts, 1975.

Schwartz, L.H. and J.L. Schwartz. *The Psychodynamics of Patient Care*. Englewood Cliffs, N.J.: Prentice-Hall, Inc., 1972.

Stanford, J.A. *Between People: Communicating One-to-One*. New York: Paulist Press, 1982.

Stanwyck, D. Self-esteem through the life span, *Family Community Health*, 6: 11–28, 1983.

Travelbee, J. *Interpersonal Aspects of Nursing* (2nd. ed.). Philadelphia: F.A. Davis Company, 1971.

Ujhely, G. What is realistic emotional support? *American Journal of Nursing*, 68 (4): pp. 758–762, 1969.

Ujhely, G. When adult patients cry, *Nursing Clinics of North America*, 2 (4): 726, 1967.

Wu, R. *Behavior and Illness*. Englewood Cliffs, N.J.: Prentice-Hall, Inc., 1973.

PART III: CONCLUSION

Part III has focused on the self-concept mode as described in the Roy Adaptation Model of Nursing. Chapter 13 provided an overview of the self-concept mode and its two subareas: the physical self and the personal self. The theoretical bases providing direction for the assessment of behaviors and stimuli in the mode was identified and a general description of the nursing process as applied to the self-concept mode was provided. More thorough exploration of the components of the mode and the related adaptation problems were the focus of Chapters 14 and 15.

Specifically, Chapter 14 dealt with positive adaptation of the physical self in terms of physical sensations, body image, and the sexual self. Adaptation problems of sexual dysfunction, rape trauma syndrome, body image disturbance, and loss were examined. In Chapter 15, the personal self was discussed relative to self-consistency, self-ideal, and the moral-ethical-spiritual self. Adaptation problems of anxiety, powerlessness, guilt, and low self-esteem were described.

Part III concludes with further development of the case study situation provided at the conclusion of Part II to illustrate application of the Roy Model to a patient care situation involving the self concept mode. As with the previous case study, the structure of the discussion is centered around the six steps of the nursing process.

The Self-Concept Mode—Case Study
Donna M. Romyn

In applying the nursing process, as described by the Roy Adaptation Model, the nurse assesses behaviors and stimuli related to both the physiological and psychosocial modes. A case study was utilized earlier to demonstrate application of the nursing process in the physiological mode. Here, the same case study will be developed further to demonstrate application of the nursing process in the self-concept mode.

CASE STUDY

ASSESSMENT OF BEHAVIOR—SELF-CONCEPT MODE
In assessing behaviors related to the self-concept mode, the nurse gathers behavioral data related to both the physical and personal components of self concept. Data may be collected by interviewing and interacting with

the individual and his significant others and by observing behaviors related to the individual's self concept.

In this case study, behavioral data were collected primarily during interactions with Mr. K. In addition, some data were obtained from his wife who spent most of her time with him and participated in providing some of his care. Assessment of Mr. K.'s self-concept behavior is summarized in Table III–1.

TABLE III–1. ASSESSMENT OF MR. K.'S SELF-CONCEPT BEHAVIOR

Physical self
  Body sensation:
"...have severe pain at times and frequent episodes of nausea and vomiting... I get angry at the pain and nausea and vomiting... sometimes it gets so bad that I would like to yell out."
"...tired all the time... rarely have enough energy or strength to do things like washing, dressing and feeding myself... feel frustrated"

  Body image:
"...thin... feel I look much older than I did even a few months ago." "...the colostomy and urinary drainage tubes are ugly.... I know that they are necessary but wish I didn't need them"

Personal Self
  Self-consistency:
"I tried to keep doing the things I always did for as long as I could but slowly I had to give up more and more of them... now I can hardly do anything... it makes me feel frustrated and helpless... feel like a burden." "Sometimes I regret not going for treatment when I was first diagnosed... it was all so scary... I couldn't imagine going... now I try to make the best of things."
"I know that I do not have long to live and accept that but thinking about dying makes me sad. I've never really thought about it before."

  Self-ideal/Self-expectancy:
"I try to endure the pain, nausea and vomiting without complaining but they make it difficult to enjoy the time I have with my wife."
"I have always been a very independent person... I don't want to become a burden to my wife."

  Moral-ethical-spiritual self:
"I have always been an honest, hardworking man... no matter what came my way I tried to deal with it the best I could... like this illness—I try to be honest about my feelings but sometimes its hard to talk about it." "We always went to church but I have not been able to lately... I really miss it... I'm not afraid to die because of my belief in God."

After assessing the individual's behavior related to each aspect of the self concept the nurse judges whether the behaviors are adaptive or ineffective in promoting psychic integrity. In this case study, it is evident that some of behaviors assessed are adaptive while others are ineffective. For example, Mr. K.'s acceptance of his impending death is adaptive in promoting psychic integrity while his feelings of frustration and of being a burden could, over time, prove to be ineffective. As behavioral data related to Mr. K.'s self concept is being collected, the factors influencing both his adaptive and ineffective self-concept behaviors also need to be identified.

ASSESSMENT OF STIMULI

In assessing the stimuli influencing Mr. K.'s self concept, the nurse identifies the factors which influence the physical and personal self behaviors assessed. To facilitate this process the nurse considers six general categories of stimuli: perception, growth and development, learning, reactions of others, stage of maturation, and coping mechanisms. These stimuli are described in detail in chapters 14 and 15. Table III–2 summarizes the stimuli influencing Mr. K.'s self-concept behaviors.

TABLE III–2.   ASSESSMENT OF STIMULI INFLUENCING MR. K.'S SELF CONCEPT

Perception:
"I am a strong person with firm beliefs... I can usually find a way to handle anything that comes my way... I can't change my illness but try to cope with it as best I can."

Growth and development:
68-year-old retired farmer
   physically unable to complete independently activities of daily living because of his fatigue, severe intermittent pain, nausea and vomiting
   colostomy and urinary drainage tube present

Learning:
"...men should be strong and endure discomfort without complaining." "...independence is important"
   "...death is part of living..., when it's your time to die you cannot change the outcome."

Reactions of others:
"...wife very supportive and brave about my illness... tries not to show her sadness... makes me wish I could take away her sorrow."
   "...wife encourages me to do what I can... helps me with what I cannot do for myself... tries not to let me feel that I am a burden."

Stage of maturation:
stage of ego integrity versus despair
   anticipates and accepts inevitability of own death but having difficulty accepting help from others as illness progresses
   attempting to maintain satisfying relationship with wife in spite of illness and impending death

Coping mechanisms:
tries to remain strong in face of adversity
   trusts in God

Once the stimuli influencing the individual's behavior are identified the nurse makes a judgment as to whether each is a focal, contextual or residual stimulus to the behaviors assessed. It is important to note that the focal and contextual stimuli influencing the physical self behaviors may differ from those influencing the personal self behaviors. In addition, some stimuli may exert a positive effect on the individual's self concept while others may exert a negative effect. Thus, it is important to identify the effect each stimulus has on the self concept in order to identify the focal and contextual stimuli which will be managed in planning nursing interventions. These focal and contextual stimuli also may be included in the statement of nursing diagnoses as is noted in the following examples.

NURSING DIAGNOSIS

In formulating nursing diagnoses related to the self-concept mode, the nurse may state separate nursing diagnoses related to the physical self and the personal self or may develop an overall nursing diagnosis related to the individual's self concept.

In this case study, several nursing diagnoses may be formulated for Mr. K. For example, in relation to the physical self, the nurse could use either of the following nursing diagnoses:

Ineffective psychic integrity with physical changes related to:

- Inability to complete own care; desire to be independent
- presence of fatigue, pain, nausea and vomiting
- belief that men should be strong
- presence of colostomy and urinary drainage tubes.

Using this format for stating nursing diagnoses the nurse summarizes the physical self-concept behaviors of concern and the focal and contextual stimuli influencing those behaviors.

As an alternative, the nurse could use the typology of adaptation problems described in Chapter 2 to cluster and label the assessment data. The appropriate label related to the physical self would be selected from the typology and used as a nursing diagnosis. In this case, the nurse could select the label "loss" as a nursing diagnosis for Mr. K.

In relation to the personal self, a nursing diagnosis for Mr. K. could be stated as:

Ineffective integration of self-ideal related to:

- feels like he is a burden
- belief that men should be strong and independent
- knowledge that his illness is creating sorrow for his wife.

Or, using the typology of adaptation problems, the nurse could summarize the personal self assessment data with the label: "powerlessness."

GOAL SETTING

In setting goals, the nurse identifies the expected behavioral outcomes of nursing intervention. In this case, the nurse sets goals to maintain adaptive self-concept behaviors and to change ineffective behaviors to adaptive behaviors thus promoting psychic integrity. Goals for Mr. K. are stated as:

1. Mr. K. will demonstrate adaptive physical self-concept behaviors within 2 days as shown by:
   - stating that he has less fatigue, pain, nausea and vomiting and can participate in some of his own care.
   - stating that he feels less frustrated by his inability to independently care for himself.
2. Mr. K. will demonstrate adaptive personal self-behaviors within two days as shown by:
   - accepting assistance with his care without feeling as frustrated or feeling that he is a burden.
   - continuing to openly discuss his feelings about his impending death.

As an alternative to setting separate goals related to physical and personal self-concept, the nurse could combine the expected outcomes into one goal such as:

Mr. K. will demonstrate adaptive self-concept behaviors within two days as shown by:

- stating that he has less fatigue, pain, nausea and vomiting and can participate in some of his own care.
- stating that he feels less frustrated by his inability to independently care for himself.
- accepting assistance with his care without feeling frustrated or that he is a burden.
- continuing to openly discuss his feelings about his impending death.

Note that each of the goals set identifies behaviors which promote psychic integrity.

NURSING INTERVENTION

In planning nursing interventions, the nurse formulates plans to manage the focal and contextual stimuli which influence the self-concept behaviors assessed. Thus, in planning interventions for Mr. K., the nurse considers the stimuli identified in the nursing diagnoses and establishes plans to maintain or alter the effects of these stimuli to promote psychic integrity.

To promote an adaptive physical self concept, Mr. K. is encouraged to discuss his desire to be independent and the meaning that "being strong" holds for him in view of his present illness. Nursing interventions are implemented to control Mr. K.'s fatigue, pain, nausea and vomiting and to conserve energy. Some of these interventions include comfort measures to reduce pain and promote rest, providing uninterrupted periods for rest, implementing measures to conserve energy and providing an environment conducive to eating. As a result, he will be able to participate in his own care to a greater extent and thus gain a measure of independence.

To prevent feelings of discomfort related to the appearance of his colostomy and urinary drainage tubes, the nurse assists Mr. K. to conceal them with dressings, clothing and bedcovers as much as possible. Thus, nursing interventions are implemented to promote psychic integrity by assisting him to deal with some of the losses he is experiencing related to his physical self concept.

To promote adaptive personal self-concept behaviors Mr. K. is encouraged to discuss his illness, his desire to be independent and his feelings of being a burden. His perceptions of his wife's sorrow and ways that he feels he could provide emotional support for her are discussed. The nurse reinforces his belief that he can cope with his illness and encourages him to maintain his trust in God. Thus, Mr. K. is able to feel like he has more control and psychic integrity is promoted by managing both the positive and negative factors influencing his personal self concept.

EVALUATION

Following nursing intervention, the nurse evaluates the effectiveness of the care provided by reassessing the individual's self-concept behaviors to determine whether or not the goals set were achieved. If the goals are met, the nurse chooses to either discontinue nursing intervention or continue to intervene to maintain the adaptive behaviors achieved. If the goals set are not met, the nurse determines whether further assessment of stimuli and modifications to the nursing diagnosis, goals or nursing interventions are required.

The extent to which Mr. K.'s fatigue, pain, nausea and vomiting are controlled vary from day to day as does his ability to participate in his own care. While he is not able to complete all of his own care independently, he does express satisfaction at being able to do "at least some things" for himself.

Mr. K. tries to provide emotional support for his wife by smiling, touching her hand and verbally expressing his gratitude for the care she provides. He maintains his belief that he would be able to cope with his illness and his faith in God.

Thus, the goals set for Mr. K. are achieved, in part. It is decided that no modification will be made to the nursing diagnosis, goals or interventions other than an extension of the time period established for goal achievement.

SUMMARY

In this chapter the case study introduced in Part II was utilized to demonstrate application of the nursing process, as described by the Roy Adaptation

Model, in the self-concept mode. Behavioral data related to each of the aspects of the physical self and the personal self were collected and the focal, contextual and residual stimuli influencing the assessed behaviors were identified. Nursing diagnoses related to both the physical and personal self concept were formulated and goals were set identifying behavioral outcomes of nursing care which would promote psychic integrity. Nursing interventions were planned and the process of evaluation was described.

Part IV

The Role Function Mode

As emphasized previously in this text, inherent in the view of a person as an adaptive and holistic system is the understanding that problems in one area of the person's functioning will affect performance in another. In addition, people interact with other persons in groups and societies. The philosophical assumptions of a common purpose for human existence (Roy 1988) also speak to the social nature of the person. Therefore, social adaptation is as much of a concern to the nurse as psychological and physiological adaptation. For this reason, the nurse must have an indepth knowledge about the role function mode in order to assess behaviors and stimuli in the mode and to assist people in dealing with the problems they are encountering.

The following two chapters address adaptation as related to the role function mode described in the Roy Adaptation Model. Chapter 16 provides an overview of the role function mode including description of the mode as it is defined in the model and identification of the theoretical bases providing direction for assessment of behaviors and stimuli. Application of the nursing process is illustrated.

Chapter 17 focuses on three common adaptation problems of the role function mode: role transition, role distance and role conflict. The nursing process again provides the framework for discussion of these problems.

Part IV concludes with a case study situation illustrating application of the role function mode in practice.

Chapter Sixteen

Overview of the Role Function Mode

Heather A. Andrews

The role function mode is one of two social modes; it focuses specifically on the roles the person occupies in society. The basic need underlying the role function mode has been identified as *social integrity*—the need to know who one is in relation to others so that one can act.

Nurses interact with individuals who occupy a wide variety of primary, secondary, and tertiary roles. Each role has associated with it expected instrumental and expressive behaviors. Similarly, there are certain disruptions or problems that are shared by all roles.

If a person is experiencing problems concerning the role he or she occupies, the effects may be manifest in the ability to heal and maintain health. Health and illness experiences, in turn, affect once's role performance. In applying the nursing process to the role function mode, the nurse assesses, diagnoses, and intervenes to promote adaptation and assist with problems. For this reason, the nurse must have an in-depth knowledge about the role function mode in order to assist people in dealing with the problems they are encountering.

In this chapter, the role function mode is defined and described, the theoretical basis providing direction for assessment of behaviors and stimuli is identified, and related nursing activities are discussed.

OBJECTIVES

After studying this chapter, the reader will be able to do the following:

1. Define *role*.
2. Describe the role function mode.
3. State the difference between primary, secondary, and tertiary roles.

4. State the difference between instrumental and expressive behavior.
5. Recognize requirements of instrumental and expressive behavior.
6. Identify behaviors that manifest adaptation in the role function mode.
7. Identify stimuli that influence adaptation in the role function mode.

KEY CONCEPTS DEFINED

- *Expressive behavior:* the feelings, attitudes, likes, or dislikes that a person has about a role or about the performance of a role.
- *Instrumental behavior:* the actual physical performance of a behavior to achieve the goal of role mastery.
- *Primary role:* an ascribed role based on age, sex, and developmental stage. It determines the majority of behaviors engaged in by a person during a particular growth period of life.
- *Role mastery:* indicates that a person demonstrates both expressive and instrumental behaviors that meet social expectations associated with the assigned roles.
- *Role performance:* defines the actions taken in relation to expected behaviors of a particular role.
- *Roles:* the functioning units of society; each role exists in relation to another.
- *Secondary role:* a role that a person assumes to complete the tasks associated with a developmental stage and primary role.
- *Social integrity:* the basic need of the role function mode: the need to know who one is in relation to others so that one can act.
- *Tertiary role:* a role that is freely chosen by a person, temporary in nature, and often associated with the accomplishment of a minor task in a person's current development.

DESCRIPTION OF THE ROLE FUNCTION MODE

Roles have been defined as the functioning units of society (Parsons and Shils 1951). Each role exists in relationship to another. For example, the parent role requires that there be a child; the employer role, an employee; and the nurse role, a patient. Associated with each role is a set of expectations about how a person behaves towards a person occupying the complementary position. Persons need to know who they are (the roles occupied) and the associated societal expectations so that they can act appropriately. This is social integrity and represents the underlying need of the role function mode (Roy 1984).

A classification of roles as primary, secondary, and tertiary has been adopted for use in the Roy Adaptation Model (Randell 1976). The *primary role* determines the majority of behaviors engaged in by the person during a particular period of life. It is determined by age, sex, and developmental stage (as illustrated in Table 16–1). Examples of primary roles are 5-year-old preschool male, 16-year-old adolescent female, and 70-year-old mature adult male. The association of age, sex, and developmental stage in labelling the primary role enables the identification of specific role behaviors in relationship to the developmental stage.

Secondary roles are those that a person assumes to complete the tasks associated with a developmental stage and primary role. For example, a 25-year-old young adult male may be faced with the task of being able to nurture, support, and provide for spouse and offspring. Secondary roles that are assumed related to this task could be husband, father, breadwinner, and mechanic. Secondary roles are normally achieved positions as opposed to primary qualities and require specific role performance. They are typically stable and not readily relinquished since they are developed and mastered over a period of time (Nuwayhid 1984). Problems of role function usually occur in secondary roles.

Tertiary roles are related primarily to secondary roles and represent ways in which individuals meet their role-associated obligations (Malaznik 1976). Associated with the role of father might be that of junior football team coach or Cub Scout leader. Tertiary roles are normally temporary in nature, freely chosen by the individual, and may include activities such as clubs or hobbies. Figure 16–1 illustrates the classification of roles as discussed.

As is obvious from this discussion, the three types of roles vary throughout life reflecting stimuli such as developmental stage and associated tasks. At times, roles must be altered when special circumstances are encountered. An example involves illness and the sick role. The sick role, when temporary in nature, is classified as tertiary but it becomes a secondary role when the illness is chronic. As Nuwayhid (1984) has

TABLE 16–1. AGE-RELATED DEVELOPMENTAL STAGES[a]

Age	Developmental Stage
Birth–1½ years	Infant
1½–3½ years	Toddler
3½–6 years	Preschool
6–12 years	Schoolage
12–18 years	Adolescent
18–35 years	Young adult
35–60 years	Generative adult
60 years +	Mature adult

[a]Based on the work of Erikson (1963).

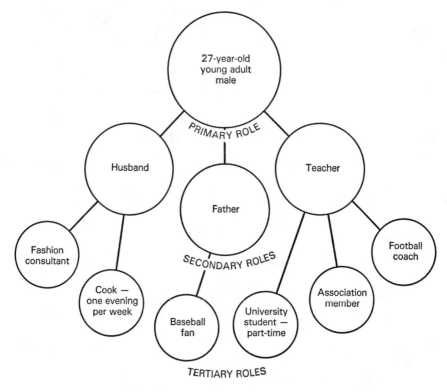

Figure 16–1. Illustration of role classification

pointed out, few persons choose to become ill; the element of choice comes in whether or not to adopt the sick role and to perform adaptive sick-role behaviors.

COMPONENTS OF THE MODE

Based on the work of Parsons and Shils (1951), two behavioral components have been identified to assist in the assessment of appropriate role behaviors. These components are termed instrumental and expressive behaviors; both apply to each role the person occupies.

Instrumental or goal oriented behaviors, are those that the person performs as part of his or her roles. The goal of instrumental behavior is *role mastery* (the demonstration of role behaviors that meet societal expectations). Instrumental behaviors are normally physical actions and usually have a long-term orientation.

Expressive behaviors involve the feelings and attitudes held by the person about his or her role and role performance. The goal of expressive behavior is direct or immediate feedback. Expressive behaviors are emotional in nature and result from interactions which enable the person to express these role-related feelings in an appropriate manner.

In addition to these two components, four role performance requirements have been described by Nuwayhid (1984), based on Parsons and Shils (1951), as necessary within the social structure to allow a person to enact role behavior, be it instrumental (that is, goal directed) or expressive (feeling based). The four role performance requirements constitute major stimuli for role behavior; their presence or absence permits the identification of expected behaviors for each role occupied by the person.

The requirements for role behavior are (1) consumer, (2) reward, (3) access to facilities/set of circumstances, and (4) cooperation/collaboration. The following example pertaining to the sick role illustrates the application of the requirements to both instrumental and expressive behaviors.

Associated with the sick role of patient is the instrumental behavior of taking medications prescribed by another. The requirements of this behavior are as follows:

1. *Consumer*—Who or what benefits from the person's performance of role behaviors. The patient himself benefits by taking prescribed pain medication.
2. *Reward*—The rewards the individual receives for performance of role behaviors. The patient's pain is alleviated and he can increase physical mobilization.
3. *Access to facilities/set of circumstances*—The availability of materials or tools to perform role behaviors. Medication is available as is appropriate equipment for its administration.
4. *Cooperation/collaboration*—The degree to which an individual is allowed time to perform role behaviors. Medication is brought to patient. Time is allowed to elapse before its effect is felt.

There are also expressive behaviors associated with the patient role as can be noted in further application of the same four requirements:

1. *Consumer*—The need for an appropriate and receptive person to relate to for immediate feedback. Nurse is available to care for patient. Physician is actively involved in patient's care.
2. *Reward*—An established network that will provide feedback on role performance. Patient receives consistent encouragement and feedback from nurse and physician.
3. *Access to facilities/set of circumstances*—The need to feel that one has what one needs to accomplish the task. Nurse provides time to discuss patient's concerns and nursing care.
4. *Collaboration/cooperation*—The positive emotional tone and belief that the setting in which the role is performed provides the circum-

stances and climate needed to fulfill the role. Patient feels that he is actively involved in decisions related to his care.

THEORETICAL BASIS FOR THE ROLE FUNCTION MODE

The description of the role function mode is based on a number of specific sociological and psychological theories and principles. These provide direction for the assessment of behaviors and stimuli relative to the role function mode and, in fact, for each of the other steps of the nursing process. The following is an identification of and brief statement relative to each of the important theoretical bases of the role function mode as described in the Roy Adaptation Model.[1]

- *Goffman* (1961)—Description of role as behaviors society expects of an individual occupying a particular role.
- *Parsons and Shils* (1951)—Description of instrumental and expressive behaviors and the requirements (also called partitions) associated with role interaction.
- *Turner* (1966)—Identification of two basic assumptions about roles; they exist in relationship to each other and are occupied by individuals.
- *Banton* (1965)—Identification of primary, secondary, and tertiary roles.
- *Erikson* (1963)—Identification of developmental tasks that provide the basis for labelling of primary role.

APPLICATION OF THE NURSING PROCESS

Since health and illness experiences affect one's role performance, the nurse, in caring for the person as a whole, considers adaptation as related to the person's role. Adaptation problems associated with the role function mode may affect the person's ability to heal and maintain health because problems in one mode may be stimuli causing ineffective adaptation in another mode.

Assessment of Behavior
The primary, secondary, and tertiary roles the person occupies and the associated instrumental and expressive behaviors form the basis for behavioral assessment of social integrity relative to the role function mode. In assessing behavior in this mode, the nurse begins by identifying the

---

[1]It is important that the reader refer to the works of the identified theorists and the following chapter if a working knowledge of the use of these theories in the Roy Adaptation Model is sought.

person's age and related primary role. From this information, secondary roles can be projected and, by purposeful questioning, secondary and tertiary roles can be determined together with their hierarchy of importance for the person. Behavioral assessment also would include the determination of instrumental and expressive behaviors associated with each role. Direct observation of the performance of specific roles can provide further information as to adaptation in the role function mode.

Consider as an example a 19-year-old young adult female who has just entered college. In addition to the secondary role of student, one can project such roles as daughter, sister, girlfriend, and participant in sports activities. Associated with the role of student are the instrumental behaviors of studying, attending classes, writing exams and papers, and participating in lab sessions. Expressive behaviors include "sounding off" with peers, complaining to parents about heavy workload, and discussing exam results with the teacher.

Following identification of the person's roles and related instrumental and expressive behaviors, tentative judgements of "adaptive" and "ineffective" are applied relative to their effect on adaptation. Adaptive behaviors are those that meet role expectations; ineffective behaviors do not meet role expectations.

Assessment of Stimuli

The four requirements of both instrumental and expressive behaviors are an important consideration when assessing stimuli influencing role function behaviors. Their presence or absence may serve as focal, contextual, or residual stimuli to the observed behaviors. Analysis of the requirements for two of the behaviors mentioned would appear as follows:

Instrumental Behavior—Studying

1. *Consumer*—Self, significant others, teacher.
2. *Reward*—Gets good grades, passes courses, receives scholarship.
3. *Access to facilities/set of circumstances*—Library is available; evenings are reserved for study time.
4. *Cooperation/collaboration*—Teachers identify important material; boyfriend calls after 9 PM; classmates study at the same time.

Expressive Behavior—"Sounding Off" with peers

1. *Consumer*—Peers.
2. *Reward*—Understanding of peers.
3. *Access to facilities/set of circumstances*—Peers have opportunity to get together after class and in residence situation.
4. *Cooperation/collaboration*—Peers are supportive of each other; all are in the same circumstances.

It is expected that a student will study; however, if one of the requirements, cooperation, is missing (boyfriend insists that the student spend all her evenings with him), it would be difficult to accomplish the prescribed behavior of studying.

In addition to the requirements, other stimuli that commonly influence behavior in the role function mode have been identified. These are listed below and illustrated with the example of the college student.

1. *Social norms*—Societal prescriptions for role behavior may vary greatly relative to culture. For example, the young woman's cultural group emphasizes the general societal expectation that students apply themselves to their study and succeed.

2. *Physical makeup and chronological age*—These influence what roles a person is suited to occupy. For example, at 19 years of age, a person's learning capabilities permit college study.

3. *Individual's self-concept*—The person must feel capable of occupying the role. For example, the young woman feels capable of undertaking and succeeding in her selected course of study.

4. *Role models*—Their number, quality, and responses. The student would look to her parents, older siblings, and other students as role models for student behaviors.

5. *Knowledge of expected behaviors*—Does the person know what behaviors are expected in performance of the role? For example, the young woman recognizes what is expected of her as a student relative to studying, obtaining passing grades, and attending class.

6. *Physical and/or emotional well-being*—This affects the individual's capacity or ability to fulfill the role. This young woman has no physical or emotional concerns that would hinder her performance as a student.

7. *Performance in other roles*—Expectations of behavior in one role may hinder performance of behaviors in another. For example, expectations associated with the role of girlfriend could possibly infringe on prescribed student behaviors.

It is possible that stimuli other than those above are relevant in an individual's situation; these should be considered as well. The context and meaning of the individual situation is taken into account. Once the stimuli influencing the person's role functioning have been identified, the behaviors, in light of the theoretical bases, are evaluated as adaptive or ineffective in maintaining social integrity. Stimuli are identified as focal, contextual, or residual and are labeled as to whether they are exerting a positive or negative influence on the person.

Nursing Diagnosis

As was described in Chapter 2, nursing diagnosis in the role function mode involves the relating of the assessment data obtained in the first two steps of the nursing process. To assist in describing and naming associated aspects within the role function mode, descriptors of effective adaptation in the role function mode have been developed. The label can take the form of summarizing the adaptive or ineffective behaviors related to the specific stimuli. An example of this method is, "Stable pattern of role mastery related to presence of requirements of all role behaviors." *Role mastery* indicates that the person demonstrates both instrumental and expressive behaviors that meet societal expectations associated with the respective roles (Schofield 1976). Periodically, throughout the lifespan, individuals are required to change roles. Associated with this task is the adaptive diagnosis of *effective role transition,* that is, the individual demonstrates adaptive expressive behaviors and a few adaptive instrumental behaviors associated with social expectations of the assigned role. The adaptive behaviors indicate positive movement toward the goal of role mastery (Nuwayhid, 1984).

As has been evident in previous chapters, in the Roy Adaptation Model, a nursing diagnosis can be worded in three ways: (1) a statement of the behaviors within one mode with their most relevant influencing stimuli, (2) a summary label for behaviors in one mode with relevant stimuli, or (3) a label that summarizes a behavioral pattern when more than one mode is being affected by the same stimuli. A nursing diagnosis illustrating method one and applying to the previous example would be "effective study habits due to participation in study group." An example of method two would be "effective role transition from high school student to college student related to encouragement and advice from high school teacher."

Three major adaptation problems associated with the role function mode have been identified: role transition, role distance, and role conflict. These are defined and addressed in detail in the following chapter.

Once the nursing diagnosis has been formulated, the nurse and patient proceed to set behavioral goals to address the maintenance of adaptive behavior or the changing of ineffective situations.

Goal Setting

Goals, set in collaboration with the person, focus on the specific role behaviors and how they will change in a given period of time. Related to the example of the college student is the following goal: "The student will increase her studying time to three hours per evening for the next week." The behavior of focus is "study time," the change expected is an increase to "three hours per evening" and the associated time frame is "for the next week."

Of initial concern would be the ineffective behaviors identified in the process of assessment although the importance of maintaining effective behaviors is acknowledged.

Intervention

As with other modes, interventions in the role function mode focus on the stimuli that are influencing the behaviors being observed. It may be necessary to change the focal stimulus or to broaden the adaptation level by managing other stimuli present by increasing, decreasing, removing, or maintaining and enhancing them.

Considering the former example, it may have been that the girl's expectations of her student role differ from social expectations. For example, her peers may believe that when one is a student, having fun is the primary objective. These expectations may differ from those of her teachers and parents. It would be important to assist the girl in identifying the appropriate role behaviors that are adaptive for her.

Similarly, interventions associated with role function and the achieving of role mastery may focus on the requirements of both instrument and expressive behaviors: the consumers, rewards, circumstances/access to facilities, and cooperation of and collaboration with others. The other stimuli commonly influencing role function adaptation may require intervention. The nurse may need to assist the patient with his or her self concept. If the person does not feel capable of fulfilling a particular role, it may be possible to provide knowledge about the role that would enhance the person's self confidence.

Perhaps it is the person's physical well being that is interfering with the ability to fulfill the expectations of the role. A person with deteriorating eyesight may have problems accomplishing the reading required in the student role. Appropriate referral by the nurse may assist in dealing with the problem.

Carrying on with the previous example and the goal stated in previous discussion, in order to increase the study time available to her, the student may have to deal with the demands her boyfriend is making. This is a change of one of the requirements for role behavior, that is, cooperation with others. Possible approaches are identified and the one with the highest probability of success is chosen for implementation.

Evaluation

As with all other modes, evaluation in the role function mode involves looking again at the preset goals to determine whether the person's behavior aligns with them. In the situation addressed previously, the goal focused on the study time and its increase to three hours per evening. Evaluation of achievement of that goal would be in a record of study time over the past week perhaps. Or, the girl may report verbally that she studied at least three hours per evening.

If the established goals are not achieved, the nurse returns to look again at the various steps of the nursing process to determine aspects for further consideration. It may be that the assessment data were incomplete or the goals were unrealistic. It must be remembered that the steps of the nursing process often occur simultaneously rather than sequentially and that the process is ongoing.

SUMMARY

This chapter has provided an overview of the role function mode including a description and illustration of primary, secondary, and tertiary roles and the associated instrumental and expressive behavioral components. The theoretical basis for the role function mode was identified and the application of the nursing process was described. Figure 16–2 illustrates the nursing process as related to the role function mode.

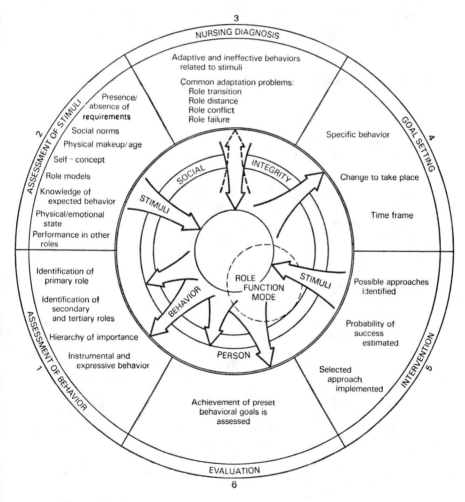

Figure 16–2. The nursing process as applied to the role function mode

Chapter 17 focuses on three selected adaptation problems of the role function mode: role transition, role distance, and role conflict.

EXERCISES FOR APPLICATION

1. Identify the primary, secondary, and tertiary roles in which you currently are involved.
2. Select one of your secondary roles and list the associated instrumental and expressive behaviors. Assess the requirements for role function of one instrumental and one expressive behavior.
3. Imagine a 45-year-old generative adult male patient. Project secondary roles for him and formulate appropriate questions or comments that would elicit information about these roles. Speculate specific behavior related to the requirements.

ASSESSMENT OF UNDERSTANDING

Questions

1. Which of the following statements apply to the description of *role* in the Roy Adaptation Model?
   a. It may be primary, secondary, or tertiary.
   b. It exists in relationship to another.
   c. It is the functioning unit of society.
   d. It is consistent throughout life.
2. In one paragraph, describe the components of the role function mode.
3. Classify the following statements as descriptive of primary roles (P), secondary roles (S), or tertiary roles (T).
   a. ____ Determined by age, sex, and developmental stage
   b. ____ Involve role-associated obligations
   c. ____ Normally achieved positions
   d. ____ Determine the majority of behaviors
   e. ____ Assumed to complete developmental tasks
   f. ____ Freely chosen
   g. ____ Require specific role performance
   h. ____ Temporary in nature
4. Label each of the following statements of behavior as to whether it is instrumental (I) or expressive (E).
   a. ____ Sending a birthday gift to a friend
   b. ____ Going to work
   c. ____ Doing housework
   d. ____ Hugging children

 e. ___ Reporting good exam results

 f. ___ Complaining about the boss

5. The list on the left represents the requirements of instrumental and expressive behavior. The list on the right represents factors that illustrate the requirements as related to the role of teacher. Label each factor with the requirement it represents.

1. Consumer	a. ___ Paycheck
2. Reward	b. ___ Class time
3. Access to facilities/set of circumstances	c. ___ Classroom and supplies
	d. ___ "Prep" time
4. Cooperation/collabora-tion	e. ___ Students
	f. ___ Curricular materials
	g. ___ Evaluation of performance
	h. ___ All students pass exam

6. Which of the following statements are behaviors in the role function mode?

 a. "I love you, Honey."

 b. "I earn two dollars an hour babysitting."

 c. Five-year-old preschool male.

 d. "I've been sick for four days."

 e. "I'm taking piano lessons."

 f. "I have four preschool children."

7. List five stimuli that commonly influence behavior in the role function mode.

 a. _____

 b. _____

 c. _____

 d. _____

 e. _____

Feedback

1. a, b, c
2. The role function mode is viewed as consisting of primary, secondary, and tertiary roles. Associated with each role are instrumental and expressive components, each with four associated requirements. The roles with their components and requirements form the role function mode with its basic need of social integrity; the need to know who one is in relation to others so that one can act.
3. a. P
 b. T
 c. S
 d. P
 e. S

    f. T
    g. S
    h. T
4. a. E
    b. I
    c. I
    d. E
    e. E
    f. E
5. a. 2
    b. 4
    c. 3
    d. 3 or 4
    e. 1
    f. 3
    g. 2
    h. 2
6. a, b, c, d, e, f
7. Any five of the following:

Presence or absence of instrumental or expressive requirements
Social norms
Physical makeup/chronological age
Individual's self-concept
Role models
Knowledge of expected behaviors
Physical and emotional well-being
Performance in other roles

REFERENCES

Banton, M. *Roles: An Introduction to the Study of Social Relations.* New York: Basic Books, Inc., 1965.

Erikson, E.H. *Childhood and Society* (2nd ed.). New York: W.W. Norton & Co., Inc., 1963.

Goffman, E. *Encounters.* Indianapolis: The Bobbs-Merrill Co., Inc., 1961.

Malaznik, N. Theory of role function, in *Introduction to Nursing: An Adaptation Model,* Sr. C. Roy, pp. 245–264. Englewood Cliffs, N.J.: Prentice-Hall, Inc., 1976.

Nuwayhid, K.A. Role function: Theory and development, in *Introduction to Nursing: An Adaptation Model* (2nd ed.), Sr. C. Roy, pp. 284–305. Englewood Cliffs, N.J.: Prentice-Hall Inc., 1984.

Parsons, T., and E. Shils, eds. *Toward a General Theory of Action.* Cambridge, Mass.: Harvard University Press, 1951.

Randell, B. Development of role function, in *Introduction to Nursing: An Adapta-*

tion Model, Sr. C. Roy, pp. 256–264. Englewood Cliffs, N.J.: Prentice-Hall, Inc., 1976.

Roy, Sr. C. *Introduction to Nursing: An Adaptation Model* (2nd ed.). Englewood Cliffs, N.J.: Prentice-Hall, Inc., 1984.

Roy, Sr. C. An explication of the philosophical assumptions of the Roy Adaptation Model, in *Nursing Science Quarterly,* 1, (1988), pp. 26–34.

Schofield, A. Problems of role function, in *Introduction to Nursing: An Adaptation Model,* Sr. C. Roy, pp. 265–287. Englewood Cliffs, N.J.: Prentice-Hall, Inc., 1976.

Turner, R.H. Role-taking, role standpoint and reference group behavior, in *Role Theory: Concepts and Research,* ed. B. Biddle and E. Thomas. New York: John Wiley & Sons, Inc., 1966.

Chapter Seventeen ──────────

Role Transition, Distance and Conflict

Kathleen A. Nuwayhid

In applying the nursing process within the framework of the role function mode of the Roy Adaptation Model, the nurse assesses, diagnoses, and intervenes to promote adaptation and handle adaptation problems. There are certain disruptions or problems that are shared by all roles although problems of role function usually occur in secondary roles.

This chapter identifies these common nursing diagnoses based on role theory. Each diagnosis is presented using the nursing process format. The maternal role has been chosen to illustrate the common disruptions of role transition, role distance and role conflict because of its universal reference, its documentation in the literature, and its relevance for nursing practice. Reference also is made to literature related to the sick role.

OBJECTIVES

After studying this chapter, the reader will be able to do the following:

1. Differentiate between role mastery and effective role transition.
2. Explain ineffective role transition.
3. Described the major contextual stimuli involved in a nursing diagnosis of ineffective role transition.
4. Describe role distance.
5. Differentiate between intrarole conflict and/or interrole conflict.
6. Describe the differences between role failure, ineffective role transition, role distance, and role conflict.

KEY CONCEPTS DEFINED

- *Role prescription:* the instrumental and expressive behaviors to be performed by an individual occupying a specific role. These may be determined by society, culture, education, or a combination of these variables.

- *Role transition:* the process of assuming and developing a new role. It is growth in a positive direction, and is compatible with the tasks of the primary role of the individual.
- *Effective role transition:* the individual adaptive processes exhibit effective expressive behaviors, and a few adaptive instrumental behaviors, that partially meet with the social expectations associated with the assigned role. However, the number or quality of the behaviors is not sufficient to formulate a diagnosis of role mastery. The adaptive behaviors indicate positive movement toward the goal of role mastery. There may or may not be some instrumental behaviors.
- *Ineffective role transition:* the individual exhibits adaptive expressive behaviors, but exhibits ineffective instrumental behaviors for a particular role. This is usually the result of an absence of role models, or lack of knowledge or education related to the role.
- *Role distance:* the individual exhibits both instrumental and expressive behaviors appropriate to a particular role, but these behaviors differ significantly from prescribed behaviors for the role (Schofield, 1976).
- *Intrarole conflict:* the individual fails to demonstrate either instrumental or expressive behaviors or both appropriate for a role as a result of incompatible expectations from one or more persons in the environment concerning the individual's expected behavior (Schofield, 1976).
- *Interrole conflict:* the individual fails to demonstrate the instrumental and/or expressive behaviors appropriate to the individual's role as a result of the occupation of one or more roles that require prescribed behaviors that are incompatible with one another.
- *Role failure:* the individual has an absence of expressive behaviors or exhibits ineffective expressive behaviors, and/or has an absence of instrumental behaviors or exhibits ineffective instrumental behaviors for a particular role.

DESCRIPTION OF THE MATERNAL ROLE[1] AND ROLE TRANSITION

The maternal role has three distinct phases: childbearing, childbirth, and child rearing. Childbearing takes place usually in nine-month incre-

[1]The maternal role is presented as occurring in the young adult stage of development, for the purposes of illustration, although motherhood can occur anywhere from adolescence through the generative adult phase of development. The secondary role of mother is most compatible with meeting the developmental tasks of the young adult. The maternal role theory presented in this chapter is used for the purpose of illustration, and in no manner is intended to be an adequate presentation of maternal role theory. The taking on of the maternal role is complex and multiphasic in nature, and provides an example that will enhance the reader's ability to learn the common role disruptions.

ments, and is spread over a period of years in a woman's life. Childbirth usually occurs over a period of hours. The average woman in the North American culture experiences childbearing and childbirth only two to four times in her lifetime. Child rearing, however, takes place over the first 18 years of the child's life. Although the expressive maternal behaviors and the instrumental maternal behaviors change as the child grows older, the secondary role of mother is permanent and is relinquished only upon death.

The transition from nonmother to mother begins in pregnancy (Rubin 1967). As with the assumption of any new role, the pregnant woman's beginning behaviors are primarily expressive behaviors (Randell 1976). She verbalizes these feelings, and they become expressive behaviors. A positive self concept is important during this phase in order for the woman to be able to think of herself as mother (Clausen 1973). The woman begins to talk about her baby as another person and to fantasize about herself as a mother. As the birth of the baby becomes imminent, she seeks out information pertaining to the role of mother from books, friends, and particularly, her own mother. She looks for role models to imitate in order to learn the instrumental behaviors of her new role (Rubin 1967). Women experiencing their second pregnancies also exhibit similar behavior, because the role of mother is mastered over a number of years and changes with the birth of each child.

The literature tells us what expressive maternal behaviors and instrumental maternal behaviors to expect the mother to exhibit after the birth of her child. In the first two to three days after birth, the mother is passive and dependent. It is a period where the majority of maternal role behaviors are expressive, and this is adaptive. Naturally, second-time mothers would exhibit instrumental maternal behaviors much sooner than would a first-time mother. During the third to tenth days after birth, the mother begins to exhibit instrumental maternal behaviors. After the second week, and until several weeks thereafter, the mother experiences a period of grief, wherein she mourns the loss of her role of nonmother, career woman, and so forth (Rubin 1967). This grief is resolved over time, and Rubin (1967) states that this usually occurs within four weeks if role transition is well in progress.

Research and descriptive literature tell us how the maternal role is attained. Society, culture, the mother's self concept, and her expectations of the maternal role tell a woman what the maternal role behaviors should be. That is, they provide *role prescriptions,* both expressive and instrumental. However, the mother's self concept, and her expectations of the maternal role, must be compatible with society's and culture's expectations, or the potential for disruption within the maternal role, and between other roles, will exist. Fortunately, there are wide variances of adaptive behaviors within the maternal role behaviors. These factors are presented later in the section discussing effective role transition.

Role Transition

The process of assuming and developing a new role is called *role transition*. By definition, role transition indicates that it is growth in a positive direction. In the case of the maternal role, a secondary and permanent role, the new role is one of a series of roles that an individual assumes to meet the developmental tasks of her primary role. It is a continuous and ongoing process. As an individual ages chronologically, the primary role changes; new developmental tasks confront the individual, and new secondary and tertiary roles are assumed in order to meet these developmental tasks. It should be noted that the transition from one secondary role to another secondary role is a much more arduous and time-consuming process than moving from one tertiary role to another. Tertiary roles, by their nature, are usually temporary and require less emotional and physical involvement than secondary roles.

It should also be remembered that an individual does not always have a conscious choice about assuming a new role. Many secondary roles can be thrust upon the individual by circumstances and the environment. For example, a man who has worked all his life as a taxi driver may have an accident that leaves him unable to drive a taxi, but he may still be able to hold another kind of job. This man, then, has to seek a new job, and even, perhaps, retraining. He did not choose to seek a new secondary role, but his ability to adapt to his new job, and make an effective transition to a new secondary role, are threats to his social integrity. It is this threat, or potential disruption, that nurses are concerned with in assessment of the role function mode of adaptation.

In assessing the role function mode adaptation of various persons with whom nurses come in contact, they will identify many secondary and tertiary roles that are in transition. Based on the data gathered and the assessment made, the nurse makes a judgment about whether the role transition is effective (that is, adaptive) or ineffective before formulating a nursing diagnosis. In order to do this, there are certain factors to identify.

APPLICATION OF THE NURSING PROCESS

As with the preceding sections of this text, application of the nursing process in situations of adaptation problems in role function, involves the six-step nursing process. By assisting the person with role concerns, adaptation in all modes is promoted.

Since the nursing process applied to the role function mode was presented in the previous chapter, the major focus of this discussion will be on the adaptation problems common to the mode.

Assessment of Behavior

The steps for assessing role function remain constant regardless of the individual or the situation. First, the nurse identifies the primary role according to age and sex and then documents the developmental tasks associated with the role. Next, all secondary and as many tertiary roles as possible are identified and analyzed. Table 17–1 gives a synopsis in column two of all behaviors to be assessed relative to primary, secondary and tertiary roles.

Of particular relevance to the nurse are the roles associated with the nurse/patient relationship and the particular social position termed the sick role (Wu 1973). Analysis of the sick role in terms of the nursing process provides insight into important factors associated with the roles of patient and nurse. Table 17–1 suggests behaviors of relevance to the person occupying the sick role.

As the nurse gathers behavioral data, the compatibility of the secondary and tertiary roles with the primary role is addressed. Problems of role function usually occur in secondary roles. Theoretical knowledge of the role prescriptons associated with many different roles has been developed.

The behaviors associated with the secondary role of mother have been described previously.

Assessment of Stimuli

The assessment of stimuli was described in detail in the previous chapter. In addition to the role performance requirements of consumer, rewards, access to facilities/set of circumstances, and collaboration/cooperation, other common influencing stimuli were identified. Table 17–1 illustrates some of these in column three together with some relevant questions. For example, in assessment of the person's knowledge about the role, the nurse assesses the persons knowledge about and experience with performing the activities involved in the role. For the mother of a new baby, previous experience with other children would be an asset and a positive stimulus in the achievement of role mastery.

After the nurse has assessed the behaviors and stimuli for each role that the person occupies, a systematic process of judging both expressive and instrumental behaviors as either adaptive or ineffective is undertaken. Then the stimuli and the effect that they have on each behavior are addressed. Combining this data enables the nurse to formulate a nursing diagnosis. In the role function mode, three categories of diagnosis have been described: role transition, role distance, and role conflict. Ideally, the nurse would make a nursing diagnosis for each role, behavior both adaptive and ineffective.

Nursing Diagnosis

Examples of adaptive nursing diagnoses relative to the role function mode were provided in the previous chapter. A diagnosis of role mastery indicates that an individual demonstrates both expressive and instrumental behaviors that meet social expectations associated with the role. In *effective role transition,* the individual adaptive processes exhibit effective expressive behaviors, and a few adaptive instrumental behaviors, that

TABLE 17–1. ASSESSMENT OF ROLE FUNCTION BEHAVIORS AND STIMULI

Factors to Assess	Behaviors	Factors to Assess	Stimuli
Roles			
Primary	Client's age, sex, developmental stage	Developmental Stage	What is the client's developmental stage?
Secondary	What activities take up most of the client's time?	Consumer	Who benefits when client accomplishes the task?
Tertiary	What other activities does the client engage in, eg, more temporary in nature? What does the client say about maintaining or modifying existing roles or adopting new roles?	Reward	What reward does the client get from accomplishing activites related to role?
	How many roles does the client perform?	Access to Facilities	Does the client have all that he needs to accomplish his activities?
Sick Role	What activities does the client do while in the hospital?	Cooperation/Collaboration	Can the client get cooperation/collaboration from people with whom he accomplishes the activity of a role?
	What are the tasks associated with the sick role?	Social Norms	What are other's/society's expectations regarding activity the client is performing? What is the client's perceptions of the role expectations imposed by others?
	Can the client perform the tasks related to the sick role?	Client's Expectations	What are the client's expectations of his role performance?
	What are feelings and/or attitudes of client related to activities of role?		What is the client's perception of self in relation to expected role behaviors?
	What does client say about activities of role?		
	What is the client's mood, emotional responses related to activities of the role?	Role Models	Is there a role model(s) in his enviranment to help client perform his role?
	Is the client exempt from normal social role responsibilities?		
	Does the client accept medical and nursing help?		
	Does the client want to get well?	Knowledge, Education and Experience	Does the client have the necessary knowledge, education and experience to perform activities related to role?

Dept. of Nursing Vanier College 1989 (used with permission)

partially meet the social expectations associated with the role. These are the two nursing diagnoses applicable to adaptive role behaviors. However, there are four possible nursing diagnoses for ineffective role behaviors: ineffective role transition, role distance, role conflict, and role failure. Ineffective role transition is dealt with first. In order to develop a clear understanding of the common adaptation problems associated with role transition, however, it is necessary to take a closer look at effective role transition.

Effective Role Transition. In *effective role transition,* the individual exhibits adaptive expressive behaviors, and a few adaptive instrumental behaviors, that partially meet with the social expectations associated with the assigned role. However, the number or quality of the behaviors is not sufficient to formulate a diagnosis of role mastery. The adaptive behaviors indicate positive movement toward the goal of role mastery.

In the initial phase of effective role transition, the behaviors will primarily be expressive behaviors. However, this occurs for a very short period of time. Almost immediately, some instrumental behaviors are observable. If the transition is effective, the number and quality of instrumental behaviors will increase over time. As noted in the literature on role theory, for role transition to occur, certain factors must be present in the environment. These factors are the requirements described in Chapter 16. Also, the expressive and instrumental behaviors are usually affected by the seven major stimuli described in that chapter.

Ineffective Role Transition. In *ineffective role transition,* the individual exhibits adaptive expressive behavior but exhibits ineffective instrumental behaviors for a particular role. Unlike the other three disruptions, which usually arise from some sort of conflict, ineffective role transition is usually the result of a lack of knowledge, education, practice or role models.

Ineffective role transition resembles effective role transition in that all of the expressive behaviors are adaptive and all of the partitions or contextual stimuli for the expressive behaviors are present. The individual experiencing ineffective role transition-maternal role has the self concept of mother, wants to be a mother, and may even know what a mother is expected to do, but she does not know how to accomplish the tasks.

Role Distance. The individual experiencing *role distance* at first appears to be experiencing ineffective role transition. However, a detailed assessment reveals that the individual's instrumental behaviors in role distance vary greatly in degree and in type of response from the individual experiencing ineffective role transition. For example, the individual has the knowledge and experience to perform the instrumental behaviors associated with a role, but does so only when absolutely necessary or when there is no one else around to perform the tasks. The individual functions at a point just short of role failure by performing the minimal number of prescribed instrumental behaviors for the role. In role distance the individual exhibits both instrumental and expressive behaviors appropriate to a particular role, but these behaviors differ significantly from prescribed behaviors for the role (Schofield 1976).

Perhaps the most significant difference between role distance and the other role function mode nursing diagnoses is that the role is incompatible with the individual's self concept. The individual feels uncomfortable because the role is undesirable, either in part or as a whole. This is important to consider because the individual may not reject an entire role, but rather certain behaviors associated with the role that the individual perceives as undesirable. The individual seeks to alleviate this discomfort by exhibiting expressive behaviors which make the role seem unimportant or unworthy. Individuals occupying complementary roles for the role are made to feel uncomfortable in their positions. The individual makes derogatory remarks about the role, jokes, belittles, and constantly speaks out about the role in negative terms, as if she is suited only for something better. It should be kept in mind that this occurs in degrees. The more undesirable the role, the more numerous, severe, and pronounced are the expressive behaviors exhibited.

Role Conflict. Whenever an individual fails to perform the prescribed behaviors for a role, for whatever the reasons, a disruption exists. The focal stimulus or immediate cause for the behavior varies according to the disruption. In ineffective role transition, it was the absence of knowledge, lack of education, or scarcity of role models that caused the disruption. In role distance, the performance of prescribed role behaviors was a threat to the self concept. However, in role conflict, the two major focal stimuli for the behaviors are different in nature, therefore, role conflict is divided into two major disruptions: intrarole conflict and interrole conflict.

In *intrarole conflict,* the individual fails to demonstrate either instrumental or expressive behaviors, or both, appropriate for a role, as a result of incompatible expectations from one or more persons in the environment concerning the individual's expected behavior (Schofield 1976). For example, Judy M. comes from a traditional Italian Catholic family. She maintains a very close relationship with her mother and is in mastery of her daughter role. Judy is now the mother of a 6-week-old baby girl. She has read and taken classes about baby care and is up to date on the current trends. Judy's mother, however, is old-fashioned, and still believes in dressing babies in three layers of clothing in the middle of summer. Judy's mother's praise and approval are very important to Judy. In performing her role as mother, Judy finds herself performing behaviors that try to meet her own perceptions of the maternal role, and then trying to meet her mother's expectations. As she vascillates back and forth, Judy applies all of her energy trying to accommodate two opposing views of the maternal role. Given this conflict, Judy will not achieve role mastery.

Interrole conflict occurs when an individual fails to demonstrate the instrumental and/or expressive behaviors appropriate to the individual's role as a result of the occupation of one or more roles that require pre-scribed behaviors that are incompatible with one another. In this situa-tion, the individual is occupying roles that are in competition with one another.

An example of interrole conflict would be the case of Louise B. Louise is an electrical engineer who was just promoted at work. She works 10 to 12 hours per day and is in role mastery. Louise delivered a baby boy eight weeks ago, and she now considers her life total chaos. She wants to be at work to maintain her position and control. At the same time, she wants to be with her baby and be involved with as much of his care as possible. As a result, she is torn between the two roles and is not experiencing mastery in either one.

Role Failure. *Role failure* differs from all the other role mode diagnoses in that the individual fails to exhibit adaptive expressive behaviors. In the beginning of the chapter, it was noted that the individual must want to assume the role. In role failure the individual does not want to assume the role, and any expressive behaviors that are observed are usually ineffective because they are aimed at pleasing the consumers for the role. The individual has an absence of expressive behaviors, or exhibits ineffec-tive expressive behaviors, and/or has an absence of instrumental behav-iors, or exhibits ineffective instrumental behaviors for a particular role. The key element in role failure is the individual's desire. If the individual exhibits any adaptive expressive behaviors concerning a role, the individ-ual cannot be in role failure.

This is important to remember because when expressive and instru-mental behaviors are ineffective, nurses too often label the client as being in role failure when really, the behavior is indicative of ineffective role transition or role conflict. Role failure does occur, but it is doubtful that the nurse in clinical practice will be confronted frequently with role fail-ure. Role failure is one of the most complex diagnoses in the role mode and usually involves one or more of the other modes of the Roy Adapta-tion Model.

Goal Setting

The nursing goal for a diagnosis of effective role transition is short term rather than long term in nature. The goal should be written in terms of what is expected of the patient, not the nurse. The person and the signifi-cant others,when appropriate, should be involved in formulating realistic goals. The goal statement identifies the behavior of focus, the change expected and a time frame for achievement. In general, the goal for effective role transition should support existing adaptive behaviors and increase the number of adaptive behaviors.

A goal for a person experiencing ineffective role transition could be, "The patient will demonstrate both satisfaction with her mothering role and effective infant care activities with six weeks." The general goal for both types of role conflict is conflict resolution, and integration of primary, secondary and tertiary roles. The general goal for a nursing diagnosis of role distance is to decrease the perceived or real threat to the client's self concept. This is a long-term goal because the process cannot be accomplished in a short period of time. In a diagnosis of role distance, the client is experiencing a threat to self concept. This is related to the client's perception that the role is incompatible with the client's self concept. Goal achievement will be reflected in the integration of instrumental and expressive behaviors.

Intervention

While goal setting has the person's behavior as its focus, intervention addresses the management of stimuli by removing, increasing, or decreasing them.

Nursing interventions for the diagnosis of effective role transition usually involve managing the identified contextual stimuli. The most frequently identified contextual stimuli are number of role models, education or knowledge level, support system, rewards, or the person's self concept. Contextual stimuli most commonly associated with this diagnosis of ineffective role transition are knowledge level of person, reward for adaptive behavior, and presence and effectiveness of a support system.

Nursing interventions for the role distance focus on decreasing the threat or discomfort to the person's self concept. Initially, the nurse could give the person information that shows the potential compatibility between the client's perception of herself and the performance of the given role behaviors. If intellectual stimulation rewards the person, then the nurse needs to appeal to the intellect when teaching about the role. However, if intellectual stimulation does not appeal to the person, other factors perceived as rewarding would be identified. For example, the well-informed person acts in a given way; the person concerned about his or her health acts a certain way. At the same time, all other stimuli that exert a positive influence on instrumental role behaviors should be supported.

For conflict resolution, nursing interventions would include managing the identified stimuli to produce a more adaptive outcome. Interventions that may be appropriate include patient teaching, that is, relative to the problem-solving process, time management, teaching of significant others, support from the nurse, and rewards for adaptive behavior.

Both intrarole conflict and interrole conflict are complex role problems.

They require that the nurse work with multiple stimuli, from the environment and from the client. Similarly role failure is a complex problem.

Evaluation

The final step in the nursing process is evaluation. Evaluation in its most general definition simply means, did you reach the established goal? If the answer is yes, there will have been a change in the person's behavior. The whole process then begins again because the patient's situation is constantly evolving. If the goals are not achieved the process begins again, but in a different sense. If there was no change in behavior, the nurse must identify the point in the nursing process where omissions occurred or where further investigation is required. When the problem area is identified, the nursing process is modified accordingly and the plan of care is revised.

SUMMARY

The nurse is concerned with promoting the person's integrity in the role function mode in health as well as illness. This chapter presented the application of the nursing process within the context of the common adaptation problems of the role function mode. The nursing diagnoses of role transition, distance, and conflict were presented. Role theory, as introduced in Chapter 16 was integrated throughout the nursing process. The nursing diagnoses presented in this chapter represent some of the current nursing literature but not all of the possible nursing diagnoses for the role function mode.

EXERCISES FOR APPLICATION

1. Among the people with whom you come in contact in your everyday life, identify and describe an example of:
   a. Effective role transition
   b. Ineffective role transition
   c. Role distance
2. Identify the major contextual stimuli involved in each of the examples that you have described.
3. Describe your assessment of what you think would constitute student role failure. Do you know anyone like this?
4. Utilizing your student or professional role, describe an example of intrarole conflict.
5. Utilizing your student or professional role, describe an example of interrole conflict.

6. Perform a complete role assessment on someone whom you know. Try to choose someone whom you think might have a potential disruption in a secondary role. Formulate a nursing diagnosis for each of this person's secondary roles.

ASSESSMENT OF UNDERSTANDING

1. Effective role transition is a part of the process of role mastery?
   a. True
   b. False
2. Which of the following behaviors would a client exhibit with a nursing diagnosis of ineffective role transition?
   a. ineffective expressive behaviors
   b. effective instrumental behaviors
   c. ineffective instrumental behaviors
   d. none of the above.
3. Identify three major contextual stimuli involved in an assessment for a diagnosis of ineffective role transition.
4. In a nursing diagnosis of role distance, the major threat is to which adaptive mode?
   a. role
   b. interdependence
   c. physiological
   d. self concept
5. Match the label in column A with the description in column B.

Column A	Column B	
1. Role distance	a. _____	Adaptive expressive behaviors but ineffective instrumental behaviors
2. Role failure	b. _____	Absent or ineffective expressive behaviors and/or absent or ineffective instrumental behaviors
3. Role conflict	c. _____	Instrumental and expressive behaviors differ significantly from those prescribed for the role
4. Ineffective role transition	d. _____	Incompatible expectations for role behaviors within environment or prescribed behaviors in one role are incompatible with those in another.

6. Discuss the difference between interrole conflict and intrarole conflict.

Feedback

1. a. True
2. c. Ineffective instrumental behaviors
3. Lack of knowledge, absence of role models, absence of rewards or feedback.
4. d. Self-concept
5. a. 4
   b. 2
   c. 1
   d. 3
6. Intrarole conflict results from incompatible expectations from others concerning the individual's behavior while interrole conflict results from occupation of incompatible roles.

REFERENCES

Clausen, J.P., et al. *Maternity Nursing Today.* New York: McGraw-Hill Book Company, 1973.

Randell, B. Development of role function, in Sister Callista Roy, *Introduction to Nursing: An Adaptation Model,* Englewood Cliffs, N.J.: Prentice-Hall, Inc., 1976.

Rubin, R. Basic maternal behavior, *Nursing Outlook,* 9, no. 11; 683–686, 1961

Rubin, R. Attainment of the maternal role: Part 1. Process, *Nursing Research,* 16, no. 3, Summer 1967, pp. 237–245.

Schofield, A. Problems of role function, in Sr. C. Roy, *Introduction to Nursing: An Adaptation Model.* Englewood Cliffs, N.J.: Prentice-Hall, Inc., 1976, pp. 265–287.

Vanier College, Dept. of Nursing. *Assessment tool: Role Mode.* St. Laurent, Quebec, Canada Unpublished material, 1989.

Wu, R. *Behavior and Illness.* Englewood Cliffs, N.J.: Prentice-Hall, Inc., 1973.

Additional References

Banton, M. *Roles: An Introduction to the Study of Social Relations.* New York: Basic Books, Inc., Publishers, 1965.

Doenges, M., and M. Moorhouse. *Nursing Diagnoses With Interventions* (2nd ed.) Philadelphia, Pa.: F.A. Davis Co., 1988.

Goffman, E. Role distance, in *Encounters.* Indianapolis: The Bobbs-Merrill Company, Inc., 1961, pp. 85–152.

Gordon, M. *Nursing Diagnosis: Process and Application.* New York: McGraw-Hill Book Company, 1982.

Gross, N., A. McEachern, and W. Mason. Role conflict and its resolution, in *Role Theory: Concepts and Research,* Bruce Biddle and Edwin Thomas, eds., New York: John Wiley & Sons, Inc., 1966.

Hardy, M.E., and M.E. Conway. *Role Theory: Perspectives for Health Professionals.* New York: Appleton-Century-Crofts, 1978.

Malaznik, N. Theory of role function, in Sister Callista Roy, *Introduction to Nursing: An Adaptation Model.* Englewood Cliffs, N.J.: Prentice-Hall, Inc., 1976.

McFarland, M., and J.B. Reinhart. The development of motherliness, *Children,* March/April 1959, pp. 48–52.

Parsons, T. *The Social System.* New York: The Free Press, 1964.

Parsons, T. Role conflict and the genesis of deviance, in *Role Theory: Concepts and Research,* Bruce Biddle and Edwin Thomas, eds., New York: John Wiley & Sons, Inc., 1966.

Pinnell, N.N., and M. de Meneses. *The Nursing Process, Theory, Application and Related Processes.* E. Norwalk, Conn.: Appleton-Century-Crofts, 1986.

Reeder, S. Becoming a mother-nursing implications in a problem of role transition, in *ANA Regional Clinical Conferences.* New York: Appleton-Century-Crofts, 1967, p. 204.

Reeder, S., et al. The family in a changing world, in *Maternity Nursing,* 14th ed. Sharon J. Reeder, Luigi Mastroianni, and Leonide L. Martin, eds., Philadelphia: J.B. Lippincott Company, 1980, pp. 23–33.

Robischon, P., and D. Scott. Role theory and its application to family nursing, *Nursing Outlook,* July 1969, pp. 52–57.

Roy, Sr. C., and S.L. Roberts. *Theory Construction in Nursing: An Adaptation Model.* Englewood Cliffs, N.J.: Prentice-Hall, Inc., 1981.

Ruddock, R. *Roles and Relationships.* Atlantic Highlands, N.J.: Humanities Press, Inc., 1969.

Turner, R.H. Role-taking, role standpoint and reference group behavior, in *Role Theory: Concepts and Research,* Bruce Biddle and Edwin Thomas, eds. New York: John Wiley & Sons, Inc., 1966.

PART IV: CONCLUSION

Part IV has presented the role function mode as it is described within the Roy Adaptation Model. Chapter 16 provided an overview of the mode through description and identification of the theoretical basis and illustration of application of the six-step nursing process. Three common adaptation problems were the focus of Chapter 17: role transition, role distance, and role conflict. These were illustrated through their application to the maternal role and the sick role.

As a conclusion to Part IV, a case study illustrating effective processes of role transition is provided. Again, the maternal role is used to convey the associated concepts to the reader.

Effective Role Transition

CASE DESCRIPTION[1]

Wendy S. is a 25-year-old primipara (a woman who has delivered her first child), who delivered a healthy 7 pounds 11 ounces baby boy 4 days ago. Her pregnancy was uneventful and uncomplicated. She and her husband attended Lamaze childbirth education classes and, at the time of delivery, she received no medication. Wendy is breast feeding her baby and plans to stay home with him, perhaps returning to work when he is ready for nursery school. If their finances permit, Wendy would enjoy being at home with the baby full time.

Until one week before delivery, she worked as a hair stylist in a local beauty salon. She has been married for three years. She and her husband are both Catholic and of German descent. Wendy is close to her mother, but her mother lives far away and will not be able to come to help with the baby. Wendy also has a close relationship with her mother-in-law. Her mother-in-law will be staying with Wendy and the baby for the first two weeks after Wendy gets home. Wendy's husband will be taking a two-week vacation after his mother leaves, so that Wendy will have at least a month of help at home. The husband is a truck driver, but he is seldom away from home for extended periods of time.

Wendy told the nurse that she took a Red Cross infant care course

[1]This case study was originally developed by Kathleen A. Nuwayhid as part of the chapter Role transition, distance and conflict,in Sister C. Roy *Introduction to Nursing: An Adaptation* Model (2nd ed) Englewood Cliffs, NJ: Prentice Hall (1984): 405–427.

while she was pregnant because she wanted to have some formal preparation for baby care. She says that it is even more thrilling seeing how excited her husband is about the baby. Wendy has helped care for friends' babies, and younger cousins, but realizes that having a baby of one's own is very different.

Wendy feels that having the baby in the room with her is a tremendous way to get to know the baby. She chose to breast feed because she wanted to do everything that she could to help the baby be healthy. The nurse caring for Wendy has observed that Wendy holds the baby comfortably, asks many questions about breast feeding, and is eager to dress and bathe him. Wendy also asks her roommate, a woman with three children, many questions about babies and what it is like when you are at home.

ASSESSMENT

Wendy's primary role is that of a 25-year-old young adult woman. Developmental tasks include establishment as an independent individual, with family and friends; building a strong, mutual, affectional bond with (possible) marriage partner and family of spouse; and being able to nurture, support, and provide for spouse and offspring.

Wendy is four days postpartum. The literature tells us that a woman who is in effective role transition will begin to exhibit beginning instrumental behaviors for the maternal role around the third day postpartum. Such instrumental behaviors as feeding, bathing, and changing the baby's diapers should be exhibited by this time.

From the data given, we can identify Wendy's secondary roles as:

1. Wife
2. Mother
3. Daughter
4. Daughter-in-law
5. Hair stylist

These are tentatively ranked in order of importance. However, to be accurate, Wendy would have to rank them herself. For the purpose of learning, we will assume that Wendy has mastered all of her secondary roles, except for the maternal role. In actual practice a nurse would perform assessments on all roles occupied by the individual.

The following is a behavioral assessment of Wendy S. based on the data collected. Behaviors are marked as E/A, expressive/adaptive; E/I, expressive/ineffective; I/A, instrumental/adaptive; or I/I, instrumental/ineffective. Keep in mind that effective role transition is a point on a continuum between nonmastery and mastery of a particular role. It is in constant motion, moving in a positive direction toward role mastery.

Assessment of Behavior

Expressive Behaviors
1. Is thrilled with having a baby of her own.   E/A
2. Derives a great deal of joy and happiness from having pro-   E/A
   duced such a healthy child.
3. Husband is thrilled that she gave him a child.   E/A
4. Wants to help baby be healthy by breast feeding him.   E/A
5. Likes having baby in the room with her.   E/A
6. Likes doing things for the baby.   E/A
7. Asks the nurse many questions about baby.   E/A
8. Asks roommate many questions about baby.   E/A
9. Tells nurse that she has a close relationship with her mother-   E/A
   in-law.

Instrumental Behaviors
1. Attended Lamaze childbirth classes.   I/A
2. Had prenatal care.   I/A
3. Actively participated in her labor and delivery.   I/A
4. Attended Red Cross infant care classes.   I/A
5. Giving physical care of baby during rooming-in.   I/A
6. Learning to care for baby in baby classes.   I/A
7. Breast-feeds baby.   I/A
8. Chose to deliver in hospital and remain in hospital for care.   I/A
9. Has planned for home care of baby and help at home.   I/A

All of the expressive maternal behaviors are adaptive. Notice that the expressive behaviors are numerous, and that even though there seem to be many instrumental behaviors present, the instrumental behaviors are primarily anticipatory in nature. The instrumental behaviors are aimed at learning the new role rather than actual role performance. This is adaptive and sequential in effective role transition. First, one feels the role; second, learns the instrumental role behavior, and finally, performs the instrumental role behaviors. In the assessment of stimuli, the nurse determines if all the factors are present in the environment for this process to take place.

Assessment of Stimuli
Focal stimulus for all behaviors: pregnancy and delivery of a healthy 7 pounds 11 ounces baby boy.

All of the environmental stimuli or role requirements are present for both the expressive and instrumental role behaviors. Although the instrumental behaviors are few in number, the stimuli are present that will allow these behaviors to occur and increase in number. We have been unable to identify any ineffective behaviors in the behavioral assessment or any disruptions in assessment of stimuli. We are ready to formulate the nursing diagnosis.

The nursing goal is a short-term goal because mastery of the maternal role takes place over an extended period of time. It is better, then, to have short term, attainable goals which will lead to the end goal of role mastery.

Because there are no disruptions, the assessment data are searched for possible weaknesses in the role requirements or the potential for disruptions to occur. Again, none are found. All contextual stimuli are present and appear to be sound. Nursing interventions, therefore, are aimed at supporting existing behaviors and increasing the number of adaptive behaviors. This is done by managing the contextual stimuli, especially role modeling, knowledge or education, the support system, rewards, and self concept, as seen in the interventions.

In Wendy's case, she will be evaluated prior to discharge, and plans for her care at home will be formulated as well. It is important to realize that although Wendy has all the stimuli present that indicate effective role transition, the nurse's role is just as crucial as if there were a major disruption. The nursing research literature suggested that unless these behaviors are supported, and the stimuli maintained by nursing interventions, disruptions will occur.

Table IV–1 summarizes the assessment of stimuli and care plan.

TABLE IV–1. SECOND-LEVEL ASSESSMENT OF WENDY S. AND CARE PLAN

Behaviors	Focal	Stimuli		Residual
		Consumer	Contextual	
Expressive	Pregnancy and delivery of healthy infant	Consumer		Religion
(1)		Baby		Culture
		Reward		Intelligence
(2), (3), and (4)			Is able to think of self as mother; positive self-concept; praise of significant others	
(5) and (6)			Physical well-being of infant	
(7), (8), and (9)		Access to facilities		
			Has access to the baby in a supportive setting	
			Cooperation/collaboration	
			Husband, nurse, mother, mother-in-law, roommate	
Instrumental		Consumer		Level of health
(1), (2), (3), and (4)		Baby and self		Physical structure
				Culture
(5), (6), and (7)		Reward		
		Healthy infant		
		Self satisfaction		
		Access to facilities		
			Physical environment of hospital; role models	
			Experience with other children	
			Cooperation/collaboration	
(8)				
(9)			Mother-in-law and husband will be at home to help with the baby	

(continued)

TABLE IV–1. (Continued)

Nursing Diagnosis	Goals	Interventions
(Includes all instrumental and expressive behaviors) Effective role transition, maternal role, as evidenced by: 1. Expressive behaviors which are compatible; expressive role behaviors of a woman 4 days after delivery. 2. All requirements of the expressive and instrumental role behaviors are present. 3. Beginning instrumental maternal role behaviors; client is learning and performing behaviors of the maternal role.	1. Client will continue to exhibit effective maternal role transition behaviors as evidenced by an increase in the number of adaptive expressive and adaptive instrumental behaviors. 2. Client will continue to have a positive relationship with her husband, baby, and significant others.	1. Nurse will provide time for client to attend child care classes in the hospital. 2. Nurse will reinforce information and skills learned in child care classes by demonstration to client, her husband and any interested significant other. 3. Nurse will support and praise all efforts made by client to care for infant. 4. Nurse and nursing staff will allow client to assume independence regarding child care at her own pace. 5. Nurse will recommend reference and reading materials concerning child care for client and husband. 6. Nurse will inform client of mother's support group and community resources for new mothers. 7. Evaluate progress prior to discharge and modify interventions as necessary.

Part V
The Interdependence Mode

The second of the two social modes described within the Roy Adaptation model is the interdependence mode. This mode focuses on interactions related to the giving and receiving of love, respect, and value through relationships with significant others and support systems. The basic need of the mode relates to a feeling of security in nurturing relationships and is termed affectional adequacy.

The nurse, as a person, has interdependence needs. She or he experiences self as a more adequate and effective person when affectional needs are met by family and persons at work and in one's social life. When the nurse works in a very stressful environment, the need for supportive relationships increases.

The nurse frequently meets clients who seek interventions in the areas defined as the interdependence mode. She or he also experiences self and personal interdependence needs and recognizes that meeting of these needs can influence one's effectiveness as a person and as a nurse. Study of the interdependence mode and how to promote feelings of security in nurturing relationships is highly relevant for the adaptation nursing process.

Chapter 18 provides the reader with an overview of the mode including description, identification of the theoretical bases, and illustration of the nursing process as applied to interdependence. In Chapter 19, the common adaptation problems of separation anxiety and loneliness are addressed. The section concludes with a case study illustrating application of the interdependence mode in practice.

Chapter Eighteen ———————

Overview of the Interdependence Mode

*Mary Poush Tedrow**

The final adaptive mode to be introduced is the interdependence mode. This mode, like the role function mode, involves interaction with others. This mode, however, focuses on closer relationships than those implied in roles or positions in society. The interdependence mode is one in which affectional needs are met. The Roy Adaptation Model notes that each person strives for adequacy and mastery. In the interdependence mode, that sense of adequacy is experienced through satisfying relationships with other people.

This chapter presents the interdependence mode from a theoretical perspective and then proceeds to explore positive adaptation and the nursing process related to it. Adaptation problems associated with the interdependence mode, separation anxiety and loneliness in particular, are addressed in Chapter 19.

OBJECTIVES

After studying this chapter, the reader will be able to do the following:

1. Describe the interdependence mode according to the Roy Adaptation Model.

*The interdependence mode has evolved in a way unlike the other adaptive modes. Initially, in the early 1970s, the interdependence mode was described and operationalized with dependent and independent behaviors. By 1975, theoretical and clinical application of the content revealed that there was redundancy of this content in the self-concept and role modes. Joyce Van Landingham, Dorothy Clough, and Mary Tedrow worked to clarify the interdependence mode. Further empirical findings led to a major revision of the mode in 1977 by Joyce Van Landingham, Mary Hicks, and Mary Tedrow. This revision was further developed in teaching and practice by the author. She acknowledges the clarifications by Brooke Randell.

2. Define and give examples of adaptive giving and receiving behaviors.
3. Identify the stimuli that influence the interdependence mode.
4. Make a nursing diagnosis for adaptive interdependence.
5. Derive goals for a patient with adaptive interdependence in a given situation.
6. Describe nursing interventions used to maintain adaptive interdependence.
7. Propose approaches to determine the effectiveness of interventions.

KEY CONCEPTS DEFINED

- *Interdependence:* the close relationships of people that involve the willingness and ability to love, respect, and value others, and to accept and respond to love, respect, and value given by others.
- *Affectional adequacy:* the feeling of security in nurturing relationships with others. Basic need of the interdependence mode.
- *Nurturing:* providing growth-producing care and attention.
- *Significant other:* the individual to whom the most meaning or importance is given. It is a person who is loved, respected, and valued, and who in turn loves, respects, and values the other to a degree greater than in all other relationships.
- *Support systems:* all persons, groups, or animals that contribute to meeting the interdependence needs of the person.
- *Receiving behaviors:* the person's receiving, taking in, or assimilating nurturing behaviors from the significant other or support systems.
- *Giving behaviors:* giving or supplying nurturing as initiated by the person toward the significant other and/or support systems.

DESCRIPTION OF THE INTERDEPENDENCE MODE

Interdependence is defined as the close relationships of people. With the heritage of nursing as a caring discipline, the current development of a nursing science of caring, and the particular humanistic philosophy of the Roy Adaptation Model, close relationships and their meaning and development become a significant topic of concern. These relationships often involve the same persons that one interacts with in role performance. However, they differ from the relationships of role function because the purpose of these relationships is to achieve affectional adequacy. *Affectional adequacy* is the feeling of security in nurturing relationships.

Through such nurturing relationships, one continues to grow as a person and as a contributing member of society. These relationships involve the willingness and ability to love, respect, and value others and to accept and respond to love, respect, and value given by others. The person who has a comfortable balance of interdependence feels adequate and secure in relationships with other people. He or she feels loved and supported by others and can express love and support for other people. These persons have learned to live successfully in a world of other people, animals, and objects.

The interdependence mode is a social mode because the needs are met through social interaction. The need underlying this social mode is the need for *affectional adequacy*. Affectional adequacy incorporates the need to be nurtured and to nurture. It includes the person's needs for care and attention, affirmation, belonging, approval, and understanding. These needs are met primarily by establishing in-depth interactions with other persons. As people strive for affectional adequacy, they may experience periods of aloneness, loneliness, and alienation.

Aloneness is a chosen state, to be by oneself for personal growth, meditation, or for an inspired artistic performance or creative activities. One needs to stand alone at times to be one's own person. The ability to spend time alone is often accompanied by mutually satisfying relationships.

Loneliness is a very different experience. Sullivan (in Fromm-Reichmann 1959) defined *loneliness* as "the exceedingly unpleasant and driving experience connected with an inadequate discharge of the need for human intimacy, for interpersonal intimacy." This is a severe state unacceptable to most people. It would seem to last longer and be more profound than the state of being lonely. Loneliness as an adaptation problem is discussed in Chapter 19.

The circular nature and the processes involved in the achievement of affectional adequacy are illustrated in Figure 18–1.

Affectional adequacy, as the need underlying the interdependence mode, involves contact with and affection from others required by and from the person as a social being. To meet this need, the person seeks out contact with others. The adaptive outcome of these contacts is affectional adequacy in the form of mutually satisfying relationships and/or aloneness.

The interdependence mode, then, looks at the person's needs for affectional adequacy. Affectional adequacy is experienced in relationships with others. Relationships with different people have different meanings for the individual. In the interdependence mode, one looks at the specific relationships of significant others and support systems. A *significant other* is the individual to whom the most meaning or importance is given. It is a person who is loved, respected, and valued and who in turn loves, respects, and values the person to a degree greater than in other relationships. The significant other may be identified by asking the question: Who is the most important person in my life? The significant other may be a parent, spouse, friend or family member, God or a Supreme Being, or an animal. For most people, the significant other is relatively stable and

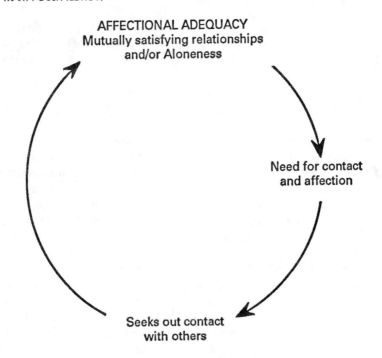

AFFECTIONAL ADEQUACY
Mutually satisfying relationships
and/or Aloneness

Need for contact
and affection

Seeks out contact
with others

Figure 18–1. Affectional Adequacy

this one remains the significant other for periods of time. The individual usually can identify one person (or possibly more) who is the significant other.

Support systems are persons, groups, or animals that contribute to meeting a person's interdependence needs. Support systems differ in intensity and meaning from significant others. An adult woman might consider her spouse as the significant other and a friend at work and her bridge club as support systems. Support systems provide the same functions of giving and receiving love, respect, and value. They contribute to affectional adequacy by their nurturing quality. However, their meaning does not carry the same intensity as that of the relationship with a significant other. Support systems include social groups and work groups that contribute to the growth of the person. The health care system may be a support system with the nurse as a particular part of that support system.

THEORETICAL BASIS FOR THE INTERDEPENDENCE MODE

Behaviors that demonstrate interdependence needs (nurturing and affection) are called receiving and giving behaviors (Randell, Tedrow, and Van Landingham 1982). Receiving behaviors are those that indicate that a person is receiving, taking in, or assimilating nurturing. Andrews and Roy (1986) further described receiving behaviors as actions, such as expressing love for another person, expressing appreciation of thoughtful actions, and allowing another to care for and protect oneself. Giving behaviors are those of giving or supplying nurturing to the other person. Andrews and Roy (1986) explained giving behaviors as including caring for another, touching, and providing physical and psychological support and performing thoughtful gestures. The diagram in Figure 18–2 illustrates the interdependence mode relationships. The arrows labeled "G" (giving) are nurturing behaviors that the person is contributing to another. The arrows labeled "R" (receiving) demonstrate the quantity and quality of behaviors received from that person.

The interdependence mode reflects the circular relationship between a person and others in the environment. It focuses on interactions related to giving and receiving love, value and respect. The person who successfully maintains relationships will have developed the ability to recognize and deal with one's own love and support needs, as well as those of other people. This process of achieving affectional adequacy includes many com-

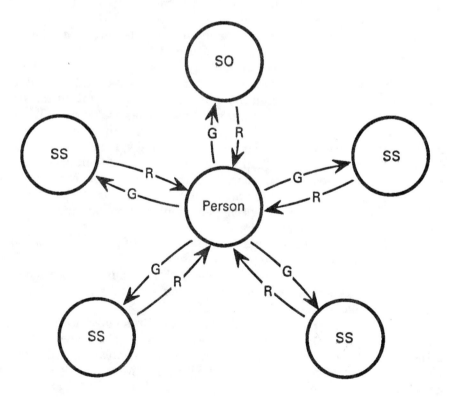

Figure 18–2. Giving and Receiving Behaviors between a Person and the Significant Other and Support Systems

ponents of interaction. These include language skills, nonverbal communication skills, and the ability to recognize the feelings and attitudes of others. The development of sympathy and caring, as well as sharing, is inherent in this process. This development begins early and continues throughout a person's life.

Friendships are important to the adaptive person and it is through friendships (with family and others) that affectional adequacy is attained. This importance is highlighted in the words of Sacajawea in Waldo (1978), "Through his life a person is content if he finds a friend. Through that one friend, a person has more contentment than he can have with hundreds of others."

The quest for affectional adequacy is part of today's culture. Intact families try to spend time together, divorced people remarry, social groups for young and old proliferate. There is a preponderance of self-help books on "satisfying relationships" and many movies and novels focus on the struggles of intimate and loving relationships. The times reflect that fewer people are married, more are living alone, and that social interaction through volunteer activities are less than a decade ago. The increasing number of elderly, especially elderly women, may mean that new ways of achieving affectional adequacy will be sought.

Randell, Tedrow, and Van Landingham (1982) believe that when a baby is born, two adaptive modes are operational—the physiological mode and the interdependence mode. Many studies document the infant's need for touch and physical contact, the bonding process and love. Out of the interactions that are primarily affectional or nurturing in nature arises the beginning of self concept, and finally roles are learned. These authors further believe that with the living out of one's life, the modes are given up in reverse sequence. For example, people who are admitted to convalescent centers in their final years give up many of their previously held roles. Sometimes even the identity of their self concept becomes less apparent if the person moves to senility or a state of coma. A form of the interdependence mode, the receptive part of interaction, and the physiological mode will remain operational.

According to this view, one begins and ends this life as a physiological and interdependent being. There are exceptions to this continuum, such as sudden death or a long productive life with minimal deterioration of functioning. A general picture of the development and relinquishing of the four adaptive modes is illustrated in Figure 18–3.

Many studies have been done and articles written elaborating on the quality and length of life. See, for example, Roy (1981), Cohen (1985), Dimond and Jones (1983), Gottlieb (1981), and Greenblatt et al (1982). Often, the factors identified with both the length of life and the "good" life are relationships with others or social support. House, Landis, and Umberson (1988) reviewed the literature noting a relationship between so-

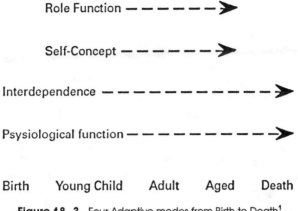

Figure 18-3. Four Adaptive modes from Birth to Death[1]

cial relationships and health. For years, it has been known that married people live longer and are healthier and often happier than unmarried people. The "social contact index" (Berkman 1978) often used in these studies takes into account whether the individual is married, has close contacts with friends and relatives, belongs to a religious group, or has organizational links. People who have contacts in only one of these categories appear to have a greater risk of dying than those who have contacts in more than one category. The classic study of Spitz (1945) showed that infants who were deprived of touch or affection simply wasted away and died.

Kane (1988) reported beginning work towards a conceptual model of family social support. She presented three interaction factors: reciprocity, advice and feedback, and emotional involvement. Kane based her work on reciprocity on the earlier work of Cobb (1976) that described an individual being involved in a network of mutual obligation. This belonging is noted by the sharing of resources with others and the giving and receiving of help. Advice and feedback relates to the quality and quantity of communication between the family and its network. She drew on the work of Caplan (1974) who emphasized the importance of relationships with significant others to work through the issues of living. Kane (1988) noted that communication is done through a process of giving advice and feedback. Emotional involvement includes the concepts of intimacy and trust. This final factor includes emotional bonds such as love, caring, warmth, and compassion.

Many sociological and psychological theorists have studied relationships and the need for affection. The works of Erikson (1963), Selman (1980), Fromm (1956), Havighurst (1953), and Maslow (1954) are used to

[1]This theoretical perspective differs from that of Dobratz (1984), as noted in Chap. 1.

provide understanding of the development and maintenance of integrity in the interdependence mode.

Erikson's eight stages of development have certain implications for the interdependence mode. For example, the developmental tasks are stimuli to behavior at some age levels. For example, the infant developing trust versus mistrust is a stimulus to the receiving behaviors in the interdependence mode.

Selman (1980) provided a description of five stages of friendship that are similar to Erikson's work but apply more specifically to affectional needs. The stages and their characteristics are listed in Table 18–1.

A friendship builds out of some commonly held beliefs, values, and interests. Some people experience the growth of a friendship from which an adult love relationship can develop. Fromm (1956) talked about love being a feeling and an action. Love has the characteristics of knowing, caring about, respecting, and feeling responsibility toward the receiver of love. Each of us has a need to be loved and supported and to love and support. The love relationship is an intense interaction with close identification with the loved one. As such, the joy and pain, as well as stresses and happiness of the other, are experienced by both people in the relationship. The love relationship includes a friendship with the other person.

Maslow (1979) identified a hierarchy of needs for individual persons. Interdependence needs were directly or indirectly represented in most levels. The first level identified food as a need, and in most societies, eating is a social event where nurturing activity occurs. At the second level, Maslow identified sex as a need, and again, sexual gratification is usually accompanied with affection. His fourth level identified love, belonging, and closeness needs, all which are interdependent in orientation.

Havighurst (1953) described developmental tasks for the infant to the mature adult. Each stage of life includes tasks related to establishing and maintaining affectional adequacy.

APPLICATION OF THE NURSING PROCESS

The nursing process as described in Chapter 2 is applied to the theoretical concepts and content of the interdependence mode. The concepts associated with interdependence have particular relevance to the nurse/patient relationship since the patient forms an interdependent relationship with the nurse as support system in specific health care situations, during hospitalization, for example.

The nurse is concerned about the interdependence mode of her clients as well as herself. Nurses frequently meet persons who are experiencing disrupted wellness or illness. People who are ill or in a state of change usually experience an increased need for love, respect, and affirmation.

TABLE 18–1. THE FIVE STAGES OF FRIENDSHIP

Stage	Age	Characteristics
0	3–7	*Monetary Playmate:* The child has difficulty distinguishing between a physical action, such as grabbing a toy, and the psychological intention behind this action. Friends are valued for their material and physical attributes, and defined by proximity.
1	4–9	*One-Way Assistance:* At this stage, the child can differentiate between one's own perspective and those of others. However, the child does not yet understand that dealing with others involves give-and-take between people. In a "good" friendship, one party does what the other party wants to do.
2	6–12	*Two-Way Fair Weather Cooperation:* The child has the ability to see that interpersonal perspectives are reciprocal, each person taking into account the other's perspective. Conceptions of friendship include a concern for what each person thinks about the other; it is much more a two-way street. The limitation of this stage is that the child still sees the basic purpose of friendship as serving many separate self-interests, rather than mutual interests.
3	9–15	*Intimate, Mutually Shared Relationships:* Not only can the child take the other's point of view, but by now he or she can also step outside the friendship and take a generalized third-person perspective on it. With the ability to take a third-person perspective, the child can move from viewing friendship as a reciprocal cooperation for each person's self-interests to seeing it as a collaboration with others for mutual and common interests. That is, friends share feelings, help each other to resolve personal and interpersonal conflicts, and help each other solve personal problems.
4	15 on	*Autonomous Interdependent Friendships:* The individual sees relationships as complex and often overlapping systems. In a friendship, the adolescent or adult is aware that people have many needs and that in a good friendship each partner gives strong emotional and psychological support to the other, but also allows the friend to develop independent relationships. Respecting needs for both dependency and autonomy is seen as being essential to friendship.

The person who has a catastrophic illness or is dying has significant affectional needs. The nurse, then, needs to know intervention approaches that will facilitate meeting the person's interdependence needs by promoting and maintaining close relationships. Nurses also practice in settings with persons who are seeking health maintenance and health promotion. The parents who bring their infant daughter to a clinic for well-child examination also need support and affirmation from the nurse regarding their efforts to form a bonding relationship with the child. Some of the situations that interfere with this relationship include: low birth weight infants that require special care away from the parents; illness, incapacity, or absence of a parent during critical stages of the child's development; and a parent's own level of security within self that allows for the giving of self in the relationship. A nurse can often be the person available to identify difficulties and to help the family deal with establishing bonding relationships, even in altered situations where such bonding is more difficult.

Similarly, parents need information about sibling relationships and friendships. It seems unusual that children need to learn to play and to share. Perhaps the nurse would not be readily aware that parents need help in teaching this to their children. The nurse will often find them very receptive to her pointing out small observations about chilren's behavior and relating it to some basic knowledge about human interaction. The titles of the stages of friendship given by Selman (1980) provide some insight into knowledge the nurse may seek out to help such families: monetary playmate; one-way assistance; two-way fair weather coopera-tion; intimate, mutually shared relationships; and autonomous interde-pendent friendships. It is particularly important to see that in sibling and playmate relationships, as in any relationship, there are stages of grow-ing and changing that are normal development. During adulthood, rela-tionships also grow and need nourishment. Couples often turn to the nurse for help in maintaining their own mutually satisfying affectional relationship.

Finally, as noted, the nurse as a person, has interdependence needs. She experiences herself as a more adequate and effective person when her affectional needs are met by her family and persons in her work and social life. Further, when the nurse works in a very stressful environ-ment, in the hospital or community her need for supportive relationships increases.

Assessment of Behavior

The nurse begins assessing in the interdependence mode when meeting the client and is keenly attuned to listen for behaviors that the person might reveal spontaneously. After creating a comfortable milieu, the nurse proceeds with an indepth assessment of behaviors and stimuli. The nurse first assesses in the two major areas of behavior under significant other and support systems (Randell, Tedrow, and Van Landingham 1982). The first group of behaviors describes the person as a recipient of love, respect, and value while the second group of behaviors describes the per-son as the contributor or giver of love, value and respect. Table 18–2 demonstrates assessment in this mode. The criteria for behavioral assess-ment are listed in the first column. Methods to elicit the behaviors, that is, interview questions and observations, are listed in the second column. Samples of behavior (the results of behavioral assessment) that represent

TABLE 18–2. ASSESSMENT OF INTERDEPENDENCE MODE

Behavioral Assessment	Methods to Elicit Behaviors	Sample of Behaviors	Possible Stimuli
Significant Other(s): The most important person(s) in one's life	Interview, using some of these questions.	Contributive: "I tell him that I love him."	Need to give and receive love, respect, and value
Giving: Nurturing behaviors that one initiates	Who is the most important person in your life? How do you express your caring to that person?	"I plan activities for us to do." Holds his hand, "I really look forward to going home and being together again."	Expectations of the relationship Awareness of affectional needs
Receiving: Nurturing behaviors from another and ones response	How does that person express affection or caring to you?	Receptive: "I love the way he rubs my back."	Nurturing ability of both people Level of self-esteem
Support System(s) Other people, groups, or animals in ones life that contribute to one's affectional adequacy	How do you feel, about the other's expression of affection to you? Observe for nonverbal behaviors.	"Look at the pretty roses he brought me." "He calls me from work several times a day."	Interactional skills Presence of other in the physical environment Knowledge about friendship
Giving: As above	Touching, looking at each other, giving gifts,		Developmental age and tasks
Receiving: As above	sharing jokes or stories, general affect, body language, etc.		

giving and receiving categories are listed in the third column. Possible stimuli are in the final column.

Assessment of Stimuli

Seven stimuli that are most important when assessing in the interdependence mode are (1) expectations of the relationship and awareness of needs, (2) nurturing ability of both persons, (3) level of self-esteem, (4) level and kinds of interactional skills, (5) presence of the other in the physical environment, (6) knowledge about friendships and relationships, and (7) developmental age and tasks.

The *expectations* of the persons that are involved in the relationship affect the quality of the relationship. If the person expects that affection is expressed by physical proximity, by spending time together, by physical contact, and by remembering birthdays, it is important that the other person in the relationship be aware of and respond to these expectations. When two people in a relationship can define their expectations clearly and communicate them, the relationship is enhanced. Once each person is aware of expectations and needs of self and the other, it is essential that both act on this information in a consistent fashion.

The *nurturing ability* of each person in the relationship also contributes to the quality of the relationship. Nurturing involves providing growth-producing care and attention. A person who experienced early bonding as an infant and tactile and verbal loving as a child will usually be able to move into adult love relationships with ease. He or she has experienced a high-quality love relationship and knows what it feels like and what the characteristics are. An adult who experienced delayed bonding or minimal bonding with a parent-child relationship that was characterized by distance, separation, and verbal negating will probably need help in learning how to build a friendship or love relationship. Likewise, traumatic experiences in the early school years, for example, loss of a parent, may interfere with later effective nurturing ability.

The *level of self-esteem,* as related to the self-concept mode, is an influencing factor for interdependence relationships. People tend to choose friendships and love relationships with persons who have a similar level of self-esteem; that is, people who have low self-esteem choose as friends people with low self-esteem. They then are reinforced in the feelings of negative self-worth and the circular process continues. Similarly, when two people, both of whom experience high self-esteem, develop a caring relationship, the reinforcement from the other serves to enhance the already high level of self-esteem. A person's level of self esteem influences the degree to which the person feels that he or she can go out to others. Likewise, self esteem will be a basic contextual factor for the person to handle the circumstances in life in which the opportunities for receiving love, value, and respect change, for example, the permanent absence of one who has been a significant other for the person.

The level and type of *interactional skills* are closely related to the level of self-esteem. If the person has open communication, is flexible, can articulate clearly, and is sensitive to the other's verbal and nonverbal behavior, the relationship is facilitated. If one of the partners does not have the interactional skills at the level desired, those skills can be learned with help. Learning may begin with recognizing that one needs to learn better skills. Many self help books are available and can make enjoyable reading. However, the person will often want feedback from a knowledgable person as he or she makes the changes which are desired.

The *presence* of the other in the physical environment influences the relationship. If friends or a couple are separated often and for long periods, it is more difficult to maintain the relationship. The presence needed for maternal bonding is an area of relationships that is being studied. Attachment occurs more readily when mother and baby have frequent and early access to each other. Any relationship is maintained more easily when proximity is possible.

Knowledge about friendship and how to build or maintain a relationship is an important stimulus. There are many theoretical discussions of friendship available. McGinnis (1980) described five activities that can deepen a friendship: (1) to put friendships or relationships first or give them top priority; (2) to talk about and express your affection for the other person; (3) to create space in the friendship so that both people can maintain their identity and autonomy; (4) to cultivate the art of affirmation, making sure that the other person knows what you value about him or her as a person; and (5) to accept your own and the other person's anger on a temporary basis. When a person has developed nurturing ability and has significant knowledge regarding the dynamics of friendship, there is a greater possibility of an indepth relationship.

The final influencing factor noted here is *developmental age* or developmental tasks or crisis. A number of theories of human development have been described. Three such theories that are particularly relevent to understanding how interdependence behavior develops are those described by Erikson (1963), Havighurst (1953) and Selman (1980). The reader is encouraged to consult the primary sources for further information. The common stimuli affecting the interdependence mode are listed in Table 18-2. In summary the degree of influence of each stimuli varies at different stages of the lifespan.

Nursing Diagnosis

The next step in the nursing process is to make nursing judgments about the data collected. This judgment reflects whether or not the behaviors indicate that the need underlying the mode is being met. In the interdependence mode, that means that the person is experiencing affectional adequacy and that the needs for love, respect, and value are being met. If this is so, the diagnosis might be stated: The patient is experiencing affectional adequacy due to (focal and contextual stimuli), for example, significant other's presence and nurturing ability, and mastery of the developmental task of maintaining a strong and mutually satisfying relationship with another. If the person is not experiencing affectional adequacy, the diagnostic statement would include relevant stimuli such as the absence of a significant other, not having learned how to communicate effectively, and/or not having learned how to nurture others.

Examples of nursing diagnoses illustrating ineffective adaptation in the interdependence mode using the three ways of stating these are provided in Chapter 19.

Goal Setting

Goals are set in collaboration with the client whenever possible. They may be general or specific. An example of goals in the interdependence mode might be: "Within two weeks, the patient will state that she feels loved and supported," or "Before the next visit, the patient will discuss with her significant other the nature of her nurturing needs"; or "The person will join a club and develop one friendship within the next month." Goals in the interdependence mode may be either short term or long term, and focus on achieving affectional adequacy. Each of the examples above identifies a specific behavior, the change expected and the time frame for achievement of the goal.

Intervention

Nursing interventions are implemented after the goals have been mutually set with the person. Interventions manage the stimuli to allow the person to maintain or make an adaptive response. Stimuli frequently involved in intervention within this mode are the seven influencing factors discussed earlier and listed in Table 18–2. The nurse generally uses herself purposefully to explore with the person, and possibly the significant other, understanding of nurturing needs, communication skills and knowledge about the self and others in close relationships. The nurse, in initiating, maintaining, and terminating a relationship with a person, has rich opportunities to provide a model of the process of developing a relationship. The nurse also can use herself therapeutically in the area of physical touch. A backrub or sitting and holding a person's hand while the person is in pain are both nurturing activities. The ultimate goal of intervention is to help the person learn how to elicit from others the nurturing they need and to reciprocate love and caring (Brown 1984 and Tedrow 1984).

Evaluation

The final step in the nursing process is to evaluate the effectiveness of intervention. This means that behaviors are reassessed and the behaviors are compared with the behavioral goals. In the interdependence mode, the behaviors that are assessed are giving and receiving behaviors. The person is the best judge of whether affectional adequacy has been attained through mutually satisfying relationships. Depending on the evaluation, the process either ends here or revision and further planning are instituted as needed.

SUMMARY

This chapter has defined and discussed the interdependence mode of the Roy Adaptation Model for nursing. The mode is social in nature and has as its goal affectional adequacy. This is accomplished through relationships with significant others and support systems. Examples of the development of this mode in friendship and love relationships were discussed. The adaptation nursing process as is summarized in Figure 18–4 was

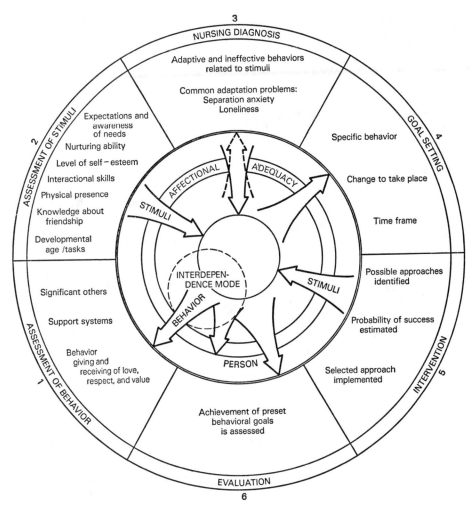

Figure 18–4. The nursing process applied to the interdependence mode

applied to the interdependence mode. Seven common stimuli affecting interdependence behaviors were explored.

Nurses frequently meet persons who are experiencing disrupted wellness or illness. People who are ill or in a state of change usually experience an increased need for love, respect, and affirmation. The nurse is concerned about the interdependence mode of her clients as well as herself.

EXERCISES FOR APPLICATION

1. Relative to your own interdependence behavior and using Figure 18.2 as a guide, identify your significant others and support systems.

    2. In your relationship with one significant other, identify your own giving and receiving behaviors.

    3. Identify at least five stimuli that influence the relationship that you identified and describe how they influence the relationship.

ASSESSMENT OF UNDERSTANDING

Questions

    1. Which of the following statements directly apply to the interdependence mode?
      a. It relates to the psychological integrity of the individual.
      b. It involves the giving and receiving of love, respect, and value.
      c. It focuses on relationships with significant others and support systems.
      d. It involves meeting needs through social interaction.
      e. It involves nurturing relationships.
      f. It has as its basic need the need to know who one is in relation to others.

    2. Which of the following descriptions of behavioral data relate to the interdependence mode?
      a. 40-year-old generative male.
      b. Support system-extended family.
      c. "I love my wife very much."
      d. "Have a chocolate. My husband brought them."
      e. "Joe has always been such a help to me."
      f. "I really appreciate all the time you spend with me."
      g. Occupation-teacher.

    3. List the eight stimuli that were identified in this chapter as commonly influencing adaptation in the interdependence mode.
      a.
      b.
      c.
      d.
      e.
      f.
      g.
      h.

Situation: Joe Russell is a 32-year-old man. He has been married to Sophia Lopez for three years. He works as an accountant for the telephone company. Joe is active in his church, belongs to a theology study group, and is a counselor for the senior high youth group. An interview with Joe reveals that his best friend is Sophia. His other friends are the six people in the theology class, the minister of education at the church, and the accountant, Arthur, with whom he shares an office. His parents live about 2 hours away, and he likes them. He has no siblings. Sophia's mom lives an hour away, and Joe thinks "she's a crazy but neat lady."

4. Derive a nursing diagnosis reflecting Joe's adaptive interdependence.
5. Identify a goal related to Joe's support systems.
6. Interventions associated with Joe's affectional adequacy, according to the approach presented, could be directed at maintenance of which of the following stimuli?
   a. nurturing ability
   b. communication skills
   c. moral-ethical-spiritual self
   d. giving behaviors
7. Identify two factors that would indicate the maintenance of affectional adequacy in Joe's situation.

Feedback

1. b, c, d, e (a relates to self concept and e to roles).
2. b, c, d, e, f (a and g are both roles).
3. a. The need to give and receive love, respect, and value
   b. Expectations of the relationship and awareness of needs
   c. Nurturing ability of both persons
   d. Level of self-esteem
   e. Level and kinds of interactional skills
   f. Presence in the physical environment
   g. Knowledge about friendship
   h. Developmental age and tasks
4. Examples: Mutually satisfying relationship with significant other evidenced by his statement that she is his best friend.
   Affectional adequacy as evidenced by multiple support systems and mutual satisfying relationship with significant other.
5. Joe will continue to maintain his relationships with his support systems over the ensuing months.
6. a and b.
7. Examples: Continued satisfying relationship with significant other. Continued maintenance of support systems.

REFERENCES

Andrews, H., and Sr. C. Roy, *Essentials of the Roy Adaptation Model*, East Norwalk, Conn., Appleton-Century-Crofts, 1986.
Berkman, B. Mental health and the aging: A review of the literature for clinical social workers, *Clinical Social Work Journal*, 6; pp. 230–245, 1978.

Brown, S.A. Loneliness, in *Introduction to Nursing: An Adaptation Model* (2nd ed.), Sr. C. Roy, pp. 442–457. Englewood Cliffs, N.J.: Prentice-Hall, 1984.

Caplan, G. (ed) *Support Systems and Community Mental Health.* New York: Behavioral Publications, 1974.

Cobb, S. Social support as a moderator of life stress, *Psychosomatic Medicine,* 38:300–312, 1976.

Cohen, S.S.L.: *Social Support and Health.* New York, Academic Press, 1985.

Dimond M., and S.L. Jones. Social support: A review and theoretical integration, in *Advances in Nursing Theory Development,* ed. Chinn, P.L. Rockville, Md, Aspen Publishers, 235–249, 1983.

Dobratz, M.C. Life closure, in *Introduction to Nursing: An Adaptation Model* (2nd ed.), Sr. C. Roy, pp. 497–518. Englewood Cliffs, N.J.: Prentice-Hall, 1984.

Erikson, E.H. *Childhood and Society.* New York: W.W. Norton & Company, Inc., 1963.

Fromm-Reichmann, F. Loneliness, *Psychiatry,* 22: 3, 1959.

Fromm, E. *The Art of Loving.* New York: Harper & Row, Publishers, 1956.

Gottlieb, B.H. (ed): *Social Networks and Social Support.* Beverly Hills, Calif.: Sage, 1981.

Greenblatt, M., R., Becerra, and E.A. Serafetinides. Social networks and mental health: An overview, *American Journal of Psychiatry,* 8:977–984, 1982.

Havighurst, R.J. *Human Development and Education.* New York: Longman, Inc., 1953.

House, J., K. Landis, and D. Umberson, Social relationship and health, *Science* vol. 241 (July 29) 540–545. 1988.

Kane, C.F. Family social support: Toward a conceptual model, *Advances in Nursing Science,* 10 (2): 188–225, 1988.

McGinnis, L. *The Friendship Factor: How to Get Closer to the People You Care For.* Minneapolis: Augsburg Publishing House, 1980.

Maslow, A.H. *Motivation and Personality.* New York: Harper and Row, 1954.

Randell, B., M. Tedrow, and J. Van Landingham, *Adaptation Nursing: The Roy Conceptual Model Applied.* St. Louis: The C.V. Mosby Co., 1982.

Roy, Sr. C. A systems model of nursing care and its effect on quality of human life, in ed. G.E. Lakser, *Applied Systems and Cybernetics,* vol. IV, New York: Pergamon Press, pp. 1705–1714. 1981.

Selman, R.C. *The Growth of Interpersonal Understanding: Development and Clinical Analyses.* New York: Academic Press, Inc., 1980.

Spitz, R. Hospitalism: An inquiry into the genesis of psychiatric conditions in early childhood, in *The Psychoanalytic Study of the Child,* eds. Feinichel et. al., vol. 1, 0. New York: International Universities Press, 1945.

Tedrow, M.P. Interdependence: Theory and development, in *Introduction to Nursing: An Adaptation Model* (2nd ed), Sr. C. Roy, pp. 306–322. Englewood Cliffs, N.J.: Prentice-Hall, 1984.

Waldo, A.L. *Sacajawea.* New York: Avon Books, 1978.

Additional References

Antonucci, T.C., Social support networks: A hierarchal mapping technique, *Generations* X, 10–12, 1986.

Antonucci, T.C., and J.S. Jackson. The role of social support in health promotion and illness prevention, *Generations* X, 10–12, 1987.

Buchda, T. Loneliness in critically ill adults, *DCCN* 1987, November–December (6), 335–340.

Capel, L.C. Loneliness: A conceptual model. *The Journal of Psychosocial Nursing Mental Health Services,* January; 26 (1) 14–19, 36, 38, 1988.

Freed, Alvyn. *Transactional Analysis for Tots.* Sacramento, Calif.: Jalmar Press, Inc., 1973.

Greenwald, J.A. Self-induced loneliness, *Voices: The Art and Science of Psychotherapy,* 8: 17–21, 1972.

Kalish, R.A. *The Psychology of Human Behavior.* Belmont, Calif.: Wadsworth Publishing Company, Inc., 1966.

Klaus, M., and J. Kennell. *Parent-Infant Bonding* 2nd ed. St. Louis: The C.V. Mosby Company, 1981.

Leininger, M.M. *Caring: An Essential Human Need.* Thoroface, N.J.: Charles B. Slack, Inc., 1981.

Lowry, R.A. *The Journals of A.H. Maslow,* vols. I & II. Monterey: Brooks/Cole Publishing Company, 1979.

Mahler, M.S., F. Pine, and A. Bergman. *The Psychological Birth of the Human Infant.* New York: Basic Books, Inc., Publishers, 1975.

Moustakas, C. E. *Loneliness and Love.* Englewood Cliffs, N.J.: Prentice-Hall, Inc., 1972.

Toffler, A. *Future Shock.* New York: Random House, Inc., 1970.

Chapter Nineteen ───────────

Separation Anxiety and Loneliness*

*Jane Servonsky and
Mary Poush Tedrow*

As was presented in Chapter 18, the interdependence mode is the mode in which affectional needs are met. Affectional needs represent the person's striving for relationships in life that provide the individual with a feeling of security in being nurtured, that is, in receiving growth-producing care and attention. The reciprocal nature of the mode is demonstrated by the person's willingness and ability both to give and to receive love, respect, and value within the relationship. Problems arise that stem from the interdependence mode when affectional needs are not met. Two such problems that occur frequently in North American society are termed separation anxiety and loneliness.

This chapter provides a theoretical overview of separation anxiety and loneliness and demonstrates how the nursing process based on the Roy Adaptation Model is used in meeting the needs of those who have this kind of unmet affectional need. The nurse, knowing that there are crisis periods for separation from the significant other, can reinforce or bring about a change in stimuli to decrease the intensity of the effect of the separation from a significant other and the effect of loneliness on the person's adaptation.

OBJECTIVES

After studying this chapter, the reader will be able to do the following:

1. Describe separation anxiety and loneliness as adaptation problem of the interdependence mode.

*The original work on loneliness as it relates to the Roy Adaptation Model was done by Sue Ann Brown in the chapter "Problem of Interdependence: Loneliness," in the first edition of *Introduction to Nursing: An Adaptation Model*, Sister Callista Roy, Englewood Cliffs, N.J.: Prentice-Hall, 1976, pp. 342–356.

2. Identify behaviors associated with separation anxiety and loneliness.
3. Describe common stimuli contributing to separation anxiety and loneliness.
4. State nursing diagnoses for ineffective adaptation in the interdependence mode.
5. Given a situation, construct a goal related to separation anxiety or loneliness.
6. Suggest nursing interventions commonly used in situations of separation anxiety and loneliness.
7. Describe the evaluation of the effectiveness of nursing interventions in the interdependence mode.

KEY CONCEPTS DEFINED

- *Alienation:* A condition or feeling of being estranged or separated from self or others.
- *Aloneness:* A chosen state of being by oneself.
- *Bonding/Attachment:* A reciprocal joining or unity between two persons.
- *Loneliness:* The exceedingly unpleasant and driving experience connected with an inadequate discharge of the need for human intimacy, for interpersonal intimacy.
- *Lonely:* Missing the contact of another who is far from one either by death, other physical separation or emotional separateness.
- *Separation anxiety:* The painful uneasiness of mind experienced by a person who is separated from a significant other.
- *Separation-Individuation:* The process by which the person is separated from the primary care giver and becomes an individual self.

DESCRIPTION OF SEPARATION ANXIETY AND LONELINESS

There is a saying: "If you can't make it with people, you can't make it." Moustakas (1972) pointed out its corollary, "If you can only make it with people and not alone, you can't make it." This precept points out some of the problems that exist in the interdependence mode of adaptation.

Separation Anxiety
Separation anxiety is the painful uneasiness of mind related to separation from a significant other. Since the focal stimulus for this condition is the actual or threatened separation from a significant other, it is isolated as a problem of the interdependence mode. Separation anxiety is first experienced in infancy and the person then has the potential for experiencing it

throughout the life span. There are developmental crises in the person's life that create a vulnerable period for anxiety related to separation. These developmental crises are addressed in the works of Mahler (1979), Bowlby (1969, 1973), Robertson (1953), and Erikson (1963).

The infant is separated physiologically at birth from the mother with the cutting of the umbilical cord. The beginning of emotional separation occurs during later stages of development. Before emotional separation can occur, emotional bonding or attachment with the significant other must occur (Klaus and Kennel 1981). *Bonding* is a term that describes a reciprocal joining or unity. It begins for the woman as she experiences pregnancy and proceeds through the tasks of pregnancy. Bonding probably begins for the fetus during this time, but is accelerated during and immediately following birth. By the time the child is ready to enter school, a process of bonding and attachment followed by a stage of separation and becoming a distinct separate individual has occurred. It is after that attachment phase and during the *separation-individuation* phase that separation anxiety first occurs and is most intense.

Mahler (1979) described three phases of the attachment-separation process that are experienced in sequence. The first phase, *autism,* occurs during the first few weeks of life. The infant does not differentiate the self from the environment, but does learn to differentiate between pain and pleasure. The second phase, the *symbiotic* phase, refers to the attachment to the mother. At this time, about one month of age, the infant does not differentiate the self from the nonself but does attach to the mother. Mahler's third phase, the *separation-individuation* process, begins soon after the symbiotic or attachment phase.

There is a four-part progression that occurs during the separation-individuation process. *Separation* refers to separation from the constant care giver (usually the mother). *Individuation* refers to clearly becoming a self. The first subphase is termed *differentiation* and emerges as the infant becomes mobile by creeping, walking, climbing, and exploring self and the environment. The infant stays near the mother and enjoys playing games with objects and people that repeatedly disappear and reappear, such as "where did it go?" and "peek-a-boo." The next subphase is termed *practicing,* during which the child explores the environment near the mother and develops motor skills. The child in this stage accepts strangers readily as long as mother is near and the stranger does not approach. The next subphase, *rapprochement,* is one in which the child actively resists separation. It is manifested by the toddler using negative behavior, such as repeatedly saying "no," or self-identity behavior such as saying "me" and "mine." There is an intense period of growth in the formation of the self-concept mode during the rapprochement phase. The separation from the mother is for longer periods, but the toddler continues to return to her frequently. The self-concept and interdependence modes are interconnected closely at this point of the toddler's life. The final subphase, *object constancy,* occurs from 18 to 36 months of age. The child develops intrapsychic symbols for the significant other. This development enables the child to begin separating without the overwhelming fear of abandonment.

Early work in separation anxiety was done by Robertson (1953) and Bowlby (1969). These authors described the infant between 3 and 6 months of age as recognizing the mother as an individual. They defined the period of 18 to 24 months as a time of peak dependency on the care giver. The child at this time is possessively and passionately attached to the mother. The child is overwhelmed when the mother is separated from him or her. Bowlby and Robertson documented on film the behavior of children who were separated at the time of hospitalization. They defined three stages of separation anxiety through which the children proceed if their significant other is separated from them: protest, despair, and denial (detachment).

In the *protest stage,* children are acutely aware of their need for their mothers. They will do anything and do it vigorously to recapture their mothers. They do believe that their energetic protesting behaviors will, in fact, return their mothers to their sides.

The next stage of separation that children move to in a few hours or days is the stage of *despair.* During this stage, children are actively mourning the loss of the significant other and they withdraw. While mourning, each child remains preoccupied with the loss of the mother and remains vigilant for her return. It is the quiet phase of separation anxiety. The child is passive and will perform self-comforting activities such as thumb sucking or clinging to a favorite toy.

The final phase of *denial (detachment)* is moved into slowly. At this point, children repress the need for their mothers and begin to be interested in the environment. Children begin to seek comfort in food and support from anyone who will give it to them. A stranger viewing a child at this stage would tend to remark on how well adjusted the child has become.

When the parents return, the child who has gone only as far as the stage of despair will usually reject the parents initially and then respond to them slowly. The attachment is reestablished slowly as the child and significant other are reunited. Passing through these stages to a resolution hopefully will lead to a more comfortable separation another time. Although separation experiences are essential to the development of the individual, they should be minimized during periods of increased stress, such as hospitalization. These early works of Robertson and Bowlby have been helpful in the movement of extending visiting hours in pediatric hospitals and instituting policies of rooming-in for parents and families so that they may stay with the child at this time.

Erikson (1963) identified eight developmental crises (stages) that are to be mastered sequentially through the life span. These were identified in Chapter 16. The tasks of infancy and early childhood relevant here are building trust and achieving autonomy. Thus another theorist described the attachment and separation through which the child must proceed to attain a separate identity.

Ainsworth (1977) and Mead (1971) explored child behavior in other cultures. Ainsworth studied children and parents in Uganda and Mead, in Samoa. Both cultures have extended family units with many adults in the child's environment. Both researchers documented that the infant did not attach as intensely to the mother and therefore did not experience the degree of separation anxiety that children do who are reared in a society without extended families.

Another crisis period for separation anxiety occurs for the school-aged child with the beginning and the end of the school year. Phenomena identified as "school phobias" are frequently separation anxiety. Ezor (1980) studied the separation anxiety related to school. The adolescent experiences separation anxiety with high frequency. This chaotic period is not unlike the toddler period, with an emphasis on clarifying one's identity and again separating from one's parents. Separation from the peer group also causes anxiety.

The adult may experience separation anxiety. Some examples of adult separation anxiety are the couple who is separating for a long period for a business or a family commitment. During the process of saying "goodbye," the stages of protest, despair, and denial (detachment) may be experienced. Protest is manifested by such statements as "I wish you weren't going" or "I'd like to be going with you." Feelings related to the protest stage are feelings of anxiety surrounding the actual separation and the projected time alone. The despair state may be manifested by behaviors of listlessness and lack of interest in the environment or anger behaviors. Many couples experience feelings and behaviors of anger that are unexpected and disturbing to them as they separate. Most adults move into detachment quickly, maintain the relationship in whatever way is possible, and look forward to being reunited and the resolution stage.

When living in a highly mobile society, adults and children terminate from their support systems with some frequency. Stanford's (1977) work with groups, especially cohesive groups, reported on separation anxiety as a group comes to a closure. If a person has given importance to the group, he or she probably will demonstrate many of the behaviors identified by Stanford.

Although Stanford's work was with students, it appears that his observations may relate to individuals in the general population who are terminating with a group. Stanford's behaviors of termination anxiety are:

1. *Increased conflict.* Students may start bickering with one another for no apparent reason, or at least no significant reason. It is almost as though they were trying to prove to themselves that "I

don't really like these people, else I wouldn't be fighting with
them. And since I don't like them, it won't be painful for me to
leave them."

2. *Breakdown of group skills.* Working together on a task, the group
may suddenly exhibit what appears to be a complete lack of skills,
and they may violate all the norms that were established previously. It is almost as though they were saying to themselves and
the teacher, "You see, we really didn't change much this year.
We're still like every other class. And since this is like every other
class, it won't be so hard to leave."

3. *Lethargy.* Some students begin to show less and less interest in
their work, as if to say, "What does it matter any more? If we're
going to have to break up, what's the use of continuing to work?"
Their lethargy may also be a symptom of depression indicating
feelings of sadness about the imminent breakup of the group.

4. *Frantic attempts to work well.* Conversely, some groups may actually increase their productivity, taking on more and more projects
and rushing to do everything they can before the term ends. They
may display impeccable group skills, working far more effectively
than ever before. Implicit in this behavior may be the message, "If
we're a model class, maybe the teacher will like us so much we
won't have to leave. Maybe our group can continue forever."

Thus separation anxiety can be demonstrated throughout the life
span, all caused by a temporary separation from the significant other or a
support system.

The nurse using the Roy Adaptation Model needs to understand
clearly the developmental tasks of the life span as they relate to affectional integrity. As nurses work with people in various health situations,
they assess and intervene frequently in the interdependence mode. This
is especially true with the newborn infant, the young child, and the significant others. The quality of the child's later life in the area of affectional adequacy is strongly related to what occurs in the infant and the
young child periods. Through intervention, the nurse can help the child or
adult reach higher levels of adaptation and integrity in the interdependence mode. Because of the particular vulnerability of the child to separation anxiety and the more extensive knowledge available in this area,
separation anxiety in the child is the example used to demonstrate use of
the nursing process according to the Roy Adaptation Model.

Loneliness

From the aged individual to the infant, from the economically privileged
person to the more deprived, loneliness exists as a common adaptation
problem. No one is immunized against loneliness; it is a lifelong struggle
for everyone to maintain affectional adequacy. The person who has mutu-

ally satisfying relationships, experiences periods of loneliness and alienation as illustrated in Figure 19–1.

The person who does not attain affectional adequacy and who, for the greater part, may have no or very few satisfying relationships suffers great emotional pain. *Alienation* is a condition or feeling of being estranged or separated from self and others. One develops alienated feelings when significant others are not meeting what is expected as one's supplier of affiliation. This deprivation of presence or contact leads to a feeling of not being needed, valued, or appreciated by others, and therein lies the roots of loneliness.

Alienation is a serious problem in contemporary society. Many social theorists have written on its pervasiveness in North American life and on the contextual factors that affect this pattern. Among these are computerization, diminishing of the family as the basic unit of society, mobility, and urbanization. Early childhood experiences of affectional adequacy or inadequacy can further contribute to interdependence adaptation. Socially, friends seem to be transient, families are physically separated, and after all, "Who does care what happens to me?" Many more persons end up living in the streets because they have no human ties that can be of help in a housing crisis. That alienation exists is undeniable. Particularly

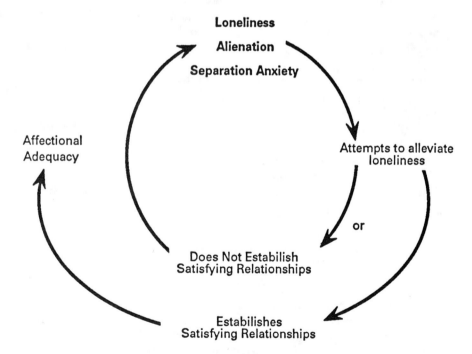

Figure 19–1. Affectional inadequacy *Seeks out friendships, rebellion, acceptance of loneliness, withdrawal, ritualistic behavior, chemical or sexual abuse.*

because of the contemporary situation, people in our society have a good to excellent chance of developing one of the variants of alienation. The major types of alienation were described by Seeman (1959) as powerlessness, meaninglessness, normlessness, isolation, or self-estrangement. Any of these types of alienation can cause the individual to feel further separated from others.

Some individuals can handle these alienated feelings by innovative ways of building relationships. An example of this is the young adult who appraises the situation and says that things are not good, not the way one would like to have them, but recognizes that they do not have to remain as such. The individual proceeds to become involved in changing things and building relationships.

Persons will use less positive means to deal with alienated feelings. These avenues involve a dependency on things or others to ward off alienated feelings. There is a pattern of using "something" to act as a bridge to relationships. These patterns include: (1) dependency on a lifestyle that emphasizes withdrawal and retreatism to feel secure; (2) dependency on performing ritualistic behaviors to deal with anxieties of alienation (chain smoking, over eating, psychosomatic illness, or any activity that is done in excess to stay busy); (3) rebelling against society by joining an alternate cultural group with subsequent dependency on it (drug culture, alcoholic state, sexual variancy groups, for example); and (4) dependency on situations retaining the status quo. This individual sees no possibility for change and considers turning against the world as the only way to deal with alienation.

Some of these alternatives can be so ineffective as to stimulate self-concept disruption. An example of this would be the individual who chooses to withdraw from the real world and stay in a fantasy existence. This condition is referred to as *self-alienation* and can involve a total collapse of one's self concept.

Alienated feelings lead to ideas of not being accepted, valued, or appreciated by others. To develop lonely feelings is the next logical step for the alienated person. The cycle of events in affectional inadequacy is demonstrated in Figure 19–1.

APPLICATION OF THE NURSING PROCESS

The nurse using the Roy Adaptation Model views each person as a whole, integrated human being. When needs are not being met in one mode or component, a decreased level of adaptation is experienced. In responding to the needs of patients, the nurse anticipates stimuli that might decrease the level of adaptation or works with a person after they have experienced a decreased level of affectional adequacy. The nurse's goal is to promote the highest level of adaptation and integrity that the person can attain.

Assessment of Behavior

The first step in assessment focuses on behavioral manifestations of separation anxiety and loneliness. For example, the child experiencing separation anxiety will present behaviors as identified by Robertson (1970) for the states of protest, despair, and denial (detachment). Behaviors associated with loneliness, such as inattention to physical appearance, may be difficult to differentiate initially from self-concept problems. This presentation of assessment focuses on each of the problems individually.

Separation Anxiety. Each person is unique in his or her response to separation. Therefore, the discussion of behavioral manifestations of these stages serves only as a general guideline for the expected behaviors.

In the initial stage of *protest,* the child has a strong desire for the significant other and expects the significant other to respond to the protesting behavior. The child may present with restlessness, crying, screaming, and physical clinging as the significant others depart. The child will grieve and is inconsolable, constantly calling for the significant others and watching eagerly for their return. Since the child is unable to comprehend this experience, he or she will feel truly deserted by the significant others. Comforting and attention given to the child by another person at this time may be rejected. For example, when two-year-old Elizabeth was hospitalized, her mother, a single parent, was unable to stay due to her work schedule. Elizabeth cried, screamed, and protested constantly for her mother during her three-day stay in the hospital. She rejected all care and attention given to her by the nursing staff.

During despair, the second stage of separation anxiety, the child may present behaviors of depression and withdrawal. The child will appear quiet, less active, and without sensation or feeling. The child mourns the loss of the significant other and feels increasing hopelessness. It is important during this stage not to mistake the behaviors of apathy as a sign of adaptation to the stress of separation. There may be disinterest in play or food. Behaviors demonstrating regression of developmental tasks previously mastered may be exhibited. These might include bed wetting, loss of established vocabulary, and other learned skills. Self-comforting coping mechanisms may be initiated by the child such as thumb sucking or clinging to a favorite toy or blanket. At the sight of the significant other, the child may again present protest behaviors. Care administered by the substitute care giver may no longer be resisted during this stage.

Denial, the third stage of the separation response, is also referred to as detachment. During this stage, superficially it appears that the child has adapted to the loss of the significant other. The child will show more interest in the surroundings, appear happy, and begin to play with others. The child detaches from the significant other, and the behaviors of this stage are a result of resignation because the child can no longer cope with the emotional distress of separation. The response of the child is not a sign of contentment, but rather is based on repression of feelings for the significant other. The child copes during this stage by establishing shallow relationships with substitute care givers, but avoids closeness with any one person. The child will become increasingly self centered and may no longer react when the significant other comes or leaves. A typical pattern is that the child will not respond to the significant other at first, but then gradually reestablishes contact.

Loneliness. With the adaptation problem of loneliness, the predominant theme is one of not being able to extend oneself to another for contact. Since the person sees one's own actions as ineffective, motivation to do anything decreases. Nothing matters enough to the individual to require attention. One begins to identify ineffective behaviors in other modes— self esteem diminishes, role failures begin to develop, and physical appearance may be neglected. Symptoms of anxiety, that is, the emotional pain a person suffers from viewing one's own dilemma with tunnel vision, are manifest in different ways by each individual.

Another group of behaviors revolves around depressive behaviors. How, then, can loneliness as an interdependency problem be distinguished? Once assessment of behavior and stimuli have been accomplished, the problem and the source of it become evident. Anxiety and depressive behaviors may not be the chief concern when it is identified that loneliness is occurring and is the cause of the anxiety or depression.

Behaviors of loneliness may be contentment to let others care for one; abuse of another person's attempt to help such as monopolizing a staff person's time; a clinging love relationship; a lack of a broad range of interests; and only tacit acceptance of those that could be satisfying. Loneliness behaviors are categorized often in the "receiving" category and these may be few in number. There are few or no "giving" behaviors. The person who is lonely has learned how to take the nurturing given by others but, for some reason, has not learned how to give nurturing effectively or to maintain the relationship (Brown 1984).

Assessment of Stimuli

In the second step of the nursing process, the nurse assesses the factors affecting the identified behaviors related to separation anxiety and loneliness.

Separation Anxiety. The focal stimulus contributing to the separation behaviors is separation or absence of the significant other. The nurse identifies the **length in time** that the separation will or has occurred and assesses if the separation is only temporary or will continue for some time. For example, the mother who has to be away from a young child while she is giving birth to a new baby will be absent for a much shorter time when compared to the mother who will be hospitalized for many months due to a serious illness.

Other stimuli that the nurse assesses include the **degree of attachment** or bonding to the significant other that has occurred. This factor will depend, in large part, on the age of the child. The amount of usual separation and the extent of social contacts within and outside of the immediate family are further important stimuli. For example, if the child has had an exclusive relationship with the significant other and has not been given the opportunity to deal with separation, the response may be more severe. The nurse assesses the child's **preparation for the separation** and identifies what the significant other has told the child about the separation. The child's coping abilities are identified and these will depend on the child's cognitive and maturational levels.

One of the most important stimuli is the **age and developmental level** of the person. Separation anxiety is a major stress from middle infancy throughout the preschool years. The age and developmental level of the child greatly influence emotional and physical response to the separation and the ability to adapt and cope with the stress. In general, infants by the end of the first six months are able to recognize their significant others and indeed are strongly attached to them. When separated from the significant other the infant will display displeasure with cries and screams, and reject the attention of strangers.

Infants and toddlers are not yet able to comprehend that objects continue to exist even though they are out of sight. Toddlers will present behaviors of protest, despair, and denial as outlined in the preceding section. Preschoolers can tolerate brief periods of separation from their significant other and are able to establish trust in another significant person. If preschoolers are stressed with illness and are unable to cope, they will manifest the behavioral stages as described earlier. However, the protesting stage will be less aggressive and more passive in this age group. The school-age child will experience separation from the significant other as well as peers. However, as the child matures and coping abilities increase, the child will be better able to deal with the separation. When separation does occur, the school-age child may demonstrate behaviors of displaced anger, hostility, loneliness, boredom, frustration, depression, eating problems, or withdrawal. As the child becomes older and more verbal, the need to act out feelings is decreased. The adolescent group will experience separation especially from the peer group. The adolescent may manifest a response to separation through behaviors of depression, loneliness, withdrawal, or boredom.

The nurse also assesses if the person is **ill, hospitalized, or in pain,** for the separation response may be enhanced by these additional stimuli. For example, a five-year-old child may present behaviors of the protesting stage if he or she is separated from the significant other when ill and/or in pain.

Assessment of the significant other's **knowledge level** regarding the separation behavioral response is important since the participation in and understanding of the situation will enhance or delay the child's coping abilities.

The **environment** where the separation is taking place is important to identify. Strange surroundings with unfamiliar sights and sounds will create additional stress during the separation experience.

Loneliness. When the behaviors that are assessed indicate loneliness, the following stimuli and their considerations are representative. In considering contextual stimuli, it is often the case that, although one is not physically removed from others, one may feel lonely in a crowd. The individual may not be able to make contact with anyone. If an individual is a member of many different groups, the chances of finding someone with whom to establish true contact may be increased. Both adolescents and adults seem to get into ruts of doing everything with the same people. These are some of the contextual stimuli that tend to contribute to loneliness.

Other stimuli one may see in the lonely person are usually related to the development of **ineffective interactional skills.** One important stimulus is interactions tending toward withdrawal from others. As was pointed out in Chapter 16, roles exist only when they are identifiable by the other's presence. For example, a mother cannot be a mother without a child. Consequently, if a person withdraws or society at large withdraws from the person, the individual cannot exist in relationship with the one withdrawing. One has difficulty being in contact with a removed person or thing. **Lack of contacts** could be an aspect in developing loneliness.

An example of such withdrawal by society could be a person who is imprisoned. Contact is lost with the majority of the population and things that establish feelings of belonging are not available. This type of withdrawal is overt. Society also can unconsciously and covertly withdraw. Examples of this are seen in reactions of some to terminal illness, disfigurement, or the physically or mentally disabled.

Nursing Diagnosis

Once assessment of behavior and stimuli relative to the interdependence mode has been accomplished, nursing diagnoses are formulated. As has been illustrated previously, nursing diagnoses are statements that relate behaviors with the factors influencing them. In the Roy Adaptation Model, these can be stated in three ways: (1) a statement of the behaviors within one mode with their most relevant influencing stimuli, (2) a summary label for behaviors in one mode with relevant stimuli, or (3) a label that summarizes a behavioral pattern when more than one mode is being affected by the same stimuli.

In situations of separation anxiety, the nursing diagnosis should reflect the stage of separation response that has been assessed. An example of this could be: "The child is in the protest stage of separation anxiety related to the prolonged absence of the ill mother." This diagnosis illustrates method two. For method one, specific behaviors would be identified with the stimulus(i) influencing them: "Crying, screaming, and physical clinging related to mother's impending departure" is an example.

In a situation where loneliness has been identified, a diagnosis using the third method could be: "Loneliness due to existence as a recluse." Conveyed in the term "loneliness" are a multitude of behaviors associated with that common adaptation problem including low self esteem, role failure, neglected physical appearance, and the absence of "giving" behaviors.

Goal Setting

In establishing goals associated with the adaptation problems of separation anxiety and loneliness, the same principles as have been emphasized in previous chapters apply. Goals will identify a specific behavior, the change expected, and the associated time frame.

The goals for a person experiencing separation anxiety will depend on the stage of response. The child who is protesting is allowed to protest. An example of a stated goal is: "The child will remain in the protest stage for one more day." The long term goal may be for the child to accept love, support, care, and reestablishment of a trusting relationship with a substitute care giver within the next two weeks.

In loneliness, the goals would relate to developing and maintaining a mutually satisfying relationship(s). To this end, a short term goal could include: "By tomorrow, the patient will be able to describe the principles of a friendship relationship." Or, "Within two weeks, the person will select and attend two groups where friendships might be established."

It is evident, in the nature of the loneliness goals, that they must be developed in consultation with the person. In the illustration related to separation anxiety, it may be appropriate to involve the significant other(s) in the formulation of goals.

Intervention

Once the goals have been established, the nurse and the patient (where appropriate) select interventions that will assist in the achievement of the goals. As has been pointed out previously, nursing interventions are directed at the stimuli in an effort to manage the ones that are having a negative effect on the individual. It also may be appropriate to maintain or enhance stimuli that are positively affecting adaptation.

In the situation of **separation anxiety,** it is necessary for the substitute care giver to intervene to help the child cope with feelings of helplessness and anger when a separation has occurred. During the protesting stage, the care giver stays with the child, has close contact, and allows the child to protest, even though this comforting and attention is rejected. With the stage of despair, the care giver shows by verbal and nonverbal communication that the child is worthwhile and loved. The child is encouraged to express feelings of despair and become more mobile in the environment. To promote a sense of security, the care given can be as similar to that given by the significant other as possible. Familiar toys and special objects from home are left with the child at this time. The child's usual mealtime and bedtime rituals are incorporated into the plan of care. The child's most immediate need during the stage of denial is the establishment of a trusting relationship with one person. To accomplish this, a primary care giver is assigned to be responsible for establishing consistent routines. With the young child, frequent meaningful contacts are essential to accomplish the goal of forming a trusting relationship. Since the young child has not yet mastered the concept of time, the frequent contacts for short periods enable the child to deal with separation and increase a sense of trust that the primary care giver will return.

Significant others need education regarding the response of children during critical stages of development and during the stages of separation anxiety. They need to understand that these reactions are normal and acceptable, and the only way a child can express and cope with the situation. As an infant develops, he or she will learn how to cope with anxiety during the gradual separation process from the significant other. The infant is given opportunities to develop a sense of trust and deal with anxiety. To help the child master the concept that people and objects continue to exist even when out of sight, interventions such as peek-a-boo games are helpful for infants, and hide-and-seek for the toddler. The school-age child and adolescent may be helped to cope with separation by exploring new interests and finding comfort in peers. They are to be encouraged to verbalize their feelings regarding the separation experience.

When dealing with the young child, it is best to expose the child first to separation in a familiar environment in which constant reminders of the significant other, such as pictures or possessions, can be seen. This helps to reassure the child that the significant other will return. When in an unfamiliar environment, it is ideal to bring in pictures of the significant other and family and objects from home. Separation can also be made to be less traumatic if the child can be left for short periods of time with another care giver who the child knows and enjoys.

When the significant other does leave, the child should be told in simple terms that she is leaving, when she will return, and who will be the substitute care giver while she is gone. Measures should be taken to reassure the child of the significant other's return. Since young children have no concept of time, it is best to relate the return to an event familiar to the child's routine. An example would be "I'll be back after your nap time," as opposed to "I'll be back at 3 o'clock." The significant other should try to avoid leaving when the child is asleep, for this behavior would reinforce that the child cannot trust the significant other.

If the child is in a strange environment such as a hospital, it is best that the significant other make every effort to stay with the child, especially during painful or intrusive procedures. Since separation is stressful, progression to advanced developmental tasks, such as toilet training, should be avoided during this time.

The main aim of intervention in situations of **loneliness** should revolve around the person decreasing ineffective behaviors and developing instead reciprocal relationships. The person needs to develop contact with others on an adaptive basis to remove feelings of estrangement.

Active friendliness to initiate contact with a lonely person is frequently used as a nursing intervention. In using this method the nurse seeks out the patient to spend time with him or her, although the verbal interaction may be minimal. The nurse does so to increase the person's social confidence and trust in another. Once trust is established by the nurse's genuine concern for the individual, the person may feel free to communicate to what degree they are lonely and how helpless it feels. Using this approach, the nurse role models effective communication behaviors and ways of establishing a relationship. Although the one-to-one relationship is the nurse's basic tool, the nurse also encourages rapport with families, neighbors, other patients, or significant persons. This may be done by exploring ways to increase contact in the person's present situation—what happens to make a contact a rewarding or a happy one, what makes it a failure, what does the individual have to offer others, what or for whom is the person lonely, and why.

If an individual is using any distractions (for example, keeping busy, joking off interactions, or using any dependent crutches) to ward off loneliness, this can be worked with by the nurse and the whole health team. The person probably is not aware consciously of using these mechanisms.

Evaluation

Evaluation involves judging the effectiveness of the nursing interventions in relation to the person's behavior. When working with the child experiencing separation anxiety, the nurse evaluates if the goal was met. That is, was the child able to reestablish a trusting relationship with the significant other or substitute care giver while accepting love and support?

In situations of loneliness, evaluation is accomplished by observing and talking with the individual about the attainment of goals. With the diagnosis of loneliness, the goals may be reached easily, but more often there are a series of short-term goals that are related to the long-term goal of affectional adequacy.

SUMMARY

Separation anxiety and loneliness are experienced by many people in our society. The incidence is even greater with hospitalized persons or the very young person and those whose suffer stigma in society. Nurses can play a vital role in minimizing the discomfort of the person by using their theoretical understanding of the processes involved to plan care based on assessment of behaviors and the factors that influence these behaviors. As distress is relieved or prevented, persons maintain greater integrity and conserve energy for health and growth.

This chapter has presented a description of these two common adaptation problems associated with the interdependence mode. Application of Roy's six-step nursing process as it pertains to the two problems was explored.

EXERCISES FOR APPLICATION

1. Visit a day-care center for young children in the early morning. Assess behaviors of both the child, the significant other, and the substitute care giver during the separation process.
2. Recall an experience in which you felt anxiety related to the separation process. What coping strategies did you find effective?
3. Think of a time when you have experienced loneliness and identify the feelings (behaviors) that you experienced as well as how you resolved the loneliness.

ASSESSMENT OF UNDERSTANDING

Questions

1. Separation anxiety may be defined as the
   a. process of separating from the care giver to become an individual self.
   b. reciprocal separation between two persons.
   c. painful uneasiness of mind experienced by one separated from a significant other.
   d. stimuli to promote adaptation during separation from a significant other.
2. Identify the following behaviors as most characteristic of separation anxiety (S) or loneliness (L).
   a. _____ a clinging love relationship
   b. _____ physical clinging to significant other
   c. _____ regression of previously mastered developmental tasks
   d. _____ neglected physical appearance
   e. _____ rejection of care and attention
   f. _____ absence of giving behaviors
3. What is the focal stimulus associated with separation anxiety?

Situation

A second grade child, upon transferring to a new school, breaks into tears upon being left in her new classroom by her mother.

4. Formulate a nursing diagnosis for the above situation using two methods: the first and second.
   Method I _____
   Method II _____
5. Construct a goal for the child described in the above situation.
   _____
6. Label the following nursing interventions as most appropriate for either separation anxiety (S) or loneliness (L).
   a. _____ remain with the person even though rejected
   b. _____ incorporate usual rituals into plan of care
   c. _____ use active friendliness
   d. _____ frequent contact with the person for short periods
   e. _____ explore ways to increase contact with others
7. How would you evaluate achievement of the goal you established in item 5?
   _____

Feedback

1. c
2. a. L
   b. S
   c. S
   d. L
   e. S
   f. L
3. Separation from or absence of the significant other.
4. Method I - Crying related to strange environment and departure of significant other.
   Method II - Separation anxiety related to being left by mother in a strange setting and absence of support system in new class.
5. Example: During lunch hour, the child will make friends with two girls from her class.
6. a. S
   b. S
   c. L
   d. S
   e. L
7. At lunch time, the child is playing with other children and no longer appears upset.

REFERENCES

Ainsworth, M.D.S. Attachment theory and its utility in cross-cultural research, in *Culture and Infancy: Variations in the Human Experience,* P.H. Lerderman, S.R. Tulkin, and A. Rosenfeld, eds. New York: Academic Press, 1977.

Bowlby, J. *Attachment and Loss,* vol 1: *Attachment.* New York: Basic Books, 1969.

Bowlby, J. *Attachment and Loss,* vol. 2: *Separation: Anxiety and Anger.* New York: Basic Books, 1973.

Brown, S.A. Loneliness, in Sister Callista Roy *Introduction to Nursing: An Adaptation Model* (2nd. ed.). Englewood Cliffs, New Jersey: Prentice-Hall. 1984, pp. 442–457.

Erikson, E. *Childhood and Society.* New York: W.W. Norton, 1963.

Ezor, P.R. Student teacher: Separation anxiety, unpublished manuscript, Mount St. Mary's College, Los Angeles, 1980.

Klaus, M.H., and J.H. Kennel. *Parent-Infant Bonding* (2nd ed.). St. Louis: The C.V. Mosby, 1981.

Mahler, M.S. *The Selected Papers of Margaret Mahler,* vol. 2: *Separation-Individuation.* New York: Jason Aronson, 1979.

Mead, M. *Coming of Age in Samoa.* New York: William Morrow, 1971.

Moustakas, C.L. *Loneliness and Love.* Englewood Cliffs, N.J.: Prentice-Hall, 1972.

Robertson, J. Some responses of young children to loss of maternal care, *Nursing Times,* vol. 49, 1953.

Robertson, J. *Young Children in Hospital* (2nd ed.). London: Tavistock, 1970.

Seeman, M. On the Meaning of Alienation, *American Sociological Review,* 24(6): December 1959.

Stanford, G. *Developing Effective Classroom Groups.* New York: Hart, 1977.

Werner, E.E. *Cross-Cultural Child Development: A View from the Planet Earth.* Monterey, Calif.: Brooks/Cole, 1979.

Additional References

Buhrmester, D., and W. Furman. The development of companionship and intimacy, *Child Development,* 58: 1101–1113, 1987.

Page, R.M. Adolescent loneliness: A priority for school health education, *Health Education* 19 (3): 20–21, 1988.

Ruddy-Wallace, M. Temperament: Assessing individual differences in hospitalized children, *Journal of Pediatric Nursing* 2(1): 30–36, 1987.

Ryan, M.C. Loneliness in the elderly, *Journal of Gerontology Nursing,* 12 (11); 22–27, 1986.

Seyster, K. A lesson in therapeutic relationship, *Imprint,* 34 (3); 56–57, 1987.

Welt, S.R. The development roots of loneliness, *Archives of Psychiatric Nursing,* 1(1): 25–32, 1987.

PART V: CONCLUSION

Part V has presented the last of the four modes described within the Roy Adaptation Model—the interdependence mode. Chapter 18 provided an overview of the mode and dealt with its description and the theoretical bases underlying the mode as well as application of the nursing process in situations of effective adaptation. Chapter 19 presented and illustrated two common adaptation problems associated with interdependence, those being separation anxiety and loneliness.

As with the other parts of this textbook addressing the various modes of the model, Part V concludes with a case study illustrating application of the Roy Model in a patient care situation.

Part VI of this textbook departs from the "essentials" topics presented to this point and focuses on application of the Roy Model in the nursing practice setting and in research related to the model.

INTERDEPENDENCE MODE—CASE STUDY

Mary Poush Tedrow[1]

The purpose of this case study and nursing process care plan (See Table V–1) is to demonstrate how the nurse may prevent an adaptation problem by changing the environment in relation to developmental age.

Maria is an 18-month-old girl. She lives with her father, mother, 10-year-old sister Lupe, and 5-year-old brother, Anthony. Maria is hospitalized for repair of a club foot. The surgery was yesterday, and she has a cast on her left foot extending from her toes to below the knee. She awakened three times during the night following surgery, crying because her foot hurt. Her postoperative course has been uneventful otherwise. It is morning, and Maria is sitting up in bed eating breakfast. Her mother, Irma, is feeding her while sipping a cup of coffee. After breakfast, Irma holds Maria on her lap while they watch Sesame Street, and Maria holds and drinks her bottle of milk (this is a morning routine at home). Maria appears secure, calls "mommy" while Irma leaves the room to go to the bathroom, holds her toy doggy out for the nurse to see and hold, and snuggles up to her mommy every chance that she gets. Irma, in turn, strokes Maria, tickles her, and talks about Daddy and Lupe

[1]Tedrow, Mary Poush, "Separation Anxiety Case Study," in *Introduction to Nursing: An Adaptation Model*, by Roy, Sister Callista. Englewood Cliffs, N.J.: Prentice-Hall, pp. 438–440. 1984.

and Anthony and what they are probably doing right now. She also mentions occasionally that she will be happy when tomorrow arrives and she and Maria may go home. Manuel, the father, brings Lupe and Anthony to visit every evening. The admitting assessment reflects that Irma, her husband, and all three children had participated in the hospital's preadmission class one week before surgery. The class emphasized maintaining the family unit during hospitalization and provided suggestions about how to make the hospital stay more comfortable and less traumatic for the child and family.

Thus we see a child who is at an age to be high-risk for experiencing separation anxiety, hospitalized for surgery and not experiencing separation anxiety. Nursing interventions have prevented problems in the interdependence adaptive mode.

TABLE V–1. ADAPTATION NURSING PROCESS CARE PLAN FOR CHILD WITH SEPARATION ANXIETY: INTERDEPENDENCE MODE

Behaviors	Stimuli
Significant other(s) Mother (Irma)	*Focal:* nurturing significant other constantly present in the environment (rooming-in)
Receiving	*Contextual:* developmental tasks, autonomy and
Mother feeds Maria breakfast	becoming a separate person
Mother holds Maria while they watch Sesame Street and Maria drinks from her bottle	The degree of attachment is intense (this is Irma's "baby" and last child)
Mother strokes, tickles	Previous separations, none; oldest child babysits when necessary
Mother talks about family unit	Preparation for hospital preadmission class attended
Mother tells Maria that they will go home soon and be with the family	by entire family, with concrete sugestions to decrease trauma of hospitalization
Giving	Homelike environment, favorite dog and blanket
Calls "mommy"	brought from home as well as a recent picture of
Snuggles up to her mommy	the complete family taken in the living room of
Support system(s)	their home
Father, brother, and sister	
Receiving	
Come to visit at hospital every evening	
Picture of family in living room to look at	
Giving	
No interaction seen	

Nursing Diagnosis: Maria's affectional needs are being met and separation anxiety has been averted due to the mother's rooming-in; articles brought from home and the family's involvement in the hospital's preadmission class.

Goal: Maria's affectional needs will continue to be met by her mother and family during this hospitalization.

Interventions:

A. Dealing with the stimuli of the nurturing significant other
  1. Provide support to Irma and reinforce what a good job she is doing at mothering during this stressful time.

2. Supply Irma with any equipment she needs.
3. Encourage Irma to have a break while the staff or other family members stay with Maria.

B. Dealing with the stimuli of preparation for the hospital
1. Play out the story of Maria's hospitalization with animals and equipment (begin with the doctor's visit, proceed through the preadmission class, surgery, and conclude with Maria being discharged). Include the mother and, if possible, the rest of the family in this activity. (While this intervention relates to taking on of the sick role, it is useful in this case for its efforts in making the situation more familiar to the child, and thus potentially lessening the effects of the strange environment.)

Evaluation: Assess behaviors and decide if they are congruent with Maria as assessed earlier.

Part VI

The Roy Adaptation Model in Practice and Research

The Roy Adaptation Model has been described throughout this text as a systematic framework for nursing activities. That is, it guides the activities of the nursing process which include assessment, nursing diagnosis, goal setting, intervention and evaluation. Furthermore, the model is a basis for knowledge development.

Andrews (1989) observed, "As nursing matures as a profession and as nurses become increasingly aware of the importance of theory-based practice, the advantages of implementing a nursing conceptual model as the basis for that practice become increasingly attractive." Research regarding the implementation of nursing models in practice (Rogers and Smith 1988, for example) demonstrated positive results associated with their implementation. These results included enhanced patient care, more comprehensive, consistent, and accurate nursing assessment and diagnosis, and more attention to the psychosocial needs of patients. Communication within nursing and with other health care professions increased and documentation improved. Nurses reported increased ability to function as a patient advocate. They reported their jobs were more interesting and the result was increased levels of professional self esteem.

The following section explores in further detail applications of the Roy Adaptation Model in the practice setting and in research. In Chapter 20, Joanne Gray describes the particular implementation projects involving the model in which she has been involved. Sister Callista Roy provides, in Chapter 21, an overview of research related to the model both from the perspective of the structure of knowledge based on the Model, and examples of studies with qualitative and quantitative designs. Both of these topics are viewed as beyond the "essentials" level presented previously in this text. For this reason, the format of the chapters is altered. Key concepts have not been extracted nor have exercises and questions been provided at the end of the chapters. The chapters are intended to provide the reader with a beginning understanding of the application of a nursing model, the Roy Model in particular, in practice and research.

REFERENCES

Andrews, H.A. Nursing models and their application in the practice setting, *NUVO: The Nurses' Voice*. (August), pp. 5–9, 1989.

Rogers, M.E., and I. Smith. Evaluation of the Implementation of the Roy Adaptation Model, Unpublished research. Mount Sinai Hospital, Toronto, 1988.

Chapter Twenty

The Roy Adaptation Model in Nursing Practice

Joanne Gray

Through the years, nursing has strived to improve the quality of patient care through education, practice and research. The development of nursing theories and models has been a part of this endeavor. Such theories, however, primarily have been in use in nursing education programs and in the work of graduate students. It is important to the professional growth of nursing that nursing theories and models move from the educational setting and be implemented by the clinical nurse in order to assess their practicality and full impact on patient care.

This chapter will focus on the use and implementation of the Roy Adaptation Model over the past ten years in five practice settings.

OBJECTIVES

After studying this chapter, the reader will be able to do the following:

1. Describe the purpose and use of one nursing model, the Roy Adaptation Model, in the practice setting.
2. Describe the change process involved in implementing a nursing theory into the practice setting as presented in this chapter.
3. List the necessary steps, according to the change process presented in this chapter, in the implementation of a nursing model into the practice setting.
4. Identify the specific outcomes that can be expected from the use of the Roy Adaptation Model in the practice setting.

PURPOSE OF A NURSING MODEL

The purpose of a nursing model is to provide direction to the practice of nursing. Direction can be provided by describing the four metaparadigm phenomena: environment, health, person and nursing (Fawcett 1989). Also, a model or theory will show relationships between the phenomena of nursing that is useful for purposes of prediction and control (Chinn and Jacobs 1978).

The nursing model selected by a nursing department can be incorporated into the structural standards of the department and become an organizing principle around which the philosophy, goals, objectives, job descriptions and documentation of the nursing process and patient care are developed. The selection of a nursing model will assist a heterogeneous group of nurses to identify their private images of nursing as well as the differences and similarities with their co-workers.

The Roy Adaptation Model has demonstrated its usefulness in providing direction to the nursing process, especially in the first three steps: two levels of assessment and development of a patient diagnosis (Fig. 20–1).

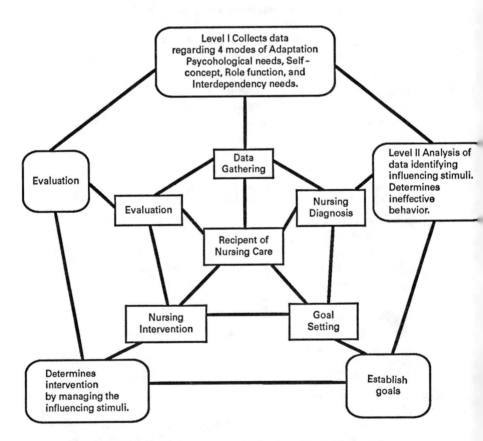

Figure 20–1. Nursing process and the Roy Adaptation Model

As noted in earlier chapters, the Roy Model becomes a guide for identifying the patient behaviors to be assessed. The second level of assessment, as described by Roy (1976, 1984), identifies the stimuli influencing the patient's behavior. Identifying the behavior and stimuli provides a systematic method for developing a nursing diagnosis. Identifying the etiology of a specific nursing care diagnosis will assist the nurse in establishing realistic goals with the patient/family and in initiating the appropriate interventions.

PROBLEM STATEMENT

The lack of written care plans that document and facilitate the use of the nursing process is still a major problem in the practice setting even though the requirements for using the nursing process have been in existence since the early 1950s. This deficiency is a serious problem, first because of implications for quality of patient care and also for the implications in accreditations, third party payment, and the fiscal drain on the nursing education department budget. Accrediting bodies, such as the Joint Commission on Hospital Accreditation of Health Care Organizations in the United States (1989), the Canadian Council of Hospital Accreditation (1986), as well as state and provincial laws, such as Title 22 in the State of California, address the requirements of individualizing patient care through utilization of the nursing process and documentation of a plan of care. In the United States, hospital accreditation is necessary in order to receive third party reimbursement for the patient's hospital bills.

The fiscal drain to the nursing department budget is found in the hours devoted to improving written patient care plans. This preparation includes the education of staff, development and implementation of appropriate forms, and frequent monitoring of the performance by quality assurance staff.

This author became aware of the scope of the problem with documentation of the nursing process while serving in the role of an inservice educator during the past twenty years. Initially, nurses were expected to state a short-term and long-term patient goal on the Patient Care Kardex and the failure to do this was a minor problem. The required documentation has become several pages of forms that include patient history and assessment and a patient care plan that includes the nursing diagnosis, goal, interventions, and evaluation. Now, a major percentage of the time of the inservice education department is spent in trying to improve the written care plans. The lack of written plans is often perceived to be related to the lack of knowledge by the nursing staff, or documentation forms not large enough or the care plan being kept in the wrong place. Therefore, there is always a need for new, innovative ways to teach the nursing process.

New and innovative ideas are also needed to design a patient care plan form that will enhance the documentation of the nursing process. All of this work is done only to find, the night before the accreditation body arrives, that there is the need for the inservice educators and the nurse administrators to go to the nursing units to write patient care plans. This was effective for several years until the accreditation surveyors began to look at the content of the nurses' notes to see if the charting reflected the nursing diagnosis listed on the patient care plan.

In this author's experiences in working to improve care plans, a common thread was noted. This common thread was that all nurses recognized and used the term "nursing process," but there was an obvious difference in interpretation of the meaning of the term. Differences were found in the terminology used to express each step and the data identified to be collected during the initial patient history and assessment. Each nurse varied in knowledge level and skills in assessment. The interpretations of the data appeared to be heavily influenced by the educational background of the nurses and their previous work experience.

Huckabay and Neal (1979) raised an important question in their search for an explanation of why care plans were not written. Their research offered several plausible explanations, but one that correlated with the observations of this author was that nurses who received positive reinforcers from their peers and supervisors when they wrote care plans tended to write more care plans than nurses who did not receive positive reinforcers. It was rare to find a supervisor who gave positive feedback to the staff nurse on written care plans because of their differing views on what constituted a patient problem.

The question raised by this author is: Can nurses give each other positive reinforcement when there is an unrecognized disagreement over what goes into the plan of care? In two subsequent descriptive research studies of the utilization of the nursing process by senior nursing students and practicing nurses, this unrecognized disagreement was validated. In a study by Gray (1986) to examine how senior nursing students utilized the nursing process, it was found that they assessed less than forty percent of the behaviors predicted. Sirski (1990) replicated this study and found that nurses assessed less than fifty percent of the predicted behaviors. In each study, as part of the interview process, the participant was asked to define the nursing process. Less than 20 percent of the participants were able to give an acceptable definition to the persons scoring the interview. The patient behaviors that were assessed and the definitions of the nursing process given by the nurses varied with their perceptions of the nursing process.

IMPLEMENTATION

In 1972, a 132-bed acute care, not for-profit, children's hospital was the first agency in Southern California to implement the Roy Adaptation

Model in the practice setting. Since 1982, there have been at least four additional hospitals in the Southern California area that have begun the implementation of the Roy Model in their practice setting. Roy notes that informally she has received work of several dozen health care agencies in the United States and abroad and that the actual number is likely much larger. The additional four hospitals to be described here ranged from a 100-bed proprietary hospital to a 248-bed nonprofit, community-owned hospital. Two of the hospitals terminated the project prior to complete implementation due to changes in the hospital management, philosophy and direction. However, the two terminating hospitals will be included in this discussion because they had completed several steps towards implementation and can provide further insight into the factors needed for success. The description of the implementation process that follows will be generalized to all projects.

Each of the projects was coordinated using a System of Management tool developed by Ingalls (1972). The tool is a seven-step process that translates managerial functions to programming activity. (See Figure 20–2). The purpose of this tool is to provide a sense of direction and organization to any change project by having a master plan and time line to maintain project focus. In addition to the general process of planning, organizing, motivating, and controlling, Ingalls (1972) defined the following seven steps within the system: (1) climate setting, (2) mutual planning, (3) assessing needs, (4) forming objectives, (5) designing, (6) implementing, and (7) evaluating. These seven steps are used to describe the projects and the implementation process. The activities of all five sites will be used in discussing each of these seven steps.

Climate Setting

Determining if the climate in any given institution is appropriate or conducive to change is the most difficult step in the implementation process. This step is especially difficult in today's climate of the acute care hospital which has become progressively more turbulent each year. It has become apparent that if a hospital waits for the perfect time to begin a change project, no change projects would ever be started. The key to success appears to be analyzing the climate factors and identifying those factors that can be controlled, or improved upon, or recognizing the climate that is not conducive to change at a particular time. Ingalls (1972) recommended that an agency evaluate the climate in the following three areas: physical, psychological and organizational.

Physical climate can include anything from the physical configuration of a nursing unit to a complete remodeling or renovation of the hospital or health care agency plant. In most agencies, remodeling and upgrading the facility is an on-going process and although it is distracting, it is not totally consuming. Many hospital employees view the remodeling process as a "permanent temporary" part of their environment and adapt accordingly.

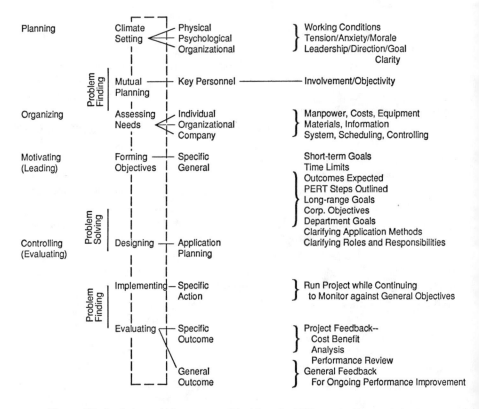

Figure 20–2. System of Management Tool (Ingalls, 1972, used with permission.)

The *psychological climate* is not as easy to evaluate because it is often the subjective opinion of the evaluator. The evaluation process is often performed by feeling or sensing the tension, anxiety, and morale of the staff. The psychological climate can make or break the successful implementation of any change and this seems especially so for implementing a nursing model.

The process of selecting a nursing model forces the nursing administrative team to look at both their own and their coworker's values and belief systems regarding the patient, nursing, environment, and health. In writing the philosophy statement and adopting a nursing model, the greatest achievements may not be the ultimate document but the interaction among fellow managers that takes place when they go through the process (Stevens 1985). If unresolved conflict existed, the selection process could be the factor that serves as a mediator to stimulate an understanding and compromise in the group. Another purpose served by using a nursing model is the orientation of the new members to the group. With the belief statement so clearly defined, it is easier to recruit and fill positions with persons holding a similar philosophy, goals, and objectives. The turnover factor in hospital administrative teams will keep the psychological climate in a state of constant change.

The *organizational climate* is determined by the ownership of the agency. It is the owners' mission statement, goals, objectives, and the top level management they select that will determine an organizational climate. The top level management determines how the fiscal resources are distributed and controlled thus affecting the utilization of the resources available to the nursing administration. For acute care settings, this determines the number of nursing care hours budgeted and how many of those hours are used in indirect or direct care of the patient.

Mutual Planning

Often a small group of people are involved in the selection of a nursing model. Thus, it is important to involve all levels of the nursing staff and hospital personnel in the implementation of the nursing model in order to gain acceptance and support.

A key issue identified in the first project was that nursing personnel are not the only employees involved in the change. The use of a nursing model created an impact on a majority of the departments with whom the nursing staff or the patient had direct contact. The medical records, purchasing and storeroom departments were affected every time a nursing form was changed. Social services personnel were affected by the change in nursing behavior in that nurses were openly and intentionally focusing on the patients' self concept, role function and interdependence needs. The social services staff immediately felt that their territory had been invaded. The schedules for other departments, such as the Lab, X-ray and Respiratory Therapy were changed when nurses began protecting the rest needs of the patients. The staff of these departments would arrive on the unit to perform a procedure to find nursing requesting not to have the patient awakened for a procedure they considered not to be life threatening if delayed. All of a sudden, nurses were verbalizing what they had felt for years: "Don't wake my patient up, he just went to sleep." Rest needs became a legitimate part of the patient's plan of care.

Assessing Needs

The assessment of needs is done at three levels: the individual staff nurse needs, the nursing department needs and the health care system needs. Characteristics of *individual nursing staff* were assessed in order to obtain general information regarding academic preparation and previous work experience. In each hospital, the nursing staff was a heterogenous group representing academic preparation ranging from unlicensed nurse aids to masters-prepared registered nurses. The nurse assistants, licensed vocational nurses, associate degree nurses, and diploma graduate nurses had a minimal exposure to the nursing process in their education and little, if any, exposure to nursing theories and models, particularly in earlier days of these projects. Nurses prepared at the bachelor degree level were more comfortable with the terms of the nursing process. However, only a small percentage of the bachelor degree level nurses utilized a nursing model. As more nursing education programs have incorporated nursing theory and models into their curricula, there has been a continual increase in the awareness and verbalization of theory terminology by nurses.

The need within the *nursing department* to improve the quality and quantity of written care plans has been the major focus of each implementation project. However, other needs within a department cannot be overlooked as these needs tend to overshadow any change project unless they are addressed. These needs include recruitment and retention of nurses to decrease the nursing shortage, staffing patterns that focus on patient-centered care, an acuity system that will accurately determine patient care hours required, and a documentation system that will reflect and support the nursing model concepts and terminology. Adequate patient care support systems such as the hours of availability by the pharmacy and central supply as well as the transport, delivery and communication systems have to be in place. A nursing model cannot improve nursing process if a majority of the nurses' time is spent in providing indirect patient care. The unmet needs within the nursing department as a whole will drain the nurses' time away from direct patient care and the time required for documentation.

The needs of a *hospital system*, or any health care agency, are driven by the needs and desires of the community in which it is located. The community needs are identified by the types of illnesses and health problems prevalent in a given geographical service area and the environment in general. There have been significant changes in the expressed desires of the consumer in the Southern California area over the past decade. Two major issues affecting the change are (1) the move from state control of master planning and the resulting specialization of hospitals to a more competitive expansion of services provided, and (2) a more affluent and informed consumer.

Orange County, California is recognized by national statistics as one of the fastest growing and higher income per capita counties in the United States. Hospitals have become competitive in the market place and focus more on the needs and desires of the consumer. Quality of patient care is important, but there is always competition within the hospital system for the fiscal resources. Issues related to this agency need could be a drawback for or could be used to the advantage of a nursing model implementation project. In Southern California, fiscal resources are heavily used in marketing the services offered by the hospital and, to date, marketing rarely includes the type of nursing services provided. Rather, a significant portion of the resources are spent in other special services to attract the patients to the hospital.

Forming Objectives

The overall goal of each project was to improve the quality of patient care through the use of written care plans. General objectives established for the project were: the Roy Adaptation Model would provide direction to the nursing process by (1) identifying the data to be gathered about each patient/family utilizing the four modes of adaptation described by Roy (1976, 1984) as a guideline, and (2) providing direction for problem identification by identifying behaviors ineffective for adaptation of patients, and determining the stimuli impinging upon the behavior. Specific learning objectives for individual nursing units and staff nurses were developed by inservice education staff as the implementation process began. Professional organizations provide guidelines for practice standards that can be influenced by the project (see, for example, College of Nurses of Ontario, Standards of Nursing Practice for Registered Nurses and Registered Nursing Assistants, Toronto, Ontario: College of Nurses of Ontario, 1987).

Designing

The design phase is the most time-consuming phase of the project. This phase encompasses the period of time involved in the clarification of roles and responsibilities of participants in the project and in the development and field testing of the patient history/assessment tools. Based on the experience of these five projects, it can be recommended that clarification of roles and distribution of responsibilities are best accomplished by a committee structure which will provide both leadership and group participation to the project.

A committee structure that has proven to be successful includes a Standards of Practice Steering Committee whose membership is composed of chairpersons or their equivalents for the following working committees:

1. Quality Assurance
2. Procedure and Protocol
3. Nursing Process
4. Professional Development
5. Patient Education

The membership of the Standards of Practice Committee and the nursing administration are responsible for selecting a nursing model that is compatible with the philosophy of nursing. The Standards of Practice Committee serves as an adviser to the Project Director in identifying and coordinating all the work to be done in the implementation process. This work will include refining the nursing department structure, standards, developing the history and assessment tools, revising nursing forms, writing procedures and on going evaluation of the project throughout the implementation process.

The Standards of Practice Committee will set the pace by developing the time line of the project and assigning tasks to specific working committees. The Nursing Process Committee is responsible for the development of the history and assessment tool that is designed around the Roy Adaptation Model. Since this may be the first exposure of the nursing staff to nursing theories and models and their application to practice, it is an important committee. Representation on this committee by each nursing unit is essential. In-depth education is necessary for this group in order to prepare the members for a leadership role and the task of involving their peers in the design and use of the unit-specific history and assessment tool. In order to minimize the resistance to change, "total participation," as described by Lawrence (1988), is used. As many people as possible are involved in setting the standards for patient assessment as the tools are developed.

Roy's nursing conceptual model serves as an outline as to what data will be gathered about each patient and to what level the assessment will be carried out. A common learning need identified in all units is related to the level of physical assessment expected by the nursing staff. If the standard included heart and lung sounds, could all nurses perform this task? If not, what content would be needed to increase the skills of the nurses to meet their standards?

The design phase of each project is not only time consuming but is often the most exciting and professionally exhilarating time for the project director. It is rewarding to see the nursing committees functioning at a high level of productivity, their sense of achievement in designing their assessment tool and beginning to utilize the model as a part of their practice. The history and assessment tool identifies the unit standards for patient assessment. An example of one such tool was developed by Rudoll, Missildine and Halasz (1988) for use in an oncology unit. The assessment components of the tool were based on the Roy Adaptation Model and examples of the nutrition and role/interdependence sections are contained in Figure 20–3.

After the history and assessment tool is developed, tested in the unit, and implemented, one can begin to utilize the second level of assessment as described by Roy (1976, 1984). In this phase, the private image of the nursing process held by each nurse begins to become open knowledge.

N U T R I T I O N

Recent Weight Gain/Loss   Yes   No | Hosp. Diet: _____   Alcohol Intake
      How Much? _____   ___   ___ | _____   Frequency
Any change in Appetite?   ___   ___ | ☐ beer _____
     If yes, Increase - or Decrease _____ | Home Diet: _____
Any special needs: Description _____ | _____   ☐ wine _____
_____ | _____   ☐ other _____
                  Follows Diet: _____

                           yes   no

Nausea/Vomiting   ___   ___
Feeder/Independent   ___   ___
Change in taste   ___   ___
Sore mouth   ___   ___
Chokes easily   ___   ___
Problem with swallowing/chewing   ___   ___

Dentures Partial/Complete _____   ☐ None

Change in Turgor, Appearance of Tongue, Condition of teeth & mucous membranes, etc.
Comments: _____
_____
_____

R O L E / I N T E R D E P E N D E N C E

1.   Marital status: ☐ single   ☐ married   ☐ divorced   ☐ separated   ☐ widowed

2.   Who are the most significant people in your life? _____

3.   Who lives in your home? _____

4.   Do you have any family and/or children in the area?   ☐ yes   ☐ no

    Who? _____

5.   What is/was your occupation? _____

6.   What hobbies or special interests are you involved in? _____

7.   Do you have friends or relatives who could help you when you go home
    needed? _____

8.   Do you have a visiting nurse: ☐ yes   ☐ no
9.   Do you desire visitor/telephone restrictions?   ☐ yes   ☐ no
    If yes, Who? _____

Figure 20–3. Examples from the nursing history and physical assessment tool Oncology Unit—Anaheim Memorial Hospital *(Rudoll, Cherie; Cheryl Missildine; and Suzanne Halasz. "History and Assessment Tool." Anaheim, California: Anaheim Memorial Hospital, 1988.)*

This is where the Roy Adaptation Model becomes a valuable tool guiding the nursing staff through the process of developing nursing diagnoses. This process is carried out in small group sessions working on a specific patient's care plan. The objective of these sessions is to assist the nursing staff in identifying behaviors and their impinging stimuli. The outcome of this exercise is a written plan of care agreed upon by the members participating in the group process.

Implementing

The work performed in the first five steps of the system management process makes the actual implementation of the model the easiest step. If the climate remained conducive to change, key people were involved in the planning, the needs assessment and objectives were on target with the needs of the system and adequate time was used in designing the tools, then the implementation phase becomes a period of revisions and refinement.

Education of the nursing staff in the use of the Roy Adaptation Model is a continual process. The process begins first with the nursing administrative staff and committee members then moves to the nursing staff of each unit as they develop and implement their history and assessment tool. The content of the Roy Adaptation Model is then incorporated into the orientation of all new employees.

Evaluating

Evaluation is done throughout the implementation process and in each step of the Ingalls Systems Management Model. An overall evaluation of the project is done after the implementation of the history and assessment tools and then again after the second level of assessment is implemented in each specific unit.

The ongoing evaluation throughout the project is based on observation, informal and formal feedback received through the committee structure and in inservice classes. For example, once the nursing staff begins to use the new history and assessment tool, many questions arise as to spacing of content and the meaning or interpretation of terms used. Corrections are made throughout the course of the implementation process. It is not uncommon for a form to be retyped six or seven times before it actually goes to the printer.

The major focus of the overall evaluation of the implementation project is the measurement of the project objectives. In each of the Southern California hospital projects, the specific goal was to improve patient care through the quality of written patient care plans. In order to achieve this goal, two specific objectives were stated: (1) the Roy Adaptation Model will provide direction to the nursing process by identifying the data to be gathered and documented on each patient, and (2) the Roy Adaptation Model will improve the quality of written care plans by providing a step-by-step method of identifying patient problems/nursing diagnosis requiring nursing intervention. Measurement of each objective was accomplished through quality assurance monitor processes as accepted by the Joint Commission on Accreditation of Healthcare Organizations.

The first objective was evaluated by doing a retrospective audit of charts prior to the implementation of the history and assessment tool with comparison of the results to a concurrent audit of charts using the Roy Model History and Assessment Tool. In each project where the tool has been completely implemented, there has been a significant improvement in the documentation of the patient's history and assessment. In the first project at Childrens Hospital of Orange County, there was a 100 percent improvement in the initiation of an assessment. In the standards established, 52 percent of all charts audited met all the criteria. In those charts not meeting one hundred percent compliance, eighty-four percent of the criteria established were met (Gray 1982).

The second objective is more difficult to measure. In order to accomplish the second level of assessment, the History and Assessment Tool needs to be fully implemented and in depth education on Roy's Adaptation Model provided to all the nursing staff. Then the reliability of using the step-by-step method of identifying non-therapeutic behaviors and determining the influencing stimuli needs to be established between the nursing administrative team and nursing staff in each unit. Measurement in each project indicated a significant improvement in the quality of the care plan while the design and implementation phase was in process. More data need to be gathered to ascertain if the change will stay in place in the positive direction or if the staff will revert to old behaviors after the implementation process has ceased.

Intangible benefits of the project are best measured through observation and verbalization of the participants. One of the observed benefits is that staff participation in the projects added a new dimension to the professional attitude toward their practice. Many nurses were participating in committee activity for the first time. Nurses began to verbalize their patient care findings using a common vocabulary. The nursing staff moved a little closer to agreement on which patient problem to document and how to prioritize the problems. Utilization of the model can be observed in the documentation forms developed following the implementation of the History and Assessment tool. One of the strongest points has been the use of the Roy Adaptation Model to assist the nursing administrative teams to coalesce their philosophy of nursing.

An example of this can be seen in the performance standards tool established in the South Coast Medical Center in Laguna Beach, California (Whitaker 1988). The first performance standards dealt with in the tool address the nursing process; the Roy Adaptation Model is named and reflected. Each of the modes and their components are addressed, the second level of assessment and the common stimuli are itemized, and are reflected in the derivation of nursing diagnoses. These performance standards, in their incorporation of the Roy Model, have the potential to become a useful employee evaluation tool as well as a tool to evaluate the effectiveness of patient care.

SUMMARY

This chapter has looked at the Roy Adaptation Model from the perspective of implementation in practice. One consultant to five implementation projects used the Roy Model, in conjunction with a seven-step process for translating managerial functions to programming activities. The experiences of these projects have been described and some general observations made about both the difficulties encountered and the benefits to be gained. The Roy Adaptation Model can be expected to make a continuing contribution to the process of making theory-based practice a reality in the daily patient care provided by clinical nurses and in the nursing service structures that support that practice.

REFERENCES

Canadian Council on Hospital Accreditation. *Standards of Accreditation of Canadian Healthcare Facilities.* June 1986.

Chinn, P.L., and M.K. Jacobs. Practice oriented theory: A model for theory development in nursing, *Advances in Nursing Science,* 1 (1) October 1978, pp. 1–11.

College of Nurses of Ontario. *Standards of Nursing Practice for Registered Nurses and Registered Nursing Assistants.* Toronto, Ontario: College of Nurses of Ontario, 1987.

Fawcett, J. *Analysis and Evaluation of Conceptual Models of Nursing.* Philadelphia: F.A. Davis, 1989.

Gray, J. The implementation of a conceptual model of nursing into the practice setting, Unpublished Masters Thesis, Los Angeles: California State University, 1984.

Huckabay, L., and M. Neal. The nursing care plan problem. *Journal of Nursing Administration,* December 1979, pp. 36–42.

Ingalls, J.D. (Ed.). *A Trainers Guide to Androgogy* (rev. ed.). Wattham, Mass.: Data Education, Inc. 1972.

Joint Commission on Accreditation of Healthcare Organizations. *Accreditation Manual for Hospitals.* Chicago, Illinois: Joint Commission of Accreditation of Healthcare Organizations, 1990.

Lawrence, P.R. How to deal with resistance to change, *People: Managing Your Most Important Asset.* Boston: Harvard Business Review, 1988.

Roy, Sr. C. *Introduction to Nursing: An Adaptation Model.* 1st ed. Englewood Cliffs, New Jersey: Prentice Hall, 1976.

Roy, Sister Callista. *Introduction to Nursing: An Adaptation Model.* Englewood Cliffs, New Jersey: Prentice-Hall Inc., 1984.

Rudoll, C., C. Missildine, and S. Halasz. Oncology unit task force history and assessment tool, Anaheim, California: Anaheim Memorial Hospital, 1988.

Sirski-Martin, K. *Utilization of the Nursing Process by Registered Nurses in the Practice Setting.* Masters Thesis, California State University, Long Beach, 1990.

State of California. Administrative Code Title 22. Social Security, Division 5. Licensing and Certification of Health Facilities and Referral Agencies, North Highland, Calif.: 1990

Stevens, B. *The Nurse as Executive* (3rd ed.) p. 25. Aspen, 1985.

Whitaker, M. Performance standards for critical care nurses. Laguna Beach, CA.: South Coast Medical Center, 1988.

Additional References

Appleton, P. and H. Chalmers. Models and theories TWO, the Roy Adaptation Model, *Nursing Times* October, pp. 45–48, 1984.

Duncan, S., and F. Murphy. Embracing a conceptual model. *The Canadian Nurse,* April pp. 24–26, 1988.

Giger, J.A., C.A. Bower, and S.W. Miller. Roy Adaptation Model: ICU Application. *Dimensions of Critical Care Nursing.* 6, (4): 215–224, 1987.

Roy, Sr. C. Adaptation: A conceptual framework for nursing. *Nursing Outlook* March 18(3): 42–45, 1970.

Silva, M.C. Research testing nursing theory: state of the art. *Advances in Nursing Science* October pp. 1–11, 1986.

Chapter Twenty-one ─────────

The Roy Adaptation Model in Nursing Research

Sister Callista Roy

Nursing as both a profession and a scholarly discipline is rooted in knowledge for nursing practice. Throughout history, family members have used their cultural traditions and understanding of the other person to help increase wellness, prevent illness, assist with recovery, and comfort the distressed and dying. Today nursing has emerged clearly as the discipline that focuses on developing an understanding of the human processes that promote health (American Academy of Nursing 1985) and as a caring profession that incorporates an understanding of human experience into health care practice (Benner and Wrubel 1989).

This chapter describes how the Roy Adaptation Model contributes to nursing as a scholarly practice discipline by guiding research in these two aspects of knowledge development for clinical practice, that is, understanding basic life processes that promote health (the basic science of nursing) and understanding how persons cope with health and illness and what can be done to enhance adaptive coping (the clinical science of nursing).

OBJECTIVES

After studying this chapter, the reader should be able to do the following:

1. Describe the perspective of nursing knowledge basic to nursing research within the Roy Adaptation Model.
2. Identify a nursing research study focusing on the basic science of nursing.
3. Identify a nursing research study focusing on the clinical science of nursing.

4. Derive a list of priorities in nursing research based on the Roy Model for a given speciality area of nursing practice.

PERSPECTIVE FOR NURSING RESEARCH

Nursing is an art and a science. Science deals with understanding both how and why questions. How does something work, why does it not, and how can we help it work? Art deals with understanding and expressing the realities of life. When a child takes a small plant apart, he or she knows only the parts that make it up, not how it works. Biology looks deeper to explain how and why the plant grows. When an artist such as Monet paints a water lily, both the artist and the viewer of the art know the plant in a way not known in biological science. Through science and art one knows and appreciates oneself, others and the world.

Basic knowledge in both arts and sciences looks deeply and closely at being; such knowledge aims to understand and express the essence of what is there and how it works. Nursing has such basic knowledge just as other disciplines do. Nursing models provide a perspective from which to view and develop the basic knowledge of the discipline. The conceptual models for nursing that have emerged over the past couple decades have the task of probing the reality of nursing to add to our knowledge for practice through research, and to direct nursing education in the science and art of nursing. Each of the several widely used nursing models, for example, Peplau, Orem, Johnson, Rogers, Roy, King, Neuman, Parse, and others, is a vehicle for developing the basic science of nursing as well as the practice discipline.

Roy (1988b) has described a general perspective for nursing knowledge as including the basic science of nursing, that is, focus on human life processes from which life patterns emerge. Secondly, the perspective for nursing knowledge places emphasis on the related clinical science of nursing, including midrange theories of intervention, and strategies related to enhancing positive life processes and patterns.

According to the Roy Adaptation Model, basic knowledge is understanding people adapting within their various life situations. The model conceptualizes the person as having cognator and regulator mechanisms that act to promote adaptation in each of the four adaptive modes: physiological, self concept, role function, and interdependence. Basic nursing knowledge, then, derived from this model seeks to understand and appreciate the hows and whys of persons functioning in this way.

Nursing is also a practice discipline. Therefore nursing knowledge based on a model includes a clinical art and science. Nursing has a long tradition of caring. Through the years this has been called by various names, such as, the interpersonal process (Peplau 1952), empathy (Travelbee 1971), caring need (Leininger 1981) and now such terms as the transpersonal caring relationship (Watson 1985). The notes of a famous writer working as a nurse at the time of the American Civil War in the nineteenth century reflect the values of this tradition. Louise May Alcott wrote in *Hospital Sketches: An Army Nurse's True Account of Her Experience During the Civil War:*

> A few minutes later, as I came in again, with fresh rollers, I saw John sitting erect, with no one to support him, while the surgeon dressed his back. I had never hitherto seen it done; for, having simpler wounds to attend to, and knowing the fidelity of the attendant, I had left John to him, thinking it might be more agreeable and safe; for both strength and experience were needed in his case. . . . John looked lonely and forsaken just then, as he sat with bent head, hands folded on his knee, and no outward sign of suffering, till, looking nearer, I saw great tears roll down and drop upon the floor. It was a new sight there; for, though I had seen many suffer, some swore, some groaned, most endured silently, but none wept. Yet it did not seem weak, only very touching, and straightway my fear vanished, my heart opened wide and took him in, as, gathering the bent head in my arms, as freely as if he had been a little child, I said, "Let me help you bear it, John"

The clinical art and science of nursing according to the Roy Adaptation Model relates the basic knowledge of adapting persons to understanding persons in situations of health and illness to discover ways of enhancing adaptation. Just as understanding cognator and regulator activity and behaviors and stimuli in each of the adaptive modes is basic knowledge for the model, the basis for the clinical art and science is the knowledge of these human processes in situations of health and illness and the planning of nursing care with individual people and groups to enhance their own adaptation.

Knowledge is developed through research in many ways. Formal research can be designed to describe phenomena (what), to correlate two or more phenomena (what and how), and to experiment with the effects of one phenomena upon another (how and why). Within each of these general types of research, there are two kinds of research design that can answer a research question. A qualitative approach views reality as emerging and relative. For example, how does this pregnant woman feel and why? A quantitative approach sees reality as discovered and measured. For example, what are the body image changes of the pregnant woman and how are these being affected by various factors? Nurses increasingly use several types of research designs and are aware of the complementarity of each. Qualitative analysis of field observations may be, for example, the basis of defining the variables for a correlational quantitative study. In one study many observations and interviews of mothers with their children in the playroom of a hospital lead to the concept of role adequacy that was used in a pre and post intervention observation tool to measure changes in the level of role adequacy.

Using many approaches and with increasing resources such as the Center for Nursing Research at the National Institutes of Health, nursing research has advanced greatly in the past decade and will make even greater progress into the next century.

As noted earlier, nursing models make their contribution to knowledge development by providing a perspective for research. Furthermore, the phenomena to study and the research questions to be asked are derived from the elements and assumptions of the model. The specific elements of the Roy Adaptation Model have been described throughout this text and the philosophic and scientific assumptions are outlined in Table 1-1. The model clearly identifies persons, as individuals and groups, as the phenomena for study. Whereas the biologist views the person as a living organism with functions such as ingestion and reproduction in common with other living organisms, the nurse using the Roy Adaptation Model views the person as unique among all living organisms. Based on the philosophical assumptions of the model, the person is seen as having purposefulness and a value and meaning that transcends all other living matter. Furthermore, the model's view of person differs from psychology and sociology. As a discipline, psychology studies individual behavior as explained by cognition and feeling, whereas the view person taken by sociology is the behavior of individuals and groups explained by understanding organized groups. In looking at the philosophical assumptions of the Roy Model, one sees a broader view of person highlighted, that is, individual holism, interpersonal processes, and the unity of purpose of human life within society.

This broad perspective of nursing knowledge is basic to identifying and conducting research for nursing. The Roy Adaptation Model has a clear perspective for the basic and clinical art and science of nursing. Further specification of the model's focus for research is deliniated by descriptions of the person and environment. Research completed, in progress, and to be accomplished can be placed within this broad perspective to outline one view of the basic and clinical science of nursing.

BACKGROUND FOR KNOWLEDGE DEVELOPMENT BASED ON THE ROY MODEL

During the past 25 years, knowledge development based on the Roy Adaptation Model has integrated several strategies: model construction; theory development, including concept analysis, synthesis, and derivation and proposition statements; philosophical explication; and research, both qualitative and quantitative. The model was originally described in the literature by Roy (1970). At Mount St. Mary's College, Los Angeles, Roy worked with colleagues to elaborate the elements of the model in two widely used editions of the definitive text on the model (Roy 1976 and Roy 1984a). Specific concepts were developed through both literature review and clinical experience, as well as reviews by content experts. (See book Chapters in each edition for contributions of individual authors). This current edition of the essentials of the model is an updating and refinement of these model elements described so as to be useful to educators and students at all levels, and to nurses in clinical practice. The development of essential elements of the model is basic to each of the other strategies of knowledge development, including research.

Theory development based on the model included the concept development described above, as well as early use of inductive processes and the later classic deductive work by Roy and Roberts (1981). Originally, the four adaptive models were defined and described by sampling 500 incidents of patient behavior in all areas of nursing practice (Roy 1972). Content analysis with inductive parsimonious clustering was used to derive categories. Confirmation of label codes was sought from the literature. Then the categories, with minor revisions based on clinical experience, were subjected to 10 years of testing in nursing practice by 1500 faculty and students. Criteria of significance, usefulness, and completeness were met (Roy 1981). At the same time numerous other educational and practice institutions were implementing the basic model elements, including the four adaptive modes as organizing concepts, and persons implementing the model were reaching similar conclusions about the adequacy of the adaptive modes.

Using a format for deductive theorizing described by Burr (1973), and extensive literature review, Roy and Roberts derived a total of 97 propositions that described relationships between and among the concepts of the regulator, cognator, and the four adaptive modes. Additional theoretical work has continued as Roy (1990) has clarified her view of adaptation and of health as both processes and states. Furthermore, Roy has begun more in-depth theorizing and research related to cognator and regulator activity by post-doctoral studies and clinical research in neuroscience nursing. A nursing model for cognitive information processing has been published (Roy 1988a).

The philosophical basis for Roy's later work was begun during her baccalaureate program when she graduated with a nursing major, but a Bachelor in Arts degree, having taken significant course work in the liberal arts, including extensive sequences in philosophy and theology. The opportunity to explicate the philosophical assumptions of the model came with an invitation to give the inaugural address of a distinguished nurse lecture series (Roy 1984b) on values for science. In individual analysis, and discussion with colleague philosophers at Mount St. Mary's, Roy continued to articulate distinctions related to her work that were not clear to the early critics who equated Roy's use of term stimuli from Helson's work with the S–R connections of behaviorism. The philosophical aspect of the development of the model is most fully treated in Roy (1988b).

Each of these basic strategies has contributed to knowledge based on the Roy Adaptation Model of Nursing. In addition, however, the model has an important role in guiding research both for a basic science of nursing and a clinical science of nursing. This role is described in the remaining sections of this chapter.

EXAMPLES OF RESEARCH WITHIN THE ROY MODEL STRUCTURE OF KNOWLEDGE

Given the generic perspective for nursing knowledge described earlier, a structure for knowledge based on the the Roy Adaptation Model of nursing has been derived. Table 21–1 shows the broad categories of the basic and clinical science of nursing. Major subdivisions of the basic science of nursing are the person or group as an adaptive system and adaptation related to health. In looking at the person or group, both adaptive processes and the adaptive modes are a focus. Topics to consider within the adaptive processes are: cognator and regulator activity for the individual

TABLE 21–1. STRUCTURE OF KNOWLEDGE BASED ON THE ROY ADAPTATION MODEL

Basic Nursing Science
Person/Group as Adaptive System
Adaptive Processes
Cognator-regulator activity
Stabilizer-innovator activity
Stability of adaptive patterns
Dynamics of evolving adaptive patterns
Adaptive Modes
Development
Interrelatedness
Cultural and other influences
Adaptation Related to Health
Person and environment interaction
Integration of adaptive modes

Clinical Nursing Science
Changes in Cognator-Regulator or Stabilizer-Innovator Effectiveness
Changes within and among Adaptive Modes
Nursing Care to Promote Adaptive Processes
in times of transition
during environmental changes
during acute and chronic illness, injury, treatment, and technological threats

and stabilizer and innovator activity for a group (as described in Roy and Anway 1989); stability of adaptive patterns; and the dynamics of evolving adaptive patterns. In looking at the adaptive modes, one studies developments, interrelatedness, and cultural and other contextual and residual influences. The second major category, adaptation related to health, is divided into research related to person/environment interaction and integration of the adaptive modes.

Examples of Roy's research will be described briefly to illustrate some of the categories from the structure of knowledge based on the Roy Adaptation Model and some of the issues involved in this research.

Basic Nursing Science—Research Examples

Two examples from Roy's earlier work (1975 and 1977), are used to illustrate studies related to basic nursing science, one related to knowledge of the person as adaptive systems and one related to adaptation and health.

In the former study related to the person as an adaptive system, the general research aim was to explore how the cognator coping mechanism acts to promote adaptation and how it relates to the four adaptive modes. These methods were used to explore this basic question. Literature on coping mechanisms was reviewed from the perspective of the adaptive modes. Grids were prepared that displayed different authors' view on each of the modes in such a way that relationships among the authors' views could be synthesized. The second step in exploring cognator mechanisms was to obtain a closer view of them acting in a given context. Ten patients on a medical unit of an acute care hospital were interviewed, half of whom were scheduled for diagnostic tests the next day and half of whom had been in the hospital for at least five days. Patients were asked open-ended questions about coping with diagnostic tests and about coping with the experience of hospitalization. Then individual patient responses were analyzed and coded into categories that seemed to express the specific cognator activity, such as, "selective attention—differential focus on a good outcome" or "affective isolation." Regulator activity was also noted as reported or observed.

Lastly, within this three-way approach, an analysis was done of 36 written recordings of the process of nursing care. The recordings were made by students in seven schools using the Roy Adaptation Model of Nursing where Roy or one of her colleagues had consulted on curriculum implementation. Although the formats and length of the recordings of care differed, the common nursing framework made it possible to prepare charts for analysis of the patient data in three categories: Patient Behavior; Focal, Contextual and Residual Stimuli; and Inferred Coping Mechanism. After naming the inferred coping mechanisms for each patient incident, a count was made of the number of times the mechanism was used across the patient sample. A list of synthesized categories was devised by organizing and combining categories from the literature and the two clinical samples until the smallest number of categories was reached which represented all situations observed. At that point 41 different coping mechanisms were tentatively identified, 18 related to self concept; 16 concerned with role function; and 11 for interdependence, with four categories being repeated once or more across the modes. This was seen as a beginning effort to move the study of cognator and regulator activity beyond the descriptions presented by Roy in 1970.

In the other study used as an example here, the relationship of adaptation to health was looked at as part of a larger study of decision-making, powerlessness, and adaptation (Roy 1977). It was hypothesized that levels of wellness would be greater with higher levels of adaptation. The design of the study was systematic controlled comparisons using survey data collected by the investigator in six hospitals across the United States. Two-hundred and eight patients met study criteria and completed data collection. Instruments to measure adaptation included an Affect Adjective Check List for anxiety and a 49-item hospital events card sort and distress scale comparing how much the events bothered the patient early in the hospitalization and on the day before discharge. In addition, physiological data from the chart was collected and the patient was interviewed about usual patterns to ascertain adaptation in the physiological mode components. Wellness was described as rate of recovery and general physical welfare. Common items in the literature, such as days in hospital, prn medications used, complications, and self report of degree of independence and rate of return to work were used as measures of wellness.

Data were analyzed with Somer's D asymmetric measure of association for ordinal variables. In the total sample, some of the measures of physiological adaptation were related to levels of wellness, but there was no evidence of a relationship between psychosocial adaptation and any of the measures of level of wellness. In looking at different hospitals and at length of stays in the hospital, however, there was such a relationship in the least acute setting and for the longer stay patients. Thus it was suggested that adaptation can have an effect on level of wellness in less acute situations and over a longer period of time. It also was noted that the measures of levels of wellness were limited and not entirely appropriate to the dynamic and holistic concept of health as it has been further defined in the Roy Model.

Clinical Nursing Science-Research Examples

The clinical nursing science based on the Roy Adaptation Model is divided into changes in cognator-regulator and stabilizer-innovator effectiveness, changes within and among the adaptive modes and nursing care to promote adaptive processes. Studies in the latter category focus particularly on times of transition, during environmental changes, and during acute and chronic illness, injury, treatment, and technological threats.

Roy's more recent research is clinical nursing science research. Two examples are provided to show the process of research and knowledge development that grounds itself in understanding the basic nursing science of adaptive processes. The research first describes changes in adaptation in given situations, and then devises and tests nursing interventions to promote adaptive processes within this context. As noted earlier, to move forward the theoretical work on cognator adaptive processes (Roy and McLeod 1981), a model of cognitive information processing was developed (Roy 1988a). A program of research was initiated that aims to contribute to an understanding of basic human cognitive processes, that is, how people take in and process environmental interactions, and how nurses can help persons use these processes to positively affect their health status. Specifically, these studies purpose to develop knowledge relevant to nursing care and the recovery of head injury patients.

The two specific aims of the first study (Roy 1985) were: (1) to describe the direction and degree of change of simultaneous and successive modes of information processing in patients with mild and moderate closed head injuries at four points in time over the first six months of recovery; and (2) to identify the relationship of specific demographic and medical factors to the nature and degree of change in information processing.

The methodology involved a descriptive repeated measures design. Data were collected for each subject at times that would maximize evidence of the dynamic changes in information processing taking place during recovery from head injury, that is, when the patient was first verbally responsive, at one week, one month and six months after injury. The data included cognitive testing of simultaneous and successive information processing, clinical measures, and demographic data related to the factors that influenced information processing. Seven theoretically and empirically sound processing tests were selected and pilot tested for use at the bedside of an injured patient. Subjects included fifty patients with mild and moderate head injury as defined by scores on the Glasgow Coma Scale and the Galveston Orientation and Amnesia Test. Plotting of mean scores and analysis of variance with repeated measures show a clear pattern of change over time. Scores improve over the six months and the variance among scores decreases. Furthermore, the pattern of information processing deficits is more pronounced for successive and planning functions than for simultaneous processing. Patients with more extensive history of drug and alcohol use scored lower on all measures and these differences were significant on three of the nine measures. Still the overall pattern of change resembled the changes for the group as a whole. There was support for the notion that the first month following mild head injury is a critical period for recovery.

The second study drew upon the findings of the first. It has two aims: (1) to develop and implement information processing practice protocols, and (2) to determine whether or not there is a difference in the change of information processing scores during the first six months of recovery from mild head injury for patients who receive information processing interventions as compared with matched subjects who recover without such interventions. Criteria for admission of subjects were the same as in the initial study and the matched controls were taken from that study.

The intervention protocol was devised from the understanding of information processing and of the changes that were described in the first study. It was then submitted to a multidisciplinary review panel for review, critique, and consensus. The protocol involved information processing practice sessions, held twice a day in the hospital for 10 to 20 minutes and twice a week at home for up to one hour. At least eight practice sessions were held during the first month of recovery, with a prescribed distribution of approximately 20 percent simultaneous tasks, 30 percent successive tasks, and 50 percent planning tasks attained over time as the patient progressed. The sessions were planned individually for the patient and conducted by a neuroscience clinical nurse specialist using simple and complex exercise materials in each of the three categories of information processing. Outcome measures of information processing, time points, and conditions for testing were the same as described for the first study.

Data on the initial nine matched pairs show some promising trends. First, the intervention protocol is useful in information processing practice and appropriate for clinical use. Secondly, when matched scores are compared on graphs, the recovery curves for the treated group have steeper slopes, particularly between the first two data points, indicating greater improvement of performance. Changes in the untreated group on the other hand appear more gradual. Processing practice, developed from basic and clinical nursing science, may enhance information processing for those who have had changes in this ability through injury. Finally, the return rate of subjects to insure complete data sets has been brought to an acceptable level. As the number of subjects is increased in this study, the data can be subjected to repeated measures analysis of variance to determine difference over time and between groups, as well as to a two-stage model of regression analysis to determine differences in the slopes between scores at different times and between scores of the two groups.

ISSUES RELATED TO RESEARCH BASED ON THE ROY MODEL

In analyzing nursing research projects based on the Roy Adaptation Model, some issues are noted that effect knowledge development by way of research. First, the question can be raised as to whether an understanding of the model is being used to generate research questions, or whether some elements of the model are being used to organize certain variables, either during design of the project or data analysis. Any of these approaches can be considered valid. However, a point will be reached when the redundancy of the latter approach will be apparent; that is, each study will resemble the other with little new understanding being added. It is expected that increasingly the greater potential of the model to direct research questions will be recognized.

A second issue is that conceptual definition of variables is key to the research. Variables are defined in terms of the structure of knowledge, that is, what is important to know, and how shall it be viewed in relation to the whole of understanding adapting persons? From this will come the choice of methods to answer the research question. Current divisions of theorists' work into those using qualitative methods and those using quantitative methods are misleading. As noted earlier, and in the examples given, multiple methods are used at every stage of the work of developing knowledge based on this particular model and this is likely the case with other models. This issue is related to the next.

This model and other approaches to understanding nursing knowledge profess a belief in holism. The notion of individual patterns is strongly represented, but this presents difficulties in describing the commonalities that make for understanding beyond an experience that is too unique to communicate. Thus clinical investigators seek ways to understand infinite variety, holism and control of variables. This is particularly true with outcome measures, as was noted in the study looking at adaptation related to levels of wellness. Rather than the dimensions measured, the conceptual definition of health within the model implies a process of being and becoming whole and integrated. The metholodogy then will be designed to tap the manifestation of the experience of being whole and integrated.

In the examples given here, the need for longitudinal studies, for refinement and replication, and for programs of research is noted. Research in nursing and research based on the Roy Model structure of knowledge are beyond simply accumulating more facts. The opportunity to seek meaning and understanding is provided. The philosophical and scientific assumptions, the essential elements of the model, and initial research efforts can guide further research.

Examining current research on the model and how it fits into this structure is one way of seeing beyond the individual facts to meaningful knowledge. This is a difficult task since compiling a complete list of publications is difficult and work in progress even more difficult to identify. A report in the Bulletin of the Medical Librarians Association (Johnson 1989) noted that 75 percent of the clinical studies applying a specific nursing conceptual framework will be missed by using conventional subject/textword search in MEDLINE or CINAHL databases. The list of citations that Roy currently has numbers over 100 entries, but it is not known how many of these are research based. Other authors report on research done on the Roy Adaptation Model. Silva and Sorrell (1987) identify doctoral dissertations and Fawcett (1989) lists the instrument development work, studies of patients' responses to various clinical problems, and studies of the effects of nursing interventions on patients' adaptation.

Some topics of on-going research of Roy's doctoral students and post-doctoral fellow include: adaptation to the mothering role after breast cancer, adaptation and gynecological surgery, the effect of discrete muscle activity on stress response, and paradigm changes and a metaparadigm related to physiological nursing research in dyspnea.

SUMMARY

In this chapter, the Roy Adaptation Model in nursing research was described from the viewpoint of the theorist. A broad perspective of nursing knowledge included the relationship between a basic nursing science and a clinical nursing science. The structure of knowledge based on the Roy Adaptation Model was derived from this broad perspective. Within this, specific categories for research were identified. Several of Roy's research projects were described to illustrate knowledge development in specific categories, and also to show clinical studies related to understanding of basic nursing science. Issues were raised that look to the future of knowledge development based on the model.

REFERENCES

Alcott, L.M. *Hospital Sketches: An Army Nurse's True Account of Her Experience during the Civil War,* (1849), Concord, Mass. (edition by Applewood Books: Cambridge, Mass., 1986).

American Academy of Nursing *Setting the Agenda for the Year 2000: Knowledge Development in Nursing.* Kansas City: American Nurses Association, 1985.

Benner, P. and J. Wrubel. *The Primacy of Caring: Stress and Coping in Health and Illness.* Menlo Park, Calif.: Addison-Welsey, 1989.

Burr, W. R. *Theory Construction and the Sociology of the Family.* New York: Wiley & Sons, 1973.

Fawcett, J. *Conceptual Models of Nursing* 2nd ed. Philadelphia: Davis, 1989.

Johnson, E.D. In search of application of nursing theories: The Nursing Citation Index. *Bulletin Medical Librarians Association.* 72 (2), 176–184, 1989.

Leininger, M. *Nursing and Anthropology: Two Worlds to Blend.* New York: Wiley & Sons, 1970.

Leininger, M. *Caring: An Essential Human Need.* Thorofare, N.J.: Charles B. Slack, 1981.

Peplau, H. *Interpersonal Relations in Nursing.* New York: Putnam, 1952.

Roy, Sr. C. Role cues and mothers of hospitalized children, *Nursing Research,* **16** (2), 178–182, 1967.

Roy, Sr. C. Adaptation: A conceptual framework for nursing, *Nursing Outlook,* **18** (3) 43–45, 1970.

Roy, Sr. C. Adaptation: A basis for nursing practice, *Nursing Outlook,* 19, (4), 254–257, 1971.

Roy, Sr. C. Psycho-social adaptation and the coping mechanisms. Unpublished paper, Clinical site, Queen of the Valley Hospital, West Covina, Calif., 1975.

Roy, Sr. C. *Introduction to Nursing: An Adaptation Model.* (1st ed., with contributing authors) Englewood Cliffs, N.J.: Prentice-Hall, 1976.

Roy, Sr. C. *Decision-Making by the Physically Ill and Adaptation During Illness.* University of California, Los Angeles, (University Microfilms International, Dissertation Copies, Ann Arbor, Michigan), 1977.

Roy, Sr. C. Roy Adaptation Model: Evaluating Ten Years of Progress and Setting Future Goals. In Roy, C. (Ed) The Third International Conference on the Roy Adaptation Model in Nursing. Proceedings. Los Angeles, Calif., 1981.

Roy, Sr. C. *Introduction to Nursing: An Adaptation Model.* Englewood Cliffs, N.J.: Prentice-Hall, 1984a.

Roy, Sr. C. Values for Science: A Clinical Nurse Scholar's Perspective. Geraldine Crawford Distinguished Nursing Lecture Series, University of San Francisco, School of Nursing, San Francisco, Calif., 1984b.

Roy, Sr. C. Cognitive Processing in Patients with Closed Head Injury. Poster Session, 18th Annual Communicating Nursing Research Conference, Western Society for Research in Nursing. Seattle, Wash., 1985.

Roy, Sr. C. Information Processing: Testing Model Based Interventions. Podium Paper. International Nursing Research Conference, Council of Nurse Researchers, Washington, D.C., 1987.

Roy, Sr. C. Alterations in cognitive processing. In Mitchel, P., L. Hodges, M. Muwaswes, and C. Walleck. (Eds.). *American Association of Neuroscience Nurses: Phenomena and Practice.* E. Norwalk, Conn.: Appleton & Lange, 1988a.

Roy, Sr. C. An explication of the philosophical assumptions of the Roy Adaptation Model. *Nursing Science Quarterly,* 1 (1): 26–34, 1988b.

Roy, Sr. C. Theorist's Response to "Strengthing the Roy Adaptation Model through Conceptual Clarification," *Nursing Science Quarterly, 3* (2), 64–66, 1990.

Roy, Sr. C. and J. Anway. Roy's Adaptation Model: Theories and propositions for administration, in Henry, B., DiVincenti, Arndt, C., & Marriner, J. *Dimensions and Issues in Administration,* St. Louis; Mosby, 1989.

Roy, Sr. C. & McLeod. D. (1981). Theory of the Person As An Adaptive System. In Roy, C., and S. Roberts. Theory construction in nursing: An adaptation model. Englewood Cliffs, NJ: Prentice Hall, 49–69, 1981.

Roy, Sr. C., and S. Roberts. Theory construction in nursing: An adaptation model. Englewood Cliffs, NJ: Prentice Hall, 1981.

Silva, M., and J. Sorrell. Doctoral Dissertation Research Based on Five Nursing Models. A select bibliography. George Mason University: Fairfax, Va., 1987.

Stevenson, J., and T. Tripp-Rimer. Knowledge about Care and Caring: State of the Art and Future Developments. Proceedings of a Wingspread Conference. Kansas City, MO: American Academy of Nursing, 1990.

Travelbee, J. *Interpersonal Aspects in Nursing* 2nd ed. Philadelphia: Davis, 1971.

Watson, J. *Nursing: Human Science and Human Care.* E. Norwalk, Conn.: Appleton & Lange, 1985.

Additional References

Farkas, L. Adaptation problems with nursing home application for elderly persons: An application of the Roy Adaptation Model. *Journal of Advanced Nursing,* 6, 363–368, 1981.

Fawcett, J., and J. Buritt. An exploratory study of antenatal preparation for cesarean birth. *Journal of Obstetric, Gynecologic, and Neonatal Nursing,* 14, 224–230, 1985.

Fawcett, J., and J. Henklein. Antenatal education for cesarean birth: Extension of a field test. *Journal of Obstetric, Gynecologic, and Neonatal Nursing,* 16, 61–65, 1987.

Germain, C. Sheltering abused women: A nursing perspective. *Journal of Psychosocial Nursing,* 22 (9), 24–31, 1984.

Hoch, C. Assessing delivery of nursing care. *Journal of Gerontological Nursing,* 13, 10–17, 1989.

Leuze, M., and J. McKenzie, Preoperative assessment using the Roy Adaptation Model. *AORN Journal,* 46, 1122–1134, 1987.

Limandri, B. Research and practice with abused women: Use of the Roy Adaptation Model as an exploratory framework. *Advances in Nursing Science,* 8 (4), 52–61, 1986.

Norris, S., L. Campbell, and S. Brenkert. Nursing procedures and alterations in transcutaneous oxygen tension in premature infants. *Nursing Research,* 31, 330–336, 1982.

Pollock, S. Human responses to chronic illness: Physiologic and psychosocial adaptation. *Nursing Research,* 35, 90–95, 1986.

Shannahan, M., and B. Cottrell. Effect of the birth chair on duration of second stage labor, fetal outcome, and maternal blood loss, *Nursing Research,* 34, 89–92, 1985.

Smith, C., M. Garvis, and I. Martinson. Content analysis of interviews using a nursing model: A look at parents adapting to the impact of childhood cancer, *Cancer Nursing,* 6, 269–275, 1983.

Index*

*Page numbers are preceded by (ta-
ble) and (illus.) to indicate the location
of tables and illustrations. Page numbers followed by n indicate that a footnote appears.